The Washington Manual® Infectious Diseases Subspecialty Consult

Faculty Advisor
Linda M. Mundy, M.D.
Assistant Professor of Medicine
Department of Internal Medicine
Division of Infectious Diseases
Washington University School of
Medicine
St. Louis, Missouri
Adjunct Assistant Professor of
Community Health
Saint Louis University School of
Public Health
St. Louis, Missouri

The Washington Manual® Infectious Diseases Subspecialty Consult

Editor
Richard Starlin, M.D.
Infectious Disease and Epidemiology Associates
Omaha, Nebraska

Series Editor
Tammy L. Lin, M.D.
Adjunct Assistant Professor of Medicine
Division of Medical Education
Washington University School of Medicine
St. Louis, Missouri

Series Advisor
Daniel M. Goodenberger, M.D.
Professor of Medicine
Chief, Division of Medical Education
Washington University School of Medicine
St. Louis, Missouri
Director, Internal Medicine Residency
Program
Barnes-Jewish Hospital
St. Louis, Missouri

LIPPINCOTT WILLIAMS & WILKINS
A **Wolters Kluwer** Company
Philadelphia · Baltimore · New York · London
Buenos Aires · Hong Kong · Sydney · Tokyo

Acquisitions Editor: Danette Somers
Developmental Editor: Keith Donnellan
Project Manager: Nicole Walz
Senior Manufacturing Manager: Ben Rivera
Senior Marketing Manager: Kathleen Neely
Creative Director: Doug Smock
Production Editors: Holly H. Auten and Kate Sallwasser,
Silverchair Science + Communications
Cover Designer: QT Design
Compositor: Silverchair Science + Communications
Printer: RR Donnelley–Crawfordsville

© 2005 by Department of Medicine, Washington University School of Medicine

Printed in the USA

The Washington manual infectious diseases subspecialty consult / editor, Richard Starlin.
    p. ; cm. -- (The Washington manual subspecialty consult series)
    Includes bibliographical references and index.
    ISBN 0-7817-4373-7
    1. Communicable diseases--Handbooks, manuals, etc. I. Starlin, Richard. II. Title: Infectious diseases subspecialty consult. III. Series.
    [DNLM: 1. Communicable Diseases--Handbooks. 2. Diagnosis, Differential--Handbooks. 3. Patient Care Planning--Handbooks. WC 39 W319 2005]
RC112.W364 2005
616.9--dc21

                                                    2003051676

10 9 8 7 6 5 4 3 2 1

Contents

Contributing Authors

Anucha Apisarnthanarak, M.D.

Instructor in Medicine
Department of Medicine
Thammasart University Hospital
Pratumthani, Thailand

Hilary M. Babcock, M.D.

Instructor of Medicine
Department of Internal Medicine
Division of Infectious Diseases
Washington University School of
Medicine
St. Louis, Missouri

Michele C. L. Cabellon, M.D.

Nephrology Fellow
Department of Internal Medicine
Barnes-Jewish Hospital
St. Louis, Missouri

Rebecca E. Chandler, M.D.

Infectious Diseases Fellow
Department of Medicine
Division of Infectious Diseases
Oregon Health and Science
University
Portland, Oregon

Erik Dubberke, M.D.

Infectious Diseases Fellow
Department of Medicine
Division of Infectious Diseases
Washington University School of
Medicine
St. Louis, Missouri

Nicholas Haddad, M.D.

Attending Physician
Department of Medicine
Division of Infectious Diseases
Aleda E. Lutz VA Medical Center
Saginaw, Michigan

Catherine A. Hermann, M.D.

Resident
Department of Internal Medicine
Yale-New Haven Hospital
New Haven, Connecticut

Bing Ho, M.D.

Nephrology Fellow
Department of Medicine
Division of Nephrology
Stanford University School of Medicine
Stanford, California

Steve J. Lawrence, M.D.

Fellow
Department of Medicine
Division of Infectious Diseases
Washington University School of
Medicine
St. Louis, Missouri

Iris Liou, M.D.

G.I. Fellow
Division of Gastroenterology
University of Washington School of
Medicine
Seattle, Washington

Kristin Mondy, M.D.

Infectious Diseases Specialist
IDXPERT, P.C.
St. Louis, Missouri

Melissa L. Norton, M.D.

Hospitalist
Department of Internal Medicine
St. John's Mercy Medical Center
St. Louis, Missouri

Erin K. Quirk, M.D.

Clinical Fellow
Department of Internal Medicine
Division of Infectious Diseases
Washington University School of
Medicine
St. Louis, Missouri

Behzad Razavi, M.D.

Infectious Disease Specialist
Clark-Holder Clinic
West Georgia Medical Center
LaGrange, Georgia

Maria B. Ristig, M.D.

Clinical Fellow
Department of Internal Medicine
Division of Infectious Diseases
Washington University School of
Medicine
Barnes-Jewish Hospital
St. Louis, Missouri

David J. Ritchie, Pharm.D., F.C.C.P., B.C.P.S.

Professor of Pharmacy Practice
St. Louis College of Pharmacy
St. Louis, Missouri
Clinical Pharmacist in Infectious
Diseases
Barnes-Jewish Hospital
St. Louis, Missouri

Richard Starlin, M.D.

Infectious Disease and Epidemiology
Associates
Omaha, Nebraska

Nathan P. Wiederhold, Pharm.D.

Assistant Professor
Division of Pharmacotherapy
The University of Texas at Austin
College of Pharmacy
Austin, Texas
Clinical Assistant Professor of
Pharmacology and Medicine
The University of Texas Health
Science Center at San Antonio
San Antonio, Texas

Chairman's Note

Medical knowledge is increasing at an exponential rate, and physicians are being bombarded with new facts at a pace that many find overwhelming. The Washington Manual® Subspecialty Consult Series was developed in this context for interns, residents, medical students, and other practitioners in need of readily accessible practical clinical information. They therefore meet an important unmet need in an era of information overload.

I would like to acknowledge the authors who have contributed to these books. In particular, Tammy L. Lin, M.D., Series Editor, provided energetic and inspired leadership, and Daniel M. Goodenberger, M.D., Series Advisor, Chief of the Division of Medical Education in the Department of Medicine at Washington University, is a continual source of sage advice. The efforts and outstanding skill of the lead authors are evident in the quality of the final product. I am confident that this series will meet its desired goal of providing practical knowledge that can be directly applied to improving patient care.

Kenneth S. Polonsky, M.D.
Adolphus Busch Professor
Chairman, Department of Medicine
Washington University School of Medicine
St. Louis, Missouri

Series Preface

The Washington Manual® Subspecialty Consult Series is designed to provide quick access to the essential information needed to evaluate a patient on a subspecialty consult service. Each manual includes the most updated and useful information on commonly encountered symptoms or diseases and highlights the practical information you need to gather before formulating a plan. Special efforts have been made to organize the information so that these guides will be valuable and trusted companions for medical students, residents, and fellows. They cover everything from questions to ask during the initial consult to issues in subsequent management.

One of the strengths of this series is that it is written by residents and fellows who know how busy a consult service can be, who know what information will be most helpful, and can detail a practical approach to patient care. Each volume is written to provide enough information for you to evaluate a patient until more in-depth reading can be done on a particular topic. Throughout the series, key references are noted, difficult management situations are addressed, and appropriate practice guidelines are included. Another strength of this series is that it was written in concert. All of the guides were designed to work together.

The most important strength of this series is the collection of authors, faculty advisors, and especially lead authors assembled to write this series. In addition, we received incredible commitment and support from our chairman, Kenneth S. Polonsky, M.D. As a result, the extraordinary depth of talent and genuine interest in teaching others at Washington University is showcased in this series. Although there has always been house staff involvement in editing The Washington Manual® series, it came to our attention that many of them also wanted to be involved in writing and making decisions about what to convey to fellow colleagues. Remarkably, many of the lead authors became junior subspecialty fellows while writing their guides. Their desire to pass on what they were learning, while trying to balance multiple responsibilities, is a testament to their dedication and skills as clinicians, teachers, and leaders.

We hope this series fulfills the need for essential and practical knowledge for those learning the art of consultation in a particular subspecialty and for those just passing through it.

Tammy L. Lin, M.D., Series Editor
Daniel M. Goodenberger, M.D.,
Series Advisor

Preface

It is with great privilege that I introduce the first edition of *The Washington Manual® Infectious Diseases Subspecialty Consult* as an addition to the entire subspecialty series of consult manuals designed to present a concise review and rational therapeutic approach to common medical problems from a subspecialist's vantage point. The series has been produced primarily through the hard work of the residents and fellows at Washington University in St. Louis. The subspecialty series will carry on in the fine tradition of *The Washington Manual® of Internal Medicine* and will undoubtedly serve as an invaluable resource.

The Washington Manual® Infectious Diseases Subspecialty Consult is a comprehensive, yet concise, resource for the diagnosis and management of common, and some not so common, problems in infectious diseases. The text provides practical information in a format that is applicable to the medical wards, including background information, pathophysiology, differential diagnosis, evaluation, and treatment plans. The information will prove an invaluable resource to nonspecialists in the field who are caring for patients, as well as to residents and students preparing for morning presentations to the attending.

Infectious disease is an exciting field in constant evolution. Over the last few decades, there have been exciting new diseases and emerging pathogens, new diagnostic methods, and development of multiple-drug–resistant organisms that have led to dramatic growth in the need for and importance of specialists in this field. In infectious disease, no case is exactly the same, so there is no "cookbook" approach to these problems. This makes each case intriguing, and even the most mundane cases have appeal. It is our hope that this manual stimulates interest in infectious disease among its readers to face the challenges ahead and pursue a career in this specialty.

It should be noted that the dosing information in the text assumes normal renal function and creatinine clearance unless otherwise indicated. Dosing information for impaired renal function is available in Chap. 27, Antimicrobial Agents.

I am extremely grateful for the editorial assistance and patience provided by Lippincott Williams & Wilkins and by Dr. Tammy Lin, whose vision of a subspecialty consult series in the grand tradition and style of *The Washington Manual®* has become a reality. Of course, the series would not be possible without Dr. Daniel Goodenberger's guidance and direction. His contribution to the education of all involved in the entire series cannot be quantified. I would like to thank Dr. Kenneth Polonsky for his support of this enterprise from the day of its conception.

We would be remiss not to thank Dr. Linda Mundy, the faculty editor for this manual. She was extremely generous with her time and desired to remain "under the radar" in accepting any credit for her assistance. The manual would have never been completed without her assistance. Dr. Kristin Mondy also deserves special commendation for her efforts in reading the text and providing edits as the project neared its end.

Last but certainly not least, a word of special thanks for my family—Lisa and Makenzie—for their support and patience during this project.

R.S.

Key to Abbreviations

ACE	angiotensin-converting enzyme
AFB	acid-fast bacilli
ALT	alanine aminotransferase
ANA	antinuclear antibody
ANC	absolute neutrophil count
ANCA	antineutrophil cytoplasmic antibody
ARDS	acute respiratory distress syndrome
AST	aspartate aminotransferase
BCG	bacille Calmette-Guérin
CBC	complete blood count
CHF	congestive heart failure
CK-MB	myocardial muscle creatine kinase isoenzyme
CMV	cytomegalovirus
CNS	central nervous system
COPD	chronic obstructive pulmonary disease
CRP	C-reactive protein
CSF	cerebrospinal fluid
CT	computed tomograph, -graphy
DIC	disseminated intravascular coagulation
EBV	Epstein-Barr virus
ECG	electrocardiogram, -graphic, -graphy
EGD	esophagogastroduodenoscopy
ELISA	enzyme-linked immunosorbent assay
ENT	ear, nose, and throat
ERCP	endoscopic retrograde cholangiopancreatography
ESR	erythrocyte sedimentation rate
ETT	endotracheal tube
FEV_1	forced expiratory volume in 1 second
FFP	fresh frozen plasma
FUO	fever of unknown origin
GI	gastrointestinal
GU	genitourinary
HACEK	*Haemophilus aphrophilus*, *Actinobacillus actinomycetemcomitans*, *Cardiobacterium hominis*, *Eikenella corrodens*, and *Kingella kingae*
HAV	hepatitis A virus
HBeAg	hepatitis B early antigen
HBV	hepatitis B virus
HCV	hepatitis C virus
HDV	hepatitis D virus
HEV	hepatitis E virus
HIV	human immunodeficiency syndrome
HPI	history of present illness
HSV	herpes simplex virus
HTN	hypertension
HUS	hemolytic-uremic syndrome

ICP	intracranial pressure
ICU	intensive care unit
ID	infectious disease
INH	isoniazid
LDH	lactic dehydrogenase
MRI	magnetic resonance imaging
NG	nasogastric
NPO	nothing by mouth
NSAIDs	nonsteroidal antiinflammatory drugs, agents
PCN	penicillin
PCR	polymerase chain reaction
PID	pelvic inflammatory disease
PJP	*Pneumocystis jiroveci* pneumonia (formerly *Pneumocystis carinii* pneumonia)
PPD	purified protein derivative
PT	prothrombin time
RSV	respiratory syncytial virus
SBE	subacute bacterial endocarditis
SLE	systemic lupus erythematosus
STD	sexually transmitted disease
TB	tuberculosis
TEE	transesophageal echocardiogram, -graphic, -graphy
TMP-SMX	trimethoprim-sulfamethoxazole
TTE	transthoracic echocardiography
UA	urinalysis
URI	upper respiratory infection
U/S	ultrasound
UTI	urinary tract infection
VDRL	Venereal Disease Research Laboratory
VRE	vancomycin-resistant *Enterococcus*
VSD	ventricular septal defect
VZV	varicella-zoster virus
WBC	white blood cell

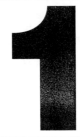

Approach to the Infectious Diseases Consult

Hilary M. Babcock

INTRODUCTION

The most wonderful and engaging aspect of the practice of IDs is also its most challenging: the great variety. Patients are of all ages and have all levels of complexity of illness. Any and all organ systems can be affected: individually, sequentially, or simultaneously. This large variety makes ID constantly interesting, rarely repetitive, and challenging to practice well. The ID consult requires a very broad approach to patients and their illnesses to attempt to ascertain what infections they are at risk for, where and how they might have acquired their infections, when and how to treat the infections, and what complications to anticipate.

Most ID consults fall into one of several broad categories: (a) assistance with a diagnostic dilemma, (b) treatment recommendations (e.g., a specific drug regimen and a planned duration of therapy), (c) management of infectious or treatment complications, and (d) infection control and occupational health recommendations (e.g., isolation guidelines or exposure management). When calling an ID consult, the caller can maximize the utility of the consult by deciding on and clearly communicating what the question is to which he or she desires an answer. For example, a consult that confirms the diagnosis of cellulitis is not helpful if the referring physician wanted a treatment recommendation for a patient allergic to PCN. Have ready for the consultant the specific question to be addressed, the patient's vital statistics (location, age, race, gender, underlying illnesses), any microbiologic diagnoses already available, and an assessment of the acuity of the problem.

Occasionally, questions to an ID consultant can be managed over the phone (e.g., simple treatment recommendations for uncomplicated illnesses and isolation policies). If the caller wishes only a phone consultation, adequate information on the patient's status, microbiology, allergies, and acuity must be provided. Some questions almost always require a full consultation, such as those involving bacteremia, resistant organisms, and high-risk patients. Some situations can be classified as ID emergencies and require immediate consultation, such as necrotizing fasciitis, rapidly progressive skin infections, meningococcemia, and epiglottitis. After consultation, it may become necessary to involve other subspecialists (e.g., surgery, orthopedics, renal, or cardiology) for assistance with a full assessment or treatment. In general, recommendations for surgical intervention or device removal should be discussed in person or by phone with the referring physician before making such a recommendation in writing.

The approach to the consult outlined below covers most aspects of a complete ID history and physical. Consults for patients with fever of unknown origin usually require most of this information. Some consults already have an infectious diagnosis and need only treatment recommendations. In that case, the consult can be tailored as needed.

HISTORY OF PRESENT ILLNESS

The HPI is the most similar to the consults of any other discipline and the most productive component of the initial evaluation. In this section, the story of the patient's primary symptoms should be told, with careful attention to their time course, nature, and severity, as well as whether similar symptoms have ever occurred before. Related symptoms should be elicited and described as well. Any previous workup should be summarized here as well, although detailed listing of prior radiologic studies and culture results can be saved for their respective sections. Ill contacts should also be noted. Based on the patient's account, numerous hypotheses for the illness will be pursued or rejected.

REVIEW OF SYMPTOMS

Any systemic symptoms not initially mentioned by the patient during the HPI should be documented. A thorough review of systems may elicit additional localizing information the patient may have forgotten or considered unrelated to the chief complaint (e.g., a transient rash). Weight loss, night sweats, and anorexia should usually be included. Fever should usually be included in the HPI. Pain of any significant impact on the patient should usually be noted regardless of location. For example, back pain is often associated with endocarditis or vertebral diskitis. Chronic complaints can also be noted here.

MEDICAL HISTORY

The medical history should include a complete list of ongoing chronic medical conditions as well as a reporting of significant illnesses in the patient's past. In evaluating recurrent infections, immune deficiencies may be a concern, and documentation of whether the patient was ill frequently as a child, had recurrent ear or skin infections, or was ever hospitalized with pneumonia can be helpful. Lack of childhood immunizations should be noted, as well as yearly influenza vaccination and pneumococcal vaccine status. Any history of illnesses that could affect immune function should be included (e.g., cancer and its treatment; autoimmune illnesses and their treatments; chronic illnesses that require treatment with immunosuppressants, such as steroids for asthma). All chronic conditions that can affect the patient's risk of infection should also be included (e.g., diabetes, with or without insulin dependence). Illnesses that reflect a risk for other infections should also be included (e.g., any patient who has had any STD is at increased risk for syphilis, HIV, and HBV). Blood transfusion history, with dates if possible, should also be included to reflect the patient's risk of having contracted HIV or HCV.

SURGICAL HISTORY

The surgical history should include any implanted devices such as joints, valves, or pacemakers, as well as splenectomy (which causes increased risk of infection with encapsulated organisms), and acid-suppressive gastric surgery (which results in increased risk of TB).

MEDICATIONS

All current medications should be listed as well as any history of immunosuppressive medications or chemotherapeutic agents. Antibiotic regimens received recently (during or immediately before the hospitalization for inpatients) should also be noted, with dates when possible. A large number of medicines are known to cause fever, most notably PCNs and cephalosporins, often without a rash or eosinophilia. Antipyretics may greatly alter the host's febrile response and should also be noted.

ALLERGIES

All allergies may be included, but particularly any antibiotic allergies must be elicited. The type of reaction should be included (e.g., rash, hives, erythema, lip swelling).

SOCIAL HISTORY

The social history can yield many important clues to a patient's illness. The patient's living situation in terms of urban or rural setting and municipal or well-water sources is often helpful. Any contact with farm animals should be noted. Other animal contacts with pets—especially cats (*Bartonella*), birds (psittacosis), reptiles (*Salmonella*), fish (*Mycobacterium marinum*), and dogs (*Toxocara canis*)—should be included. Occupational history (e.g., lab technician in microbiology lab or silo cleaner) should be noted. Recreational pursuits [e.g., cigarettes, alcohol, marijuana smoking and other drug abuse (nasal, PO, IV, skin popping), hunting (*Tularemia*), gardening (*Sporothrix*), spelunking (*Histoplasmosis*)] should be noted. Number and health status of sexual partners can also be helpful, as well as any history of male-to-male sex.

Travel history should be included here as well. Recent travel (within the last 6 mos) should be noted, as well as any distant history of travel to places where some indolent diseases are endemic (e.g., TB in Vietnam, coccidioides in the southwestern United States).

PHYSICAL EXAM

As with any specialty, a thorough and complete exam is essential. Pay particular attention to the fever curve. Temperatures >39°C (102.2°F) are more likely to be caused by an infectious etiology. However, very high fevers raise the possibility of heat stroke. A dramatic fever with rhythmic cycles is suggestive of pyogenic infection, especially an abscess, although this is not specific. Some tropical infections (e.g., malaria) have characteristic fever curves. Attention must also be paid to the cutaneous exam. Many acute infections are accompanied by characteristic rashes that greatly aid in their diagnosis (e.g., petechiae and purpura in meningococcemia). Lesions on the fingers and toes can be clues to endovascular infection. The mouth can provide important clues, especially if thrush is present (raising the possibility of HIV) or there is evidence of poor dentition (raising the possibility of endocarditis or lung abscess due to aspiration). A careful exam for lymphadenopathy is warranted initially. Focal adenopathy would direct the examiner to carefully examine the drainage area, whereas diffuse adenopathy raises questions of primary HIV, EBV, or secondary syphilis. Heart murmurs are always important, whether new or old.

LAB TESTS

The lab tests section of the consult should include dates and results of all current lab studies as well as past lab tests that reflect a history of renal or hepatic insufficiency. Recent results of CBC, basic chemistries, liver function tests, and UA should be noted. The WBC and differential trend up or down should be noted. Drug levels of antibiotics should be noted. All current cultures (positive and negative) should be listed at this time, with sites, dates, and susceptibility profiles. Blood cultures should have a notation of the number drawn and the number positive at each draw. This is vitally important in determining the significance of a positive culture. Any prior testing for HIV (including CD4 count and HIV RNA level), HBV, and HCV should be noted. Pathology reports from current or prior procedures should be reviewed and the relevant ones reported. Relevant radiologic studies should be reviewed and reported.

ASSESSMENT AND PLAN

As in all specialties, a thorough but concise summary of pertinent findings from the history and physical exam should be presented. A ranked list of possible etiologies, from likely to rare, and a plan for evaluating those possibilities should follow. The decision to initiate treatment is based on the acuity of illness of the patient, the need for further diagnostic evaluation before treatment, the likelihood of a particular illness, the concern for potential adverse events and drug interactions, and the patient's agreement with the plan. The choice of appropriate antibiotics is discussed in Chap. 27, Antimicrobial Agents.

TOP TEN FREQUENTLY ASKED QUESTIONS FOR INFECTIOUS DISEASE INPATIENT CONSULTATIONS

1. My patient has *Candida* in a urine culture. What should I do?

There are two key issues: (a) Does the patient have evidence of a UTI (consistent symptoms such as dysuria, fever with no other obvious source, lower abdominal pain, *and* pyuria, with an increased number of WBCs in the urine sample)? (b) Does the patient have a urinary catheter?

If the patient has evidence of a UTI with symptoms and pyuria, then treatment may be indicated [fluconazole (Diflucan)]. If there are no consistent symptoms and little or no pyuria, then treatment is not indicated. *Candida* is often present on perineal skin, and contamination of a urinary collection is common.

If the patient has a urinary catheter in place, it should be removed or at least changed. In patients with chronic urinary catheters, symptoms are the best guide to the need for therapy. Many of these patients have persistent colonization without infection, and the irritation from the catheter may give them chronic low levels of pyuria as well. Treatment should be reserved and cultures only obtained when the patient complains of UTI symptoms [1].

2. My patient has VRE in the urine. What should I do?

Place the patient on contact isolation. See item number 1 for determination of whether the patient has a UTI. If the patient does have evidence of a UTI, any catheters should be removed or changed, and treatment can be initiated with nitrofurantoin (Macrodantin) if the isolate is susceptible to it. Nitrofurantoin reaches high enough concentrations in urine to eradicate most VRE infections. Chloramphenicol (Chloromycetin), quinupristin/dalfopristin (Synercid), and linezolid (Zyvox) should be reserved for systemic infections.

3. My patient has diarrhea and VRE in the stool. What should I do?

Put the patient on contact isolation and look for a cause of the diarrhea, especially *Clostridium difficile*. *Enterococcus* is a normal colonizer of the GI tract, regardless of whether it is resistant to vancomycin (Vancocin). It is not a cause of diarrhea and does not require treatment.

4. My patient has a bad cellulitis but has anaphylaxis to PCNs and cephalosporins. What can I use for treatment?

Clindamycin (Cleocin) is an often-overlooked agent for treating skin infections. It has excellent gram-positive coverage.

5. I just admitted a patient with HIV on antiretroviral treatment (ART). Should I hold his medicines until we figure out why he's sick?

In general, ART should be continued if at all possible, although exceptions do occur. If the patient is unable to take any oral medications, then *all* ART should be held at once and restarted at once when symptoms resolve. If the patient is on abacavir (Ziagen) and has symptoms of hypersensitivity (e.g., rash, abdominal pain, nausea and vomiting, or fever), all medications should be stopped. If the patient has evidence of symptomatic hyperlactatemia (shortness of breath, abdominal pain), all medications should be stopped.

Never stop or start only one medicine at a time, as this can induce viral resistance to medications.

6. My patient has *Candida* in her blood culture. How serious is that?

Very serious. *Candida* bloodstream infections always require treatment. Any intravascular catheters should be removed and treatment initiated as soon as possible. *Candida albicans* is the most common cause of candidal bloodstream infections and is almost always susceptible to fluconazole (Diflucan), so this is reasonable therapy to initiate while awaiting speciation of the isolate. Evaluation for septic complications should be considered in all patients without rapid clinical and microbiologic improvement on therapy. Ophthalmologic evaluation of the retina and hepatosplenic U/S may be indicated [1].

7. Can I keep this central line?

In patients with intravascular access and positive blood cultures, the desire to preserve the access is always strong. If the access can be removed, it should be.

A great review by organism and type of central venous access can be found in reference 2.

8. Who needs meningococcal prophylaxis?

When a patient is admitted with meningococcemia or meningococcal meningitis, there is always a rush for prophylaxis. The only people who need prophylaxis are (a) immediate family or household members of the patient and (b) health care workers who had intimate contact with respiratory secretions of the patient (i.e., those who intubated the patient without wearing a mask).

9. When should I treat chronic decubitus ulcers with antibiotics?

Chronic decubiti are universally colonized with multiple microorganisms. Treatment should only be initiated when there is a change in the wound (e.g., significantly increased drainage, more purulent drainage or more foul-smelling drainage) or when the patient develops symptoms of infection (e.g., fever, malaise, pain).

10. Our patient with neutropenic fever is still neutropenic, still has fever, and has been on vancomycin and cefepime for 4 days. What do we do now?

This can be a very difficult management issue. A thorough evaluation is indicated, starting with a very careful physical exam looking for unrecognized or undrained sources of infection. Noninfectious causes (e.g., thromboemboli) should be considered. Testing for *C. difficile* may be helpful. Empiric antifungal therapy is sometimes warranted [3].

KEY POINTS TO REMEMBER

- Be thorough!
- Be thoughtful!
- If the phone story is unclear, uncommon, or uncertain, a full consult is needed before rendering an opinion.

REFERENCES

1. Rex JH, Walsh TJ, Sobel JD, et al. Practice guidelines for the treatment of candidiasis. *Clin Infect Dis* 2000;30:662–678.
2. Mermel LA, Farr BM, Sheretz RJ, et al. Guidelines for the management of intravascular catheter-related infections. *Clin Infect Dis* 2001;32:1249–1272.
3. Hughes WT, Armstrong D, Bodey GP, et al. 2002 guidelines for the use of antimicrobial agents in neutropenic patients with cancer. *Clin Infect Dis* 2002;34:730–751.

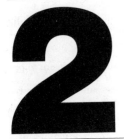

Febrile Syndromes

Michele C. L. Cabellon
Erik Dubberke

FEVER OF UNKNOWN ORIGIN

The classic definition of **fever of unknown origin** (FUO) is a temperature of ≥38.3°C (101°F) for a period of >3 wks for which a cause is not diagnosed after 1 wk of intense in-hospital investigation. This definition has been extended to the outpatient setting, as many of these patients do not require hospitalization anymore. Infection is usually the cause of approximately one-third of all cases of FUO, with neoplasm at 20–30%, collagen-vascular diseases at 10–20%, miscellaneous causes at 15–20%, and the remaining cases are undiagnosed at 5–15%. Most of the time, common etiologies are still the cause but may have unusual presentations (remember, rare is rare). Several components of the diagnostic evaluation should be completed before declaring a fever as FUO. These include general lab tests such as CBC, chemistries, ESR, UA, HIV antibody, and ANA; PPD; chest x-ray (CXR); and three sets of blood cultures off antibiotics. A CT of the abdomen should also be considered depending on the presenting symptoms.

Differential Diagnosis

The differential diagnosis is broad and can be broken down into categories of some common causes of FUO.

Infectious Causes

CMV can give a mononucleosis-like syndrome with low-grade fevers for >3 wks. Mildly elevated liver transaminases may be present. A CMV IgM antibody or CMV PCR should be sent.

Disseminated TB may present with increasing infiltrates, elevated ESR, and anemia. PPD is negative in one-half of patients, and sputum is positive for AFB in only one-fourth to one-half. Bone marrow biopsy may be revealing in up to 80% when anemia, leukopenia, and monocytosis are present. Culture from bronchoscopy may be helpful, but the British antilewisite is rarely positive.

If culture-negative endocarditis is suspected, blood cultures must be held for ≥2 wks to rule out the HACEK organisms (*Haemophilus aphrophilus*, *Actinobacillus actinomycetemcomitans*, *Cardiobacterium hominis*, *Eikenella corrodens*, and *Kingella kingae*). *Bartonella* species and *Legionella* species need special agar to isolate them. If *Coxiella burnetii* is suspected, serologic testing is needed because blood cultures will remain negative. A TEE is positive for valvular vegetations in >90% of cases.

Malignant Causes

For diagnosing lymphoma, look for lymphadenopathy and splenomegaly on exam, the presence of B symptoms (weight loss, night sweats), thrombocytopenia, and anemia. A very high LDH may be a clue.

Fever may be the presenting symptom in 15% of cases of renal cell carcinoma. Search for microscopic hematuria and erythrocytosis. Metastatic disease to the liver may have corresponding persistent low-grade fever.

Atrial myxomas present with cardiac murmur and other signs that resemble subacute bacterial endocarditis.

Collagen Vascular Disease Causes

With adult Still's disease, the classic triad in a young adult includes high fever, arthritis, and a macular or maculopapular rash on the trunk and peripheral extremities. These signs appear in the evenings and may be exacerbated by skin irritation. Diffuse lymphadenopathy and an elevated ESR are almost always present.

Temporal arteritis comprises almost 15% of FUO in patients >55 yrs. Consider a temporal artery biopsy in older patients if the ESR is elevated, even if there are no temporal symptoms.

Polyarteritis nodosa may present as testicular tenderness, mononeuritis, or livedo reticularis on skin exam. An ANCA test should be sent if suspicious and an angiogram considered.

Other, often-overlooked causes include cirrhosis, alcoholic hepatitis, drug fever, uninfected hematomas, subacute thyroiditis, and sarcoidosis. Some newly discovered causes are becoming more recognized. Hypergammaglobulinemia IgD syndrome is comprised of a large joint arthritis, rash, and very high levels of circulating IgD. In Kikuchi's disease or histiocytic necrotizing adenitis, leukopenia, liver transaminitis, splenomegaly, and lymphadenopathy usually are seen. The diagnosis is made by lymph node biopsy.

Clinical Manifestations

A thorough history and physical exam are essential to obtaining diagnosis, and the history should be repeated until the answer is found. Things to ask about include medications, previous illnesses, alcohol ingestion, travel or occupational exposures, pets (e.g., birds, cats, farm animals), animal or insect bites, and familial disorders. It is important to repeat a full review of systems every couple of days to uncover hidden clues.

Just as important as the history, the physical exam should be careful and thorough and should be repeated several times to follow the appearance of new findings. Pay special attention to the thyroid, teeth, skin, temporal arteries, lymph nodes, and eyes. New or changing cardiac murmurs or the presence of hepatosplenomegaly may be important clues.

Diagnosis

The most important concept for diagnosis is that there are no good algorithms or pathways to follow. Clinical judgment based on the information in each case should guide which diagnostic tests are ordered next. A good start is reviewing all available lab and study results. These facts should be pieced together with history and physical exam findings. It is important to remember that patients' complaints are usually helpful but may be misleading in many cases; a broad differential must be maintained. When you have a source to potentially obtain tissue diagnosis, it should be pursued quickly. Sometimes, an answer is never found despite a thorough investigation. If so and the patient is stable, it is reasonable to just watch the patient until the fevers resolve or some other clue presents itself.

Treatment

Treatment for FUO is the treatment for the underlying cause. Most causes of fever eventually present themselves; thus, it is important to resist the temptation of empiric antibiotics, high-dose steroids, or other treatments if the patient is clinically stable.

Key Points to Remember for Fever of Unknown Origin

- Perform a careful clinical exam and history; try to exclude any noninfectious causes.
- Pay close attention to any indwelling catheters and open wounds; culture if appropriate.
- Review any new medications or blood products received to ascertain if there is a correlation with fever.
- The likelihood of an infectious etiology of FUO decreases as time progresses and no infectious etiology is discovered.

FEVER IN THE POSTOP PATIENT

The key to looking at a surgical patient with fever is to consider the time period that has elapsed since the actual operation. One must keep in mind that a temperature of >38.5°C (101.3°F) is common in the postop patient—in approximately one-third of patients. In general, a fever at <48 hrs postop is less worrisome unless severe symptoms are associated with it (e.g., mental status changes). A fever at >48 hrs is significant and should be thoroughly investigated.

Differential Diagnosis

The classic "five Ws" of postop fever are *w*ind (atelectasis/pneumonia), *w*ater (UTI), *w*ound, *w*alking [deep venous thrombosis (DVT)], and "*w*onder" drugs (drug reaction). **Things you do not want to miss:** abscess, deep wound infections, or DVT.

<24 Hrs Postop

Fever with onset <24 hrs after surgery is almost always due to atelectasis from shallow breathing and inadequate pain control. Encouraging deep breaths with respiratory therapy can resolve the problem. If the patient is having a lot of secretions, a CXR may be helpful to rule out pneumonia. It is rare to have a wound infection at this stage, but if present, the likely organisms are *Streptococcus* and *Clostridium* (necrotizing, bronze, weeping, painful wound). Other things to consider are thyroid storm, Addisonian crisis, transfusion reactions if the patient received blood products, and intestinal leaks, depending on the type of surgery involved.

Postop Days 1–2

One must consider the same etiologies as in the first 24 hrs, in addition to other infections related to instrumentation, such as UTI if a Foley catheter was inserted and bacteremia from central lines. A CBC, UA and urine culture, blood cultures, and CXR are part of the initial workup. Remember to always think of the five Ws.

Postop Days 3–5

Postop days 3–5 are when more serious causes of fever appear. Again, consider the above sources, along with some that are not as obvious. Pneumonia may develop in this period, especially if the patient is on a ventilator. DVT can occur in both the lower extremities and the pelvic veins. Acalculous cholecystitis, especially in immobile patients or those who received large amounts of blood products, may present with fever as well as pancreatitis. Candidiasis in patients on total parenteral nutrition must be considered. Wound infections and leakage are most common, along with hematomas.

Postop Days ≥6

Again, etiology of fever tends to be more serious in this period. Anastomotic leaks, abscesses (intraabdominal sources may involve infections with both gram-negative aerobes and anaerobes), infected hematomas, and deep wound must be ruled out. New problems to consider are *Clostridium difficile* colitis for those patients who have received antibiotics and parotitis in those who have or had an NG tube. Usually, the causative organism in parotitis is *Staphylococcus aureus*. Patients at higher risk for this condition are those with poor oral hygiene, those who are NPO, and those who are dehydrated.

Pathophysiology

There are many causes of fever in a surgical patient. Intraop contamination has been reduced by the use of periop antibiotics. It is recommended that an antibiotic that covers anticipated pathogens be given before the surgery, within 60 mins before the skin is cut. This timing is critical because the antibiotic must reach the tissues before the contamination occurs. The most commonly used antibiotic for this purpose is cefazolin (Ancef).

Clinical Manifestations

In any patient, a full physical exam is warranted. It includes wound inspection and examination of all lines and drains, a full respiratory exam, and examination of the extremities for evidence of thrombosis. The array of physical presentations can be broad, so a careful history focusing on any complaint of the patient is helpful to determine the possible cause.

Treatment

Treatment of postop fever is achieved by treating the underlying cause. Analgesics and antipyretics can be used for symptomatic relief.

Key Points to Remember for Postop Fever

- Consider all sources when evaluating the patient initially: wounds, central and peripheral lines, all other drains, chest tubes, Foley catheters, and heart valves, or other hardware inserted during the surgery.
- Culture any possible existing fluids if no source is apparent but there is suspicion for infection: pleural effusions, ascites, percutaneous drains, sputum, CSF, blisters, and catheter tips. Cultures of wounds are generally not helpful unless they are obviously infected.
- If you suspect loculated collections or undrained pus, do not hesitate to obtain further imaging to help you pinpoint the diagnosis.

FEVER IN THE ICU

The approach to the febrile patient in the ICU should be systematic and comprehensive in order not to miss potentially life-threatening causes and to avoid unnecessary expense and invasive procedures. Any disease process that elicits the release of proinflammatory cytokines interleukin-1, interleukin-6, or tumor necrosis factor-alpha can produce fever. Although infections are the most common cause of fever in the ICU patient, many noninfectious inflammatory conditions cause the release of proinflammatory cytokines. Conversely, not every patient in the ICU with an infectious process mounts a fever response. 10% of septic patients are hypothermic at presentation, and 35% are normothermic. Thus, the differential diagnosis of etiologies of fever in an ICU patient is extensive, although the clinical suspicion for infection in this patient population should be high even in the absence of documented fever.

Differential Diagnosis

Infectious Etiologies

Most infections in the ICU are associated with foreign bodies [endotracheal tubes, central venous catheters (CVCs), NG tubes, Foley catheters, or prosthetic devices], previous surgical procedures, or antibiotic-associated colitis. The most common nosocomial infections in the ICU include ventilator-associated pneumonia (VAP), sinusitis, bloodstream infections, UTIs, surgical wound infections, and *C. difficile* colitis.

   VENTILATOR-ASSOCIATED PNEUMONIA. VAP can be difficult to diagnose, and no single method is ideal. 25% of patients who are mechanically ventilated develop pneumonia, with a subsequent 27% attributable mortality rate. VAP should be suspected in febrile patients with changes in the lung exam (e.g., development of crackles, consolidation, an effusion, or a change in the character of respiratory secretions). For initial evaluation, visual inspection of sputum and review of sputum Gram's stain findings and culture results are usually sufficient. It is often difficult to differentiate between a colonizing organism with a true pathogen; if the sputum appears purulent or if the Gram's stain shows a large number of neutrophils, infection is more likely than colonization. If there is a concern for VAP, a portable, upright CXR should be done while keeping in mind that if it is early enough in the course of a VAP, there may not be any radiographic changes; conversely, if pulmonary infiltrates are observed, it may be difficult or impossible to differentiate pneumonia from noninfectious etiologies (e.g., pulmonary edema, hemorrhage, atelectasis, or oxygen toxicity).

URINARY TRACT. Bacteriuria is very common in the ICU setting, especially in patients with indwelling Foley catheters, suprapubic catheters, ureteral stents, or nephrostomies, and deciding when it represents true infection versus colonization can be difficult. UA to assess for pyuria as well as urine culture and susceptibilities should be performed. Pyuria (>10 WBCs/HPF on UA) in a non-neutropenic patient with a urine culture that grows >10^4 colony-forming units/mL likely represents infection.

CLOSTRIDIUM DIFFICILE. Most patients with *C. difficile*–associated fever have watery diarrhea, although some patients may present with an ileus or toxic megacolon. Clinical features of *C. difficile* colitis include diarrheal stools that conform to the container in which they are placed, prior exposure to antibiotics, positive fecal leukocyte analysis, evidence of colitis on CT scan, or pseudomembrane formation observed on colonoscopy. Other enteric pathogens hardly ever cause fever in ICU patients, but the possibility of infectious enterocolitis should be considered in patients with a significant travel history, HIV disease, or unusual exposures. In patients with new-onset diarrhea, a stool specimen should be submitted for *C. difficile* toxin by enzyme immunoassay (sensitivity for toxin A–producing strains, 72%) and fecal leukocytes. If the enzyme immunoassay is negative, a second sample should be sent; multiple stools increase the sensitivity of the toxin assay for *C. difficile* colitis (sensitivity can increase another 5–20%). If severe disease is present, the patient should be empirically placed on metronidazole (Flagyl) while awaiting results of the tests, or endoscopy should be performed to look for pseudomembranous colitis. If two enzyme immunoassays are negative for *C. difficile*, empiric therapy is not recommended, and other causes of diarrhea should be considered.

CATHETER-ASSOCIATED INFECTION. Up to 25% of CVCs become colonized with bacteria, and approximately 20–30% of these colonized catheters result in bloodstream infections (i.e., approximately 5% of CVCs are associated with bloodstream infections). CVC infection should be suspected (a) in patients with bacteremia/fungemia without obvious source who have an intravascular device at the onset of fever; (b) if inflammation or purulence is noted at the catheter insertion site or along the catheter tunnel; (c) when there is abrupt onset of infection associated with fulminant shock; and (d) when multiple sets of blood cultures are positive for organisms that might otherwise be disregarded as contaminants (e.g., coagulase-negative staphylococci). Femoral and jugular venous catheters have higher rates of infection than subclavian venous catheters. See Chap. 15, Solid Organ Transplant Infections, for more details.

SINUSITIS. Sinusitis is often clinically silent and is an underappreciated cause of fever in the ICU. Up to 85% of nasally intubated patients develop sinusitis within 1 wk. Purulent nasal discharge is present in only 25% of ICU patients with proven sinusitis. If sinusitis is suspected, a CT scan of the sinuses should be performed. If radiographic findings are consistent with sinusitis, the diagnosis can be confirmed by paranasal sinus puncture and aspiration performed under sterile conditions for culture, although in most cases, empirical antibiotic therapy (e.g., imipenem) is administered without culture confirmation of the diagnosis. Sinusitis is best treated by removal of the NG tube.

WOUND INFECTION. The incidence of surgical wound infection varies according to the classification of the wound. Reported wound infection rates increase from clean (1–3%), to clean-contaminated (4–5%), to contaminated (6–15%), to dirty wounds (16–40%). Fevers on postop days 1–3 are generally not secondary to wound infections unless *Clostridia* or group A streptococci are involved. Defervescence often does not occur until up to 72 hrs after surgery to control an infection (e.g., abscess drainage). New fever or fever persistent >4 days after surgery should raise suspicion for a persistent undrained abscess or necrotic tissue or a new infection. All wounds should be inspected periodically for erythema, purulence, or tenderness. If infection is suspected, the wound should be opened, and purulent material should be submitted for Gram's stain and bacterial culture. Infections complicating surgical procedures involving the GI, genitourinary, or respiratory tracts often are polymicrobial with the normal endogenous microflora. Infections complicating clean surgeries are most often caused by *Staphylococcus aureus*.

Noninfectious Etiologies

Many noninfectious etiologies of fever occur in the ICU but do not typically lead to a temperature >38.9°C (102°F). The main exceptions include fever secondary to drugs and transfusion reactions.

DRUG FEVER. Drug fever should be suspected in patients with an otherwise unexplained fever, especially when antibiotics (beta-lactams), antiarrhythmics (procainamide), anticonvulsants [phenytoin (Dilantin)], antihypertensives [methyl-dopa (Aldomet)], and granulocyte-macrophage colony-stimulating factors are being used. Drug fever may be associated with leukocytosis, eosinophilia, or relative brady-cardia. The diagnosis of drug fever is based on the temporal relationship of fever starting after the suspected drug is initiated and resolution when the drug is discontinued. Life-threatening causes of drug fever include neuroleptic malignant syndrome (induced by psychotropic medications) and malignant hyperthermia. It is also important to remember that withdrawal from certain drugs (alcohol, benzodiazepines, barbiturates, and opiates) can cause fever as well.

TRANSFUSION REACTION. Fever complicates blood transfusions 0.5% of the time and is more common with platelet transfusions. Transfusion fever is usually induced by antibodies against antigens on transfused leukocytes or platelets. Febrile reactions often start 30 mins to 2 hrs after the transfusion has begun.

ENDOCRINE CAUSES. Two endocrine emergencies can present with fever in ICU patients: thyroid storm and acute adrenal insufficiency. Both of these conditions may be indistinguishable from septic shock.

OTHER CAUSES. Other potentially life-threatening causes of fever in the ICU that should always be considered in the differential diagnosis include acalculous cholecystitis, pulmonary embolism, subarachnoid hemorrhage, and fat embolism after long bone fracture.

Clinical Manifestations

Often, ICU patients are unable to give a history, so the workup of a febrile patient in the ICU should start with a review of the chart and a physical exam. Many causes of fever in the ICU may be evident on the physical exam. The exam should focus on conditions that are common to patients in the ICU. The sinuses, lungs, abdomen, urinary tract, and skin should be assessed, as well as any sites of prior invasive procedures or prosthetic material. Findings on the exam should guide the selection of appropriate diagnostic studies.

Treatment

The take-home note for fever in the ICU patient is this: If infection is suspected, empirical broad-spectrum antibiotic therapy should be initiated promptly after appropriate specimens have been obtained for Gram's stain and culture. Mortality is 10–15% lower in septic patients who are initially treated with an effective antibiotic (defined as an antibiotic to which the causative organism is susceptible *in vitro*).

Key Points for Fever in the ICU

- Perform a careful clinical exam and detailed chart review; exclude common noninfectious causes such as DVT, medications, and transfusion reactions.
- Culture any catheter or wound sites that appear to be at risk of infection; consider removal or change of catheters if possible.
- If a nosocomial infection is suspected, consider empiric antibiotic treatment to cover pathogens such as methicillin-resistant *S. aureus* and *Pseudomonas* species.

FEVER AND RASH

Rash is associated with several causes of fever and systemic illnesses, including infectious etiologies. History is crucial in obtaining the correct diagnosis. Initially, the evaluation begins by determining if the patient is hemodynamically stable and if the rash appears to be a sign of a contagious infection for which isolation precautions are necessary.

Pathophysiology

Rash may be caused by embolization of the causative organism into the distal blood vessels causing capillary burst or by the effect of toxins released into the bloodstream. The pathophysiology of the rash determines its clinical presentation.

Clinical Manifestations

Petechiae are lesions that measure ≤3 mm in diameter and may range in color from red to black. They are often palpable. Larger lesions of the same kind are called **purpura**. These lesions may coalesce to form large ecchymoses. Petechiae do *not* blanch on pressure due to the presence of extravasated RBC pigments in the lesions. This is the most ominous of all rashes, because the presence of petechiae often indicates a potentially fatal underlying etiology.

Flat, nonpalpable lesions are called **macules;** small, solid, palpable lesions are referred to as **papules.** Both of these lesions are usually associated with viral illnesses or drug eruptions, but virtually any type of infectious process may appear or present as a macular or papular rash. The differential diagnosis for these lesions is extensive.

Nodules are palpable, solid-feeling lesions deeper than the skin surface that indicate involvement of the disease in the dermis layer of the skin. These lesions may be painful and quite large.

Vesicles are small, fluid-filled, blister-like lesions. If vesicles contain purulent material, they are referred to as **pustules.** Larger lesions are classified as **bullae** and may result in sloughing of massive areas of skin.

Erythema is a widespread rash that blanches. The patient may appear flushed. Often, erythema appears only in the areas of usual sun exposure, which may then allow it to be confused with a suntan.

Differential Diagnosis

There is a wide range of both infectious and noninfectious etiologies for each type of skin lesion. Some of the most common are discussed here.

Petechiae

Petechial lesions may be found in septicemia caused by any organism, but some are more classic. *Neisseria meningitidis* septicemia must be considered in any febrile patient with a petechial or macular rash. The diagnosis can be confirmed by Gram's stain of petechial scrapings, CSF, or peripheral buffy coat smear showing gram-negative diplococci. The treatment of choice is PCN G, 300,000 U/kg/day divided into q2h doses. Third-generation cephalosporins also are effective therapy. Ceftriaxone (Rocephin), 2 g IV q24h, is a reasonable alternative to PCN in light of its ease of administration.

Streptococcus pneumoniae and *Haemophilus influenzae* septicemia are both caused by encapsulated bacteria and can be associated with profuse petechiae. These conditions may mimic symptoms of meningococcemia, especially in asplenic patients.

Gonococcemia usually causes a polymorphic rash, which includes petechiae, as well as macules, papules, and pustules that are clustered mostly around affected joints. Scraping of the lesions shows gram-negative diplococci on Gram's stain. This rash is usually associated with polyarthritis and tenosynovitis.

Rocky Mountain spotted fever is caused by *Rickettsia rickettsii* and begins with fever, chills, headache, and myalgias. A macular rash begins 1–5 days later over the peripheral extremities and then can turn petechial later as it spreads to the trunk and face. In general, this rash has a more gradual onset than meningococcemia.

Typhus, a recrudescent, louse-borne disease, may present with petechiae that are usually located in a truncal distribution and then migrate to the periphery. Typhus may present after a stressful event (e.g., surgery), and it should be considered as a diagnostic possibility in the elderly patient population from eastern Europe, where it is prevalent. Rat-bite fevers caused by *Spirillum minus* and *Streptobacillus moniliformis* can also present as a petechial rash.

Bacterial endocarditis may be associated with petechial lesions seen mostly on extremities and mucous membranes (peripheral sites), which are the result of infectious emboli. The lesions can appear and resolve, so it is helpful to circle lesions to follow their possible disappearance later.

Viral causes of petechial rash include enteroviral infections, acute HBV, Epstein-Barr virus, rubella, and dengue fever. There are several noninfectious causes of petechial rash, including allergy, Henoch-Schönlein purpura, thrombocytopenia, hypersensitivity vasculitis, acute rheumatic fever, and SLE.

Macules and Papules

A macular rash is probably the most common infectious exanthem. Macules can be caused by viral or bacterial infections. Secondary syphilis can present with a macular rash that appears between 2 wks and 6 mos after the initial chancre. It usually consists of tan to reddish-brown macules throughout, including the palms and soles of the feet. In moist areas of the body, lesions are raised and broad and are very contagious due to the high content of spirochetes in the lesions. Such lesions in the groin are called **condylomata lata.**

Another typical papular rash is seen with typhoid fever, caused by *Salmonella* species. The classic symptoms include fever, leukopenia, depression, abdominal pain, bradycardia, and constipation. The pink papules, which are called **rose spots,** usually concentrate on the trunk. These blanch on pressure and are usually few in number. The organism cannot be isolated from these lesions.

Infections from tick bites can typically result in a rash. In ehrlichiosis, only a minority of patients develop a rash, but if present, the macules involve the palms and soles.

The initial stage of Lyme disease characteristically is accompanied by a rash, called **erythema chronicum migrans,** which is an expanding lesion with central clearing ("target lesion"). The presentation of Lyme disease may be deceiving, however, as 10–15% of cases initially present with multiple macular lesions and fever.

Other conditions that are more rarely associated with a maculopapular rash include *Mycoplasma* infections and psittacosis, which may be associated with an erythematous exanthem. Murine typhus is a rickettsial infection from a rat-flea bite. The rash begins in the axillae and migrates outward, and it is often associated with a headache.

Viral causes of a macular or papular rash with fever include human parvovirus B19 [fifth disease, erythema infectiosum ("slapped cheeks" appearance that may become generalized)], human herpesvirus-6, coxsackieviruses, CMV, EBV, enterovirus, acute HIV infection, HBV, rubeola, rubella, and adenovirus.

Noninfectious causes of a macular rash with fever include serum sickness, dermatomyositis, SLE, erythema marginatum, allergy (especially drug reactions), and erythema multiforme (which may be precipitated by an infection; look for target lesions).

Other considerations in a patient with fever and a maculopapular rash include Sweet's syndrome (acute febrile neutrophilic dermatosis), which may present as high fever, headache, and arthralgias associated with tender, bluish-red papules that have irregular borders. Some of these lesions may have central clearing or pustules, and they are generally located on the face, neck, and extremities but spare the trunk. Diagnosis is made by skin biopsy, with the hallmark finding being neutrophilic infiltration into the dermis. Sweet's syndrome is associated with certain malignancies, ulcerative colitis, and monoclonal gammopathies of undetermined significance.

Phenytoin hypersensitivity syndrome may be associated with sudden fever, a macular rash, generalized lymphadenopathy, and leukocytosis, which may appear months or even longer into the treatment time with the drug.

Nodules

Fungemia may result in nodular infiltrates in the skin. Sepsis from *Candida* species may present as a sudden development of diffuse nodules. This should be considered in patients who are receiving parenteral nutrition. Histoplasmosis, blastomycosis, coccidioidomycosis, and sporotrichosis in their disseminated forms may also cause fever and a nodular rash. These findings are more common in immunocompromised hosts.

Ecthyma gangrenosum is a nodular rash that is seen in the first 12–24 hrs after onset of *Pseudomonas* sepsis. These lesions are generally painless round macules that change to bullae and slough off to leave a deep ulcer. An overlying black eschar may develop over the ulcer. Ecthyma gangrenosum is classically seen in the groin and axilla but can be widespread.

Erythema nodosum lesions are tender nodules that are typically located on the anterior portions of the legs. Many infectious and noninfectious causes may precipitate the disease and can present in association with fever. These lesions usually heal without scarring once the underlying condition is treated.

Erythema induratum consists of painful red nodules located over the posterior ankles that may suppurate. This is an unusual manifestation of a TB reaction and is a sign of reactivation after long-standing infection. No AFB organisms are found in sampling of the lesions, as this is a hypersensitivity reaction from bacilli at remote locations. The diagnosis can be made by wedge biopsy.

Vesicles

Vesicles are another common manifestation of viral infections. Primary *Varicella zoster* infection presents with a rash that begins as papules but evolves into vesicles quickly (such lesions typically are described as having a "dew drop on a rose leaf" appearance). These lesions are most heavily concentrated on the trunk. The key to recognizing this rash is that lesions of different stages are present at one time. HSV disseminated infection may also present with widespread vesicles, but this disease is usually only seen in immunocompromised hosts. Scraping of the blisters reveals multinucleated giant cells when using a Tzanck preparation (which is also positive in patients with varicella). The vesicular fluid can also be sent for viral culture to confirm the diagnosis.

Staphylococcal bacteremia and gonococcemia can be associated with widespread pustules. Rickettsial pox, although rare, presents with painless pustules that develop at the site of a mite bite and later turn to a black eschar. Later, a generalized rash of papules capped by vesicles can be seen. Disseminated *Vibrio vulnificus* causes a classic rash that consists of bullae that may become hemorrhagic. This disease is contracted by eating undercooked, contaminated seafood. It is usually seen with higher incidence in patients with underlying liver or kidney disease or with diabetes mellitus.

Other viral causes of a vesicular rash with fever include coxsackieviruses (hand-foot-and-mouth disease), parvovirus B19, and HIV. Noninfectious causes include allergy, contact dermatitis, and eczema herpeticum (HSV infection of an underlying atopic dermatitis).

Erythema

Widespread erythematous rashes are commonly seen in disseminated staphylococcal and streptococcal infections. Group A *Streptococcus* infection in the form of scarlet fever or toxic shock–like syndrome is associated with erythema produced by pyrogenic exotoxins. PCN G, 24 million U/day IV in divided doses, or a first- or third-generation cephalosporin in addition to clindamycin, 600–900 mg IV q8h (which appears to decrease toxin production), is the regimen of choice for initial treatment. Disseminated *S. aureus* infection is the cause of the classic toxic shock syndrome: fever, hypotension, erythema, and possible multisystem organ failure. This overwhelming infection can be contracted from overcolonized areas of the body or from wound infection. Staphylococcal scalded skin syndrome, another form of widespread *Staphylococcus* infection, can present with areas of sloughing skin and is more common in children. Treatment of choice for these infections is nafcillin (Nafcil) or oxacillin (Bactocill), 2 g IV q4h.

Enterovirus infections are a rare cause of erythematous rash. Noninfectious causes of fever and diffuse erythema are lymphoma, Sézary's syndrome, toxic epidermal necrolysis, and Kawasaki's disease.

Diagnostic Workup

The crucial pieces of the history must include questions about recent travel or occupational exposures, exposure to animals and pets, all drug ingestion (prescription, over-the-counter, herbal, and illicit) within the last 30 days, and insect exposures. Any history of valvular heart disease or other predisposing illnesses and immunocompetence status are important considerations. Recent exposure to other ill humans should be ascertained.

The physical exam should include a search for lymphadenopathy; genital, mucosal, or conjunctival lesions; signs of meningitis; evidence for arthritis; and hepatosplenomegaly.

To characterize the rash, the types of skin lesions, their distribution, and number are identified. The pattern of progression of the rash and the timing of onset of the rash relative to fever and other clues in the history can be helpful.

Blood cultures should be drawn on all patients who appear toxic. Sometimes, culture can be taken from the lesions themselves, especially vesicles. The rash can be biopsied if the etiology remains difficult to isolate. Additional testing is directed by clinical findings.

Treatment

For any patient with acute illness, fever, and disseminated rash, a reasonable empiric regimen to begin is ceftriaxone, 1–2 g IV q24h, and doxycycline (Monodox), 100 mg IV or PO q12h. This may be altered once more clinical information is available. Many rashes do not require specific treatment and resolve on their own, especially if viral in etiology.

Key Points to Remember for Fever and Rash

- Things not to miss: meningococcemia, pneumococcemia, and Rocky Mountain spotted fever.
- When bullous skin lesions appear in face of sepsis, consider the following infections: group A *Streptococcus*, *Pseudomonas*, *Vibrio*, and *Staphylococcus*.

NEUTROPENIC FEVER

Neutropenic fever in chemotherapy patients is a common occurrence. 50–60% of febrile neutropenic patients have an established or occult infection, and >20% of patients with an ANC of <100/mm^3 have bacteremia. **Neutropenic fever** is defined as a single temperature ≥38.3°C (101°F) or a temperature ≥38°C (100.4°F) over ≥1 hr in a patient with an ANC of ≤500/mm^3 or ≤1000/ mm^3 with a predicted decline to ≤500/mm^3. A rapid decrease in the neutrophil count and protracted neutropenia (ANC, ≤500 for >10 days) are major risk factors for infection in neutropenic patients.

Evaluation

The onset of fever should be dated from the first day of the last cycle of chemotherapy. This allows estimation of the duration of neutropenia. The history and physical exam should focus on subtle signs and symptoms of inflammation in areas commonly infected in neutropenic patients. This may not be obvious, and because the patients are neutropenic, they often have few to no signs of inflammation. The most commonly affected sites include the periodontium, pharynx, lower esophagus, lung, perineum and anus, skin lesions, bone marrow aspiration sites, the eye, vascular access sites, and tissue around the nails. Chemotherapy-induced mucosal damage may allow translocation of bacteria from the intestinal lumen to the bloodstream as the source of bacteremia and fever. Two sets of blood cultures should be obtained in all febrile neutropenic patients. Samples should be obtained for Gram's stain and culture from any of the previously mentioned areas if they appear to be infected. If the lesions are chronic, samples should be sent for fungal and atypical mycobacteria cultures. If the patient has diarrhea, stool should be tested for *C. difficile* toxin and for bacterial pathogens, viruses, and protozoa. Urine cultures are indicated if there are signs or symptoms of a UTI, a urinary catheter is in place, or the UA is abnormal (of note, pyuria is often absent in neutropenic patients). CXRs should be obtained if a lower respiratory tract infection is suspected. Skin lesions should be biopsied. CSF should be obtained only if there are signs or symptoms of an infection of the CNS. In addition, CBC, serum transaminases, Na^+, K^+, and creatinine levels should be obtained on admission and followed at least every 3 days to monitor for complications of the infectious process or drug toxicity and to plan for supportive care.

Management

Antibiotics should be initiated promptly in neutropenic patients, as overwhelming sepsis can occur in a short period of time in these immunosuppressed patients. The type, frequency, and antibiotic susceptibilities of the bacterial isolates found in similar patients at a particular institution should guide the initial antibiotic regimen, while keeping in mind potential limitations for certain antibiotics (drug allergy, end-organ dysfunction). No study has demonstrated striking differences in efficacy between monotherapy and multidrug combinations. Only broad-spectrum, bactericidal, gram-negative coverage (antipseudomonal) has influenced overall mortality; thus, carbapenems, ceftazidime, and cefepime may be used as monotherapy in most cases. Studies with quinolone monotherapy have shown both favorable and unfavorable results; therefore, quinolone monotherapy is not recommended for routine initial therapy. The most common duotherapy regimens (excluding vancomycin) include an aminoglycoside with an antipseudomonal PCN or with a cephalosporin. Again, there are no major differences in overall mortality when compared with monotherapy regimens, but duotherapy is associated with aminoglycoside toxicities. Vancomycin is indicated for initial therapy, along with appropriate gram-negative coverage, in patients with severe mucositis, prior quinolone prophylaxis, known colonization with oxacillin-resistant *S. aureus* or cephalosporin-resistant pneumococcus, obvious catheter-related infection, or hypotension. Empiric vancomycin should be discontinued if initial cultures are negative for gram-positive organisms after 3–4 days. Duration of antibiotic therapy: ≥3 days are needed to determine efficacy of the initial regimen. After 3 days, further treatment is determined by culture results, regardless of whether the fever has resolved, the ANC, the patient's risk stratification, and whether the patient's condition has deteriorated.

If the causative organism and site of infection are identified, therapy can be adjusted to the most appropriate treatment. If the patient is afebrile within 3 days and no etiology is identified, the patient can be risk stratified as follows:

- ANC ≥500/mm^3 by day 7: If the patient remains afebrile, the antibiotics can be discontinued.
- ANC ≤500/mm^3 by day 7: If the patient remains clinically well and is afebrile for 5–7 days, then antibiotics may be discontinued.
- If the patient has an ANC <100/mm^3, severe mucositis, or unstable vital signs, the patient should be continued on IV antibiotics. Antibiotics should be continued until leukocyte recovery has been present for ≥5 days.
- Persistent fever during the first 3 days of treatment: If the fever persists for >3 days in patients without an identified site of infection or causative organism, this suggests a nonbacterial infection, a bacterial infection resistant to the antibiotic(s) being used, emergence of a secondary infection, inadequate serum and tissue levels of the antibiotic(s), drug fever, or infection at an avascular site. These patients should be reassessed on day 4 or 5 and should continually be reassessed every 4–5 days if fever is persistent. If reassessment does not reveal a cause of fever, then one of four management options can be pursued: (a) stopping antibiotics if the ANC is >500/mm^3, (b) continuing current antibiotics, (c) changing or adding antibiotics, or (d) adding amphotericin B (see below).

Reassessment

Reassessment should include a review of all previous cultures, a thorough physical exam, CXRs and sinus radiographs, vascular catheter inspection, reculture of blood and specific sites of infection, and imaging of any organ suspected of infection. Special studies may be done for *Toxoplasma gondii*, HSV, CMV, Epstein-Barr virus, enterovirus, enteric protozoa, *Mycobacterium tuberculosis*, nontuberculous mycobacteria, and *Chlamydia pneumoniae* if clinical features suggest any of these disease processes.

Stopping Antibiotics

Stopping antibiotics can be considered when no evidence of infection can be found and recovery of the ANC to ≥500/mm³ has been present for 4–5 days in stable patients without mucositis. However, these patients should be reassessed for occult viral or fungal infections, as lesions may become apparent with recovery of the neutrophil count.

Continuance of Current Antibiotics

In patients with no deterioration in clinical status, continuing the initial antibiotic regimen may be considered. If vancomycin was one of the initial antibiotics and all cultures remain negative for gram-positive organisms, then vancomycin can be discontinued. This decision is strengthened if ANC recovery is expected in the next 5 days.

Changing Antibiotics

When there is evidence of disease progression, consideration should be given to either adding antibiotics or changing to different antibiotics. If vancomycin was not one of the initial antibiotics, and blood or site-specific cultures reveal gram-positive organisms or if there is evidence of life-threatening sepsis, then vancomycin should be given.

Addition of Antifungal Coverage

Fewer than 33% of febrile neutropenic patients who do not respond to a 1-wk course of antibiotics will have a systemic fungal infection, most commonly caused by *Candida* or *Aspergillus* species. Most are of the opinion that patients who remain febrile and profoundly neutropenic for 1 wk despite broad-spectrum antibiotics are candidates for antifungal therapy. Before antifungal therapy is started, evidence of systemic fungal infection should be sought (lesions biopsied, CXRs and sinus radiographs, cultures, CT scan of the abdomen). Fluconazole (Diflucan) may be considered at institutions with low rates of mold infections and drug-resistant *Candida* infections in patients without evidence of sinus or pulmonary disease who have not been on fluconazole prophylaxis. Amphotericin B and antibiotic therapy can be discontinued after 2 wks of continuous therapy if there are no lesions on exam, CXR, and CT scan of the abdomen. Voriconazole can be used as well.

Use of Antiviral Drugs

Viral infections are not common in neutropenic patients (except bone marrow transplant patients), and routine use of antivirals is not indicated. If skin or mucous membrane lesions are suggestive of HSV or VZV, treatment with acyclovir (Zovirax) is indicated even if the patients are afebrile. These lesions may provide a portal of entry for bacterial pathogens in neutropenic patients.

Granulocyte Transfusions

The routine use of granulocyte transfusions is not indicated in febrile neutropenic patients. Some clinicians believe granulocyte transfusions are useful in profoundly neutropenic patients with microbiologically documented infection that cannot be controlled with optimal antibiotic therapy or by the administration of colony-stimulating factors.

Colony-Stimulating Factors

The routine use of colony-stimulating factors is not indicated because of the high likelihood of a good outcome with standard antibiotic therapy. In addition, no study has been able to demonstrate a decrease in infection-related mortality with the use of colony-stimulating factors. Certain conditions in which worsening of the condition is predicted and a long delay in recovery of the marrow is expected may warrant the use of colony-stimulating factors (e.g., pneumonia, hypotension, severe cellulitis or sinusitis, fungal infections, and multiorgan dysfunction secondary to sepsis).

Antimicrobial Prophylaxis

The use of antimicrobial prophylaxis should be highly individualized. Considerations in the use of prophylaxis include expected duration and extent of neutropenia, mucous membrane or skin lesions, indwelling catheters, instrumentation, periodontal disease, dental procedures, postobstructive pneumonia, status of malignancy, and compromise of other immune responses as well as patient compliance, hygienic habits, and environment. Although multiple studies have shown efficacy of TMP-SMX and quinolone prophylaxis in reducing the number of infectious episodes during the neutropenic period, antimicrobial prophylaxis is not recommended (except TMP-SMX for patients at risk for *Pneumocystis jiroveci* pneumonia) because of concerns of drug toxicity, emergence of bacterial resistance, fungal overgrowth, and lack of reduction in mortality rates.

Key Points to Remember for Neutropenic Fever

- An aggressive workup should be initiated as soon as possible, including a detailed history and physical exam, blood and urine cultures, CXR, and cultures of any indwelling catheter sites.
- Serologic tests (see Reassessment section), stool cultures, and tissue cultures should be promptly obtained if clinically warranted.
- Empiric broad-spectrum, gram-negative coverage should begin after cultures have been obtained (see Management section). Vancomycin should be added initially if clinically indicated.
- Patients who remain febrile and neutropenic ≥1 week despite broad antibiotics and negative cultures should be considered for additional antifungal therapy.

FEVER IN THE RETURNED TRAVELER

Perhaps one of the more challenging diagnoses to be made by the infectious diseases practitioner is that of fever in the returned traveler. In this situation, the differential diagnosis becomes exceptionally broad, including not only the typical causes of fever not related to the patient's travel, but also a host of infectious diseases often not familiar to the practitioner. Poorly understood emerging diseases also enter the differential. Moreover, there are few primary data regarding fever in the returned traveler. In most case reports, typically 25% of patients remain undiagnosed. Accordingly, it may be most helpful for the practitioner to focus on early identification of potentially fatal and treatable disease and early identification of potential public health threats.

Approach to the Patient

History

A complete, thorough history must be performed with elucidation of the following:

- The dates of departure and return
- The date of onset of symptoms
- A complete description of symptoms including any fever pattern
- Confirmation of fever

- Countries and cities visited and the nature of the accommodations
- Activities, particularly unusual ones
- Animal exposures
- Sick contacts
- Source of food and water
- Medical history
- Medications, including those taken before and during travel
- Compliance with malaria prophylaxis
- Vaccination status before travel

When inquiring about associated symptomatology, attempts to elucidate symptoms of and potential exposure to hemorrhagic fevers are crucial given the high morbidity and mortality rates of these illnesses and their potential public health threats.

Physical Exam and Diagnostic Workup
A complete physical exam should be performed with attention to the following:

- HEENT: scleral icterus, conjunctival injection, conjunctival petechiae
- Neck and nodes: lymphadenopathy
- Abdomen: organomegaly
- Skin: icterus, rash, petechiae, purpura

The standard lab evaluation should include CBC, standard chemistries, liver function tests, and UA. Other lab orders should be targeted toward physical exam findings.

Differential Diagnosis

When assessing fever in the returned traveler, the differential diagnosis becomes exceptionally broad, including not only the typical causes of fever not related to the patient's travel, but also a host of infectious diseases often not familiar to the practitioner. It is important to remember that the travel history may be completely irrelevant to the etiology of the fever and that the fever may be an adverse effect of medicine used to protect the patient from acquiring infection or used empirically for therapy.

Infectious causes of fever acquired while traveling can be divided into three categories. Those illnesses that are common and that have a wide, international distribution include malaria, viral hepatitis, arboviral infections (including dengue fever), enteric bacterial and viral infections, and TB. Less common infections with wide distribution include acute HIV infection, amebic liver abscess, polio, brucellosis, toxoplasmosis, and filariasis. Uncommon infections with distribution limited to certain regions include yellow fever, scrub typhus, leptospirosis, plague, leishmaniasis, schistosomiasis, hemorrhagic fevers, relapsing fever, melioidosis, African sleeping sickness, severe acute respiratory syndrome (SARS), and typhus (louse-, flea-, and tick-borne) [1].

To date, three large-scale studies have been performed regarding the etiology of fever in the returned traveler. In each study, malaria was the most common cause of fever, followed in varying frequencies by respiratory infections, diarrhea/gastroenteritis, viral hepatitis, and UTI. The percent of patients who remained undiagnosed ranged from 9% in the study by O'Brien et al. of Australian inpatients [2] to 25% in cohorts of ambulatory and hospitalized patients as reported by Doherty et al. [3] and MacLean et al. [4].

In general, if the patient has traveled to a tropical region where malaria is endemic, this disease must be considered regardless of whether the patient was provided malaria prophylaxis. Several studies have shown that only 15–60% of travelers comply with the proper prophylactic regimen. Moreover, resistance to multiple agents used for prophylaxis and treatment has been described among *Plasmodium* species.

Common Etiologies Corresponding to Concomitant Symptoms

Diarrhea and Fever
Diarrhea is the most common symptom described by patients when returning from travel in a foreign country. Approximately 8% of this population suffers from diar-

rhea, which occurs approximately four times more frequently than fever alone [5]. Typically, 15% of travelers with diarrhea also complain of fever. Etiologies to consider include *Salmonella, Shigella, Campylobacter, Yersinia,* and *Escherichia coli. Shigella* infection is particularly common after travel to India and, recently, to the Mexican Yucatan peninsula. These bacterial infections frequently cause fever to 40°C (104°F)— higher than is usually observed in viral enteritis caused most commonly by Norwalk virus or rotavirus. Amebiasis, giardiasis, and cryptosporidiosis should be considered in the traveler with low-grade fever and potential exposure to contaminated water.

Jaundice and Fever

The combination of jaundice and fever is most worrisome for acute viral hepatitis. For travelers, HAV is the largest risk with its worldwide distribution. Hepatitis E should also be considered if the patient has recently returned from South Asia. Both of these viruses are typically acquired by consumption of water and food contaminated with human fecal material. HBV and HCV are less easily acquired by the average traveler. The combination of jaundice and fever also raises concern for yellow fever even in those patients who have received yellow fever vaccine, although vaccine failure is quite rare. Other etiologies include Lassa fever, Rift Valley fever, and dengue, although the hemorrhagic manifestations of these illnesses are usually more striking than icterus.

Fever, hepatomegaly, and jaundice as a sign of cholangitis are typical of liver fluke and biliary helminth infections. Signs of hepatic dysfunction may also accompany typhoid fever, legionellosis, malaria, leishmaniasis, TB, schistosomiasis, brucellosis, and histoplasmosis. Although they do not typically present with jaundice, focal hepatic infections with *Entamoeba histolytica* and *Echinococcus* and polymicrobial liver abscess are characterized by liver function tests and liver imaging abnormalities. The possibility of drug-induced hepatitis as a result of administration of prophylactic and therapeutic agents should always be considered in the patient with fever and liver function abnormalities.

Mental Status Changes and Fever

The traveler returning from Africa or other endemic areas with the combination of mental status changes and fever should immediately be evaluated for falciparum malaria, which may also present with seizures and is often life-threatening. Meningococcus should also be ruled out, as this agent is particularly common in the sub-Saharan nations of Kenya and Tanzania as well as in Nepal and Saudi Arabia, where epidemics have recently been described. Rabies, Japanese encephalitis, rickettsial infections, and typhoid fever should also be considered. A history of travel to the southwestern United States should prompt consideration of coccidioidomycosis in the patient with fever, headache, and confusion. Similar symptomatology occurs with paracoccidioidomycosis acquired during travel to South America. The classic organisms causing eosinophilic meningitis are *Angiostrongylus cantonensis* and *Gnathostoma,* which are acquired in Southeast Asia and the South Pacific islands. Fever and mental status changes are rarely signs of neurocysticercosis, which usually presents with seizure.

Diagnostic Workup

As mentioned above, lab testing and imaging should be tailored toward specific symptoms or physical exam findings. If malaria is suspected, thick and thin blood films should be examined by experienced technicians. Stool specimens from the patient with diarrhea and fever should be cultured for bacterial pathogens and analyzed for parasites and fecal leukocytes. Often, the exam of multiple samples is required, as parasites and their cysts, ova, and larvae are often present in small numbers and are not passed continually. Patients with negative stool studies and persistent diarrhea may require referral to a gastroenterologist for colonoscopy. Patients with signs of hepatic disease require liver function testing and often hepatic imaging in the form of abdominal CT and U/S. Biliary imaging and ERCP may also be required to diagnose parasitic biliary infections. Lumbar puncture is required for returning travelers with acute fever in combination with headache, seizure, or confusion. Brain imaging should also be considered in these patients to rule out focal CNS infections.

Treatment and Follow-Up

It is beyond the scope of this chapter to discuss the treatment of the illnesses listed above. It should be stressed, however, that cerebral malaria is a medical emergency requiring prompt diagnosis and proper antimalarial chemotherapy. In addition, the patient should be monitored and treated for hypoglycemia, which may potentiate falciparum malaria, and should be given the appropriate supportive treatment for fever and hemolysis. In general, the administration of antipyretic therapy is not contraindicated in tropical infections, although avoidance of acetaminophen is advised when viral hepatitis or other hepatic infections are suspected.

Ambulatory patients should be seen within 1 wk of their initial presentation for review of lab testing and to assess for persistent or evolving symptoms as well as efficacy of any treatment prescribed. Any traveler with signs of hemorrhagic fever should be reported immediately to the local health department and admitted to the hospital with appropriate isolation for supportive treatment.

Key Points to Remember for Fever in the Returned Traveler

- If traveling to a malarial region, always consider malaria in a returned traveler with fever.
- Obtain a thorough history of events before and during the patient's travels and consider incubation periods of various possibilities before narrowing the differential.

SUGGESTED READING

Arnow PM, Flaherty JP. Fever of unknown origin. *Lancet* 1997;350:575–580.

Blackbourne LH, ed. *Surgical recall*, 2nd ed. Baltimore: Williams & Wilkins, 1998.

Braunwald E, Fauci AS, Kasper DL, et al., eds. *Harrison's principles of internal medicine*, 15th ed. New York: McGraw-Hill, 2001.

Chamberlain R. *The surgical intern pocket survival guide*. Alexandria, VA: International Medical Publishing, 1996.

Cunha BA. Fever of unknown origin. *Infect Dis Clin North Am* 1996;10:111–127.

De Pauw BE, Donnelly JP. Infections in the immunocompromised host: general principles. In: Mandell GL, Bennett JE, Dolin R, eds. *Mandell, Douglas, and Bennett's principles and practice of infectious diseases*, 5th ed. Philadelphia: Churchill Livingstone, 1999:3079–3089.

De Pauw BE, Meunier F. Infections in patients with acute leukemia and lymphoma. In: Mandell GL, Bennett JE, Dolin R, eds. *Mandell, Douglas, and Bennett's principles and practice of infectious diseases*, 5th ed. Philadelphia: Churchill Livingstone, 1999:3090–3101.

Hirschmann JV. Fever of unknown origin in adults. *Clin Infect Dis* 1997;24:291–302.

Hughes WT, Armstrong D, Bodey GP, et al. 1997 guideline for the use of antimicrobial agents in neutropenic patients with unexplained fever. *Clin Infect Dis* 1997;25: 551–573.

Lawrence PF, ed. *Essentials of general surgery*, 2nd ed. Baltimore: Williams & Wilkins, 1992:143.

Magill AJ. Fever in the returned traveler. *Infect Dis Clin North Am* 1998;12:445–469.

Marik PE. Fever in the ICU. *Chest* 2000;177:855–869.

O'Grady NP, Barie PS, Bartlett JG, et al. Practice guidelines for evaluating new fever in critically ill adult patients. *Clin Infect Dis* 1998;26:1042–1059.

Schlossberg D. Fever and rash. *Infect Dis Clin North Am* 1996;10:101–110.

Schwartz SI, ed. *Principles of surgery*, 7th ed. New York: McGraw-Hill, 1999:447–448.

Weber DJ, Cohen MS, Fine J. The acutely ill patient with fever and rash. In: Mandell
    GL, Bennett JE, Dolin R, eds. *Mandell, Douglas, and Bennett's principles and
    practice of infectious diseases*, 5th ed. Philadelphia: Churchill Livingstone, 1999.

REFERENCES

1. Strickland GT. Fever in the returned traveler. *Med Clin North Am* 1992;76:1375–
   1392.
2. O'Brien D, Tobin S, Brown GV, Torresi J. Fever in returned travelers: review of
   hospital admissions for a 3-year period. *Clin Infect Dis* 2001;33:603–609.
3. Doherty JF, Grant AD, Bryceson AD. Fever as the presenting complaint of travelers returning from the tropics. *QJM* 1995;88:277–281.
4. MacLean J, Lalonde R, Ward B. Fever from the tropics. *Travel Med Adv* 1994;
   5:27.1–27.14.
5. Steffen R, Rickenbach J, Wilhelm U, et al. Health problems after travel to developing countries. *J Infect Dis* 1987;156:84–91.

Upper Respiratory Tract Infections

Rebecca E. Chandler

ACUTE PHARYNGITIS

Acute pharyngitis (commonly referred to as **sore throat**) is an inflammation of the pharyngeal cavity, most often caused by infection and manifested by sore throat, with or without dysphagia. Sore throat is the fourth most common symptom seen in medical practice. The most important decision regarding this diagnosis is whether it is attributable to group A beta-hemolytic *Streptococcus* (GABHS), as treatment of this organism limits spread of the disease and prevents both suppurative (tonsillar and peritonsillar abscesses) and nonsuppurative (rheumatic fever, poststreptococcal glomerulonephritis) sequelae.

Differential Diagnosis

The microbiology of acute pharyngitis is diverse. Viruses are the most common causes of pharyngitis in both children and adults. The viral etiologies are diverse and include adenovirus, rhinovirus, coronavirus, influenza, parainfluenza, RSV, HSV, coxsackievirus, enterocytopathogenic human orphan virus, HIV, Epstein-Barr virus, CMV, measles, and rubella. Bacterial causes are also multiple, but by far the most common (15% of all infections) and most important is GABHS. Other bacterial causes include *Chlamydia pneumoniae*, *Mycoplasma pneumoniae*, *Haemophilus influenzae*, *Corynebacterium diphtheriae*, *Treponema pallidum*, *Neisseria gonorrhea*, *Mycobacterium tuberculosis*, *Arcanobacterium haemolyticum*, *Yersinia enterocolitica*, *Yersinia pestis*, and *Coxiella burnetii*. The most important fungal cause is *Candida albicans*. Noninfectious etiologies of acute pharyngitis include Kawasaki's disease, Stevens-Johnson syndrome, and Behçet's syndrome.

Viral URIs frequently occur in mini-epidemics. They are more common in the winter (RSV, parainfluenza, influenza, varicella, and measles), with the exception of the enteroviruses, which are more common in the summer. Adenoviral infections occur year-round. GABHS infections occur more commonly in the winter.

Pathophysiology

The pathogenesis of sore throat due to pharyngitis is poorly understood. Some infections produce inflammatory mediators (rhinovirus), whereas others directly invade pharyngeal cells and induce an inflammatory response. Adenovirus and EBV produce lymphoid hyperplasia and tonsillar exudation. Streptococcal infection inflames the posterior pharynx and may produce palatal petechiae.

Clinical Manifestations

Most cases of acute pharyngitis are associated with a URI and begin with a prodrome of malaise, fever, and headache. Coryza and sore throat develop subsequently. Some infections also produce cough. Pharyngitis caused by GABHS is associated with significant pharyngeal edema, often with palatal and uvular petechiae. Tender cervical lymph nodes are common. A typical rash, **scarlet fever,** may be seen with streptococcal pharyngitis. It is an erythematous rash that typically begins in the groin and spreads over the body. It has a sandpaper quality and may be pruritic. Other bacteria and viruses may cause a similar picture, making the etiology of pharyngitis difficult to ascertain on clinical grounds. Careful exam for the presence of pharyngeal and tonsillar asymmetry is warranted to evaluate for abscess. Suppurative complications include tonsillar and peritonsillar abscesses. Such patients typically have fever, odynophagia, and muffled voice; physical findings include trismus, unilateral swelling, and deviation of uvula.

Diagnosis

The multiple etiologies of pharyngitis are difficult to distinguish on clinical grounds alone. Important factors to consider in clinical diagnosis are epidemiology, symptoms, and signs. Because of the great overlap between the clinical features of GABHS and those of other etiologic agents, lab testing should be performed to assure the diagnosis and thus prevent overuse and nonjudicious use of antibiotic therapy. Two types of testing are used in current practice: throat cultures and rapid antigen detection tests (RADTs). Throat cultures are the gold standard. The cultures are plated on blood agar plates, occasionally with the use of bacitracin discs to enhance growth of certain flora and prevent that of others. Cultures may reveal growth at 24 hrs but may require up to 48 hrs. The sensitivity of cultures approaches 95%. RADT detects the presence of group A carbohydrate on a throat swab by ELISA or latex agglutination assay. With a specificity >95%, it allows for decreased time to diagnosis and thus treatment; however, its sensitivity may be only 80–90% at best, so negative RADTs should be confirmed with a throat culture. The Infectious Diseases Society of America (IDSA) guidelines recommend that the diagnosis of GABHS be suspected on clinical grounds and then confirmed by the results of lab testing.

Treatment

As previously mentioned, the primary goal of treatment of GABHS pharyngitis is to limit spread of the disease and to prevent both suppurative and nonsuppurative complications. Although early treatment clearly decreases the risk of spread of disease, there are data to suggest that therapy may be delayed up to 9 days after the onset of symptoms and still prevent the occurrence of complications. The traditional antimicrobial for primary prevention of rheumatic fever has been IM repository PCN. More recent clinical trials have indicated that benzathine PCN is also effective in primary prevention of rheumatic fever. Other antimicrobials are capable of eradication of GABHS and thus are considered to be efficacious as well. However, some strains have been found to be highly resistant to macrolide antibiotics. Given these facts, the treatment of choice is oral PCN V (250 mg PO qid) or parenteral benzathine PCN (1.2 million units IM). Other possible choices include macrolides [erythromycin, 250 mg PO qid, is suggested for PCN-allergic patients; clarithromycin (Diaxin), 50 mg PO bid; azithromycin (Z-Pak)], ampicillin/amoxicillin, cephalosporins, or clindamycin (Cleocin). Most oral antibiotics, with the exception of azithromycin (Zithromax, Z-Pak; given for 5 days), should be given for a duration of 7–10 days to ensure eradication of the disease. Tonsillar and peritonsillar abscesses are treated with incision and drainage, procurement of specimen for microbiology cultures, and antibiotic therapy. According to IDSA guidelines, it is not necessary to perform throat cultures on or to treat asymptomatic household contacts. When a large outbreak occurs, however, cultures should be performed on all individuals, but only those with positive cultures should be treated. The preferred prophylaxis regimen is benzathine PCN G, 1.2 million units IM q4wks. Alternatively, PCN V, 125–250 mg PO bid; sulfadiazine (Microsulfon), 1g PO qd; or erythromycin, 250 mg PO bid, may be used.

The IDSA advises that follow-up cultures after appropriate therapy are not necessary in asymptomatic individuals to document eradication of infection. Persistence of symptoms after adequate treatment is not an uncommon phenomenon, nor is the presence of positive cultures after therapy. Treatment failures, defined with a positive culture at the end of therapy, occur in up to 20% of patients. Possible explanations include noncompliance and infection with a new streptococcal strain, but rarely is reinfection with the original strain the cause. Carrier states of GABHS may also occur; however, these carriers are both unlikely to spread the organism or to suffer from potential complications. Differentiating between carrier state and true recurrent infection is difficult; it must be approached with consideration of clinical characteristics and with the aid of lab tests (e.g., serotyping). For those patients with symptomatic, repeated culture–positive GABHS shortly after appropriate therapy, 10-day courses of clindamycin or amoxicillin/clavulanate (Augmentin) are recommended.

RHINOSINUSITIS: ACUTE AND CHRONIC

Acute Rhinosinusitis

Rhinosinusitis is defined as inflammation of the mucosa of the nose and paranasal sinuses. Acute rhinosinusitis is 1 of the 10 most common diagnoses in ambulatory clinical practice; in 1995, it accounted for an estimated 25 million office visits to physicians in the United States. At such visits, physicians prescribe antibiotics 85–98% of the time, making acute rhinosinusitis the fifth most common diagnosis for which antibiotics are prescribed.

Differential Diagnosis

Most cases of rhinosinusitis are caused by uncomplicated viral upper respiratory tract infections; the most common viral agents are rhinoviruses and adenoviruses. However, up to 2% of cases may be complicated by superimposed acute bacterial rhinosinusitis. Approximately 70% of cases of community-acquired bacterial rhinosinusitis are caused by *Streptococcus pneumoniae* and *H. influenzae*; additionally, up to 25% of pediatric cases are caused by *Moraxella catarrhalis*, whereas other less common bacterial causes include *Staphylococcus aureus*, other *Streptococcus* species, *Neisseria* species, gram-negative rods, and anaerobes. Fungi such as mucormycosis and *Aspergillus* may be causative in those patients immunocompromised by such conditions as diabetes, HIV, and chronic renal failure.

Pathophysiology

The paranasal sinuses (maxillary, sphenoid, ethmoid, and frontal) are outpouchings of the nasal mucosa. They are connected to the nasal cavity via ostia, which have diameters of approximately 1–3 mm, and they are lined with mucoperiosteum and cilia, which sweep mucus toward the ostia. Rhinosinusitis is the result of impaired mucociliary clearance and obstruction of the ostia. Stagnant secretions and decreased ventilation result, leading to an environment with decreased pH and oxygen tension, creating a perfect culture medium for bacteria. Predisposing factors for the development of rhinosinusitis are numerous: viral URIs, allergic rhinitis, anatomic abnormalities (e.g., deviated septum and nasal polyps), dental infections, hormonal changes (e.g., puberty and pregnancy), mechanical ventilation, NG tubes, nasal irritants, and immunodeficiency diseases.

Clinical Manifestations

Patients with bacterial rhinosinusitis describe a prolonged illness, with purulent rhinorrhea, maxillary toothache, unilateral pain that may be augmented by leaning forward, and poor response to decongestants or antihistamines. Very important in the history is the duration of symptoms: Those patients with bacterial rhinosinusitis will have had symptoms for ≥7 days; any lesser amount of time is more likely to be associated with only a viral rhinosinusitis. On examining a patient with probable bacterial rhinosinusitis, one should note the absence or presence of fever and concentrate on close exam of the sinuses. Palpation should be performed in the following areas: the maxillary floor, palpated from the palate; the anterior maxillary wall, palpated from the cheek; the lateral ethmoid wall, palpated from the medial canthus; the frontal floor, palpated from the roof of the orbit; and the anterior frontal wall, palpated from the supraorbital skull. Such manipulation may bring about tenderness in the affected area. Purulent secretions should be searched for in the nasal cavity. Transillumination is used to evaluate the maxillary and frontal sinuses. Additionally, the physical exam may be used to note any features that may be contributing to formation of bacterial sinusitis.

Diagnosis

The difficulty in diagnosis is distinguishing between viral and bacterial rhinosinusitis. Several studies have been published to attempt to identify clinical features specific to bacterial rhinosinusitis; however, none used the gold standard of aspiration and culture of sinus secretions. Considering all the studies, the following list of signs and symptoms appears to be consistent with the diagnosis: purulent nasal drainage, maxillary tooth or facial pain, unilateral maxillary sinus tenderness, biphasic nature of the illness, and duration of symptoms >7 days. Imaging modalities for the diagnosis of bacterial rhinosinusitis include plain films, U/S, and CT of the sinuses. Several studies have attempted to explore the accuracy of sinus radiography findings to predict bacterial rhinosinusitis. Findings of complete opacification and air fluid levels are the most specific, with mucosal thickening less so. It is important to note that the absence of all three has a 90% sensitivity in ruling out the disease. Current recommendation from the American College of Physicians/American Society of Internal Medicine is to make a diagnosis on clinical grounds.

Treatment

The question of treatment remains a bit controversial. Randomized, placebo-controlled trials of antibiotics using pre- and posttreatment sinus aspirates and cultures have not been performed. Rather, studies have used clinical and radiologic diagnostic modalities to measure improvement. Two metaanalyses (Cochrane Collaboration and Agency for Healthcare Research and Quality) have concluded that antibiotics are more efficacious than placebo in reducing or eliminating symptoms at 2 wks; however, the benefit is small, as most patients who receive placebo also improve (69% of patients) in the same time period. Taking these data into account, the favored decision is the antibiotic treatment of patients with moderate or severe cases and only symptomatic treatment (decongestants, mucolytic agents) of patients with mild cases. Although the incidence of beta-lactamase–producing organisms is 25% in some communities, initial antibiotic treatment should be with narrow-spectrum agents. Trials have revealed TMP-SMX (Bactrim; one DS tablet PO bid), amoxicillin (500 mg PO tid), and doxycycline (100 mg PO bid) as choice agents. Three metaanalyses have concluded that newer broad-spectrum agents are not significantly more effective than narrow-spectrum agents. In terms of duration of treatment, most older studies had a duration of 10–14 days; however, a more recent Veterans Administration study compared the effectiveness of Bactrim bid for 3 days versus 10 days; results revealed that shorter courses may be just as effective. Scheduled follow-up is not generally necessary for uncomplicated bacterial rhinosinusitis. However, 10–25% of patients have persistent symptoms despite treatment. Evaluation at that point may include imaging with plain films or CT to confirm the diagnosis. A trial of second-line therapy, such as amoxicillin-clavulanate (875/125 mg PO bid), or a PO cephalosporin for 14 days is reasonable. If symptoms continually persist, ENT referral for evaluation is preferable. Complications of bacterial rhinosinusitis include orbital infections, brain abscess, meningitis, cavernous thrombosis, osteomyelitis, and mucoceles.

Chronic Rhinosinusitis

Chronic rhinosinusitis is much more likely to be caused by such organisms as *S. aureus*, alpha-hemolytic *Streptococcus*, and anaerobes. Use of antibiotics is controversial, as controlled clinical trials are lacking. Most authorities advise refraining from treatment in absence of symptoms (e.g., fevers, pain, and purulent discharge). However, patients often find brief courses of antibiotics of great benefit.

ACUTE EPIGLOTTITIS

Acute epiglottitis is defined as the inflammation, most often caused by infection, of the epiglottis and its surrounding structures. It is a respiratory emergency, as the inflammation of these structures may lead to upper airway obstruction. It has been commonly thought of as a disease of children, usually occurring between the ages of 2 and 6. However, the epidemiology has changed as a result of the widespread use of *Haemophilus* vaccination in children. In 1980, the ratio of children to adults was 2.6:1.0; by 1993, the ratio had declined to 0.4:1.0. The incidence in adults is currently approximately 1 in 100,000/yr.

Differential Diagnosis

The differential diagnosis of acute epiglottitis includes other infectious diseases, systemic conditions, and local causes. Infectious possibilities include mononucleosis, *C. diphtheriae*, *Bordetella pertussis*, croup, Ludwig's angina, and retropharyngeal or peritonsillar abscesses. Systemic conditions include amyloidosis, sarcoidosis, pemphigus, pemphigoid, Wegener's granulomatosis, and allergic drug reactions. Local causes include foreign bodies, tumors, and inhalation irritation from substances such as hydrocarbons and even cocaine.

A variety of organisms are known to cause acute epiglottitis, with the most common being *H. influenzae* type b, *S. aureus*, and beta-hemolytic *Streptococcus* species. Other bacterial causes (e.g., *Klebsiella*, *Escherichia coli*, *M. tuberculosis*) and fungal causes (e.g., *Candida* and *Aspergillus*) may be found in those patients with underlying illness (e.g., COPD or immunodeficiency states). Although anaerobic bacteria are important inhabitants of the microbiologic milieu of the upper respiratory tract, they have only rarely been reported as significant etiologic agents in acute epiglottitis. Finally, viruses have often been believed to be a common cause of mild epiglottitis; however, only HSV has been documented histologically.

Pathophysiology

The pathophysiology of acute epiglottitis involves the infection and, most important, the resulting inflammatory process of the epiglottis and its surrounding structures. As a result of the inflammation, these structures become very edematous and erythematous. Obstruction of the glottis and thus the entrance to the bronchial tree may occur as a result.

Clinical Manifestations

The symptoms of acute epiglottitis are quite consistent. An illness with **severe sore throat** and **pain on swallowing, with associated fever** and shortness of breath is typically described. Other, less typical symptoms include anterior neck tenderness and hoarseness. The illness will likely have begun within the past 6–12 hrs, and it will not have been preceded by any kind of viral syndrome. Patients may exhibit a sense of anxiety and will likely be seated upright in a forward-leaning position. Tachycardia and tachypnea are almost invariably present. There may be evidence of **drooling**, a **muffled voice,** and **respiratory distress.** Palpation of the neck may reveal lymphadenopathy and tenderness in the area of the larynx. Auscultation of the chest may reveal crackles or bronchial breath sounds if there is associated pneumonia or pulmonary edema.

Diagnosis

Diagnosis of acute epiglottitis relies primarily on the presentation of the patient and the use of direct visualization of the supraglottic structures. Laryngoscopic evaluation should only be carried out by those individuals trained in such procedures, with equipment for immediate intubation close at hand. It will reveal the presence of a "cherry red" edematous epiglottis. Radiographs of the soft tissues of the neck may reveal an enlarged epiglottis with a normal subglottic space; however, they also may often be normal. A sensitivity of 38% and a specificity of 76% have been reported. Cultures of blood and the epiglottis frequently grow out the causative organism.

Treatment

The management of patients with acute epiglottitis involves stabilization of the airway and the prompt administration of antibiotic therapy. A staging system has been developed to aid in the decisions regarding the protection of the airway. Stage I patients are those in no respiratory distress with a respiratory rate of <20 breaths/min. They may be managed conservatively under close observation in an ICU. Stage II patients are those with mild to moderate respiratory distress with a respiratory rate of >20 breaths/min. They should be intubated or receive a formal tracheotomy in an OR. Stage III patients are those with severe respiratory distress with a respiratory rate of >30 breaths/min. These patients need immediate airway intervention with either intubation or cricothyrotomy. There is controversy on the use of steroids; their use has been advocated by many, but there are no controlled trials revealing any benefit from them. Additionally, IM epinephrine has been described as useful in a case report of two patients.

First-line antibiotic treatment for acute epiglottis are the third-generation cephalosporins [e.g., ceftriaxone (Rocephin, 2 g IV q24h) and cefotaxime (Claforan, 2 g IV q4–6h)] or the beta-lactam/beta-lactamase inhibitor combination drugs [e.g., ampicillin/sulbactam (Unasyn), (3 g IV q6h)]. The time course of therapy should be approximately 7–10 days. Patients should respond to therapy within 12–48 hrs. The average length of time of intubation is 2 days. Direct visualization is the best method for monitoring improvement and determining the time of extubation.

With expeditious diagnosis and treatment, patients with acute epiglottitis recover without sequelae, and there is no need for follow-up. Recurrent epiglottitis may occur, albeit rarely; in those circumstances, patients should be evaluated for other underlying disease, such as collagen vascular disease, sarcoidosis, or occult malignancy. Household contacts of those patients with acute epiglottitis should receive therapy with rifampin (Rifadin, Rimactane) prophylaxis for up to 4 days.

ACUTE LARYNGITIS

Acute laryngitis is defined as inflammation of the larynx leading to the loss of voice or a change in the character of voice, hoarseness. It commonly occurs in the winter in the setting of other upper respiratory tract infections, particularly pharyngitis.

Differential Diagnosis

Differential diagnosis includes voice abuse, gastroesophageal reflux disease, paralysis of the vocal cords, malignancy; infectious considerations include epiglottitis and tracheitis. The most common etiologic agents are those viruses associated with pharyngitis, including rhinovirus, adenovirus, influenza, parainfluenza, and RSV. Bacterial laryngitis is less common but can be caused by *Streptococcus pyogenes*, *M. catarrhalis*, and even *M. tuberculosis* and *T. pallidum*. Fungal causes include *Histoplasma capsulatum*, *Blastomyces dermatitidis*, and *C. albicans*.

Pathophysiology

The pathogenesis of the disease involves the infection and resultant inflammation of the larynx and surrounding structures. Edema of the vocal cords results in hoarseness or loss of voice.

Clinical Manifestations

Patients with laryngitis typically describe symptoms of upper respiratory tract infections, such as pharyngitis, along with hoarseness or aphonia. Symptoms will typically have lasted <7–10 days. Symptoms of respiratory obstruction may occur. Along with the typical signs of pharyngitis, patients with laryngitis have a diffuse erythematous and edematous larynx. Ulcerations may or may not be present. Exudates or membranes may be characteristic of pathogens such as EBV, streptococcal species, and *Diphtheria*.

Diagnosis

Diagnosis may be made based on clinical presentation alone. Plain films or direct visualization of the oropharynx may be performed to exclude the possibility of the life-threatening condition of acute epiglottitis.

Treatment

Treatment of laryngitis is mainly supportive. Saline gargles, voice rest, and air humidification are mainstays. If change of voice or loss of voice persists for >2 wks, direct visualization should be sought to exclude other causes.

COMMON COLD

The common cold, or **viral rhinosinusitis,** is defined as a mild, self-limited illness caused by infection of the upper respiratory tract mucosa by viruses. The common cold is the most common acute illness in the United States and the industrialized world. It is also the most common cause of absence from school and work. Most cases of the common cold do not present to the physician's office and are self-treated. It has been estimated that Americans spend $1 billion annually for over-the-counter medications for symptomatic relief.

Differential Diagnosis

A variety of viruses are responsible, including rhinovirus, coronavirus, RSV, influenza, parainfluenza, and adenovirus. There exists a seasonal variation among the viruses (e.g., rhinoviruses usually attack in the early fall and mid- to late spring, whereas coronaviruses predominate in the midwinter).

Pathophysiology

The basis of the common cold is simply the infection of the mucosa of the nasal and paranasal sinuses by viral pathogens, with resultant instigation of the inflammatory response. Transmission of the viruses responsible for the common cold is through both direct physical contact and, to a lesser extent, aerosolization. What is most typically involved is nose-to-hand to hand-to-nose transmission.

Clinical Manifestations

Patients with the common cold report one or more of the following symptoms: nasal discharge and congestion, sneezing, sore throat, cough, and hoarseness. Constitutional symptoms, such as low-grade fever or myalgias, may also be present. The duration of symptoms is typically <7 days. Physical exam findings are relatively lacking. Patients may have a low-grade temperature, and they may exhibit clear nasal discharge, mild erythema of the nasal mucosa and throat, cough, and hoarseness.

Diagnosis

The diagnosis of the common cold is purely clinical, given the consistency of symptoms. Identification of the exact causative virus by either clinical characteristics or lab evaluation is not possible or even necessary. More important is the diagnosis of complicating superimposed bacterial infections, such as bacterial rhinosinusitis or otitis media.

Treatment

Antiviral therapy for the common cold is not indicated. Rather, therapy is directed at symptomatic treatment, using NSAIDs and topical and oral decongestants. It is interesting to note that neither antihistamines nor expectorants have been proved to provide consistent relief of cold symptoms, but hot chicken soup has been documented to increase the clearance of nasal mucus. Zinc lozenges have received much attention; although some studies indicate that they accelerate improvement in symptoms, they must be taken q2h and have side effects of nausea and bad taste in the mouth.

KEY POINTS TO REMEMBER

- The goal of diagnosis and treatment of acute pharyngitis is determination of GABHS as the cause and initiation of appropriate antibiotic therapy to prevent complications and to limit spread of the disease.
- The most common etiologic agents of acute rhinosinusitis are viral, making antibiotic therapy unnecessary.
- Acute epiglottitis is an infectious disease emergency; rapid diagnosis on clinical grounds and protection of the airway are essential.
- Symptomatic relief is the mainstay of treatment of both acute laryngitis and the common cold.

REFERENCES AND SUGGESTED READINGS

Bisno AL, Gerber MA, Gwaltney JM Jr, et al. Diagnosis and management of group a streptococcal pharyngitis: a practice guideline. *Clin Infect Dis* 1997;25:574–583.

Carey MJ. Epiglottitis in adults. *Am J Emerg Med* 1996;14:421–424.

Fagnan LJ. Acute sinusitis: a cost effective approach to diagnosis and treatment. *Am Fam Physician* 1998;58:1795–1802.

Hickner JM, Bartlett JG, Bessner RE, et al. Principles of appropriate antibiotic use for acute rhinosinusitis in adults: background. *Ann Intern Med* 2001;134:498–505.

Koster FT, Barker LR. Respiratory tract infections. In: Barker LR, Burton JR, Zieve PD, eds. *Principles of ambulatory medicine*, 5th ed. Baltimore: Williams & Wilkins, 1999:342–362.

Virk A, Henry NK. Upper respiratory tract infections. In: Wilson WR, et al., eds. *Current diagnosis and treatment in infectious diseases*. New York: McGraw-Hill, 2001:98–117.

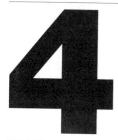

Pulmonary Infections

Rebecca E. Chandler

ACUTE BRONCHITIS

Acute bronchitis is inflammation of the lower respiratory bronchial tract characterized by the sudden onset of cough with or without production of phlegm and accompanying upper respiratory and constitutional symptoms among previously healthy adults.

Differential Diagnosis

Only very rarely is the etiologic agent causing acute bronchitis ever identified. The most common culprits are viruses, particularly influenza A and B, parainfluenza, and RSV more often than rhinovirus, coronavirus, and adenovirus. Bacterial organisms account for only approximately 10% of cases of acute bronchitis. Leading causes are *Bordetella pertussis*, *Mycoplasma pneumoniae*, and *Chlamydia pneumoniae* in healthy adults, whereas *Streptococcus pneumoniae*, *Haemophilus influenzae*, and *Moraxella catarrhalis* are more typical in those patients with underlying pulmonary disease. Recent evidence suggests that *C. pneumoniae* and *Bordetella* may be equally as prevalent as *Mycoplasma*. Noninfectious causes include asthma, gastroesophageal reflux disease, postnasal drip, smoking, toxic inhalations, and ACE inhibitors.

Pathophysiology

There is direct invasion of the epithelial cells of the tracheobronchial tree by pathogens, with resultant release of the mediators of inflammation and constitutional symptoms of fever, malaise, and myalgias. Increases in bronchial secretions and hypersensitivity of the airway epithelium result in the symptoms of cough, phlegm production, and, occasionally, wheezing. One study revealed that up to 40% of patients with acute bronchitis may have decreased FEV_1 on spirometry; another similar study revealed that patients may have a positive histamine challenge test up to 6 wks after diagnosis. This hyperresponsiveness is believed to correlate with repair of the airway epithelium after infection.

Clinical Manifestations

Symptoms include cough, often productive, in addition to other URI (coryza, rhinorrhea) and constitutional complaints (fever, myalgias) of <2 wks' duration. The clues to acute bronchitis are found on observation of vital signs and the auscultation of the lung fields. Vital sign abnormalities have been found in numerous studies to be an important feature of pneumonia, thereby making their absence more likely to favor a diagnosis of acute bronchitis. Also, 40–50% of patients diagnosed with acute bronchitis have documented abnormalities on pulmonary exam. Wheezes, rales, and rhonchi are the predominant findings. In contrast, URIs have no auscultatory findings, and pneumonia has those of fremitus, decreased breath sounds, and egophony.

Diagnosis

Imperative in the diagnosis of acute bronchitis is the determination of the absence of pneumonia, which is best determined by a chest x-ray. It has been suggested, however, that in those patients with cough in whom the index of suspicion for pneumonia is low (no vital sign abnormalities, no clear pulmonary findings), the chest x-ray may not be warranted. Serology, PCR, and cultures have been proven to be limited in their identification of pathogens, and antibiotic therapy has not been shown to alter the course of disease; thus, attempts to aid diagnosis with microbiology studies are not recommended. However, ongoing studies in Europe are looking at the use of CRP in excluding bacterial bronchitis or pneumonia.

Treatment

Multiple studies indicate that there is no role for antimicrobial therapy, even in cases of bacterial bronchitis. A metaanalysis of eight trials concluded that antibiotics do not affect the resolution of productive cough or alter the course of the disease. The only exceptions to the antibiotic rule are in the case of severe, persistent disease that causes concern for pertussis or in documented outbreaks of pertussis; even in these cases, the administration of treatment is intended to prohibit spread of disease, not aid recovery. Bronchodilators do appear to reduce the duration of cough. Additional agents for symptomatic relief may also be used, such as dextromethorphan or codeine and NSAIDs or acetaminophen. Follow-up is generally not necessary for uncomplicated cases of acute bronchitis. However, if the illness persists for >2 wks, the diagnosis of pertussis may need to be considered. Failure of improvement might also suggest other disease states on the differential diagnosis and prompt reevaluation of the patient's history and physical exam.

COMMUNITY-ACQUIRED PNEUMONIA

Pneumonia is the leading infectious disease and the sixth most common cause of death in the United States. The key to prevention of death is the identification of those patients with high risk of mortality, the successful procurement of microbial cultures, and the rapid institution of appropriate antibiotic therapy. **Community-acquired pneumonia** (CAP) is defined as an acute infection of the lower respiratory parenchyma obtained by a person not hospitalized or living in a long-term-care facility.

Differential Diagnosis

The differential diagnosis includes infectious agents of CAP and mimickers of pneumonia, such as CHF, pulmonary edema, septic emboli, malignancies, and foreign body inhalation. Infectious agents are multiple, including bacteria (*S. pneumoniae, H. influenzae, M. catarrhalis, C. pneumoniae, M. pneumoniae, Legionella pneumophila, Staphylococcus aureus, Klebsiella pneumoniae*, oral anaerobes, *Nocardia*, and, less commonly, *Chlamydia psittaci* and *Coxiella burnetii*), viruses (influenza, CMV, RSV, measles, herpes zoster, hantavirus), and fungi (*Histoplasma, Coccidioides, Blastomyces*). PCP and *Aspergillus* are important causes of CAP in immunosuppressed individuals. Agents of bioterrorism (e.g., *Bacillus anthracis, Yersinia pestis*, and *Francisella tularensis*), however, are also potential causes of CAP. Important factors to consider as clues to differentiate between these multiple agents are patient's age, comorbid conditions, occupation, and hobbies, as well as season of year, geographic location, and trends in community disease.

By far, the most common and the most lethal cause is *S. pneumoniae*. It has been found to account for roughly two-thirds of the cases of pneumonia, as well as two-thirds of the cases of pneumonia resulting in death. Current data suggest that 25–35% of *S. pneumoniae* isolates from an infected person are at least intermediately resistant to PCN. Furthermore, there is evidence to suggest that resistance extends also to cephalosporins, macrolides, and, to a small extent, fluoroquinolones.

Pathophysiology

For an organism to cause pneumonia, it must have successfully overcome the host defense mechanisms of aerodynamic filtration and cough reflex and the mucociliary clearance mechanisms of the bronchial airways and in deposit on the alveolar surfaces of the lung parenchyma. Alveolar macrophages take up the invading organisms and initiate the inflammatory response. The resulting exudate of proteins and cells appears by exam and by radiographic evidence of consolidation. When the inflammatory process involves an entire lobe of the lung, it is called *lobar pneumonia*. In contrast, *bronchopneumonia* defines a process limited to the alveoli contiguous to the bronchi.

Clinical Manifestations

"Typical" pneumonia is characterized by the abrupt onset of fever, cough productive of purulent sputum, dyspnea, and, occasionally, pleuritic chest pain. Etiologic agents of typical pneumonia are the most common causes of pneumonia, including *S. pneumoniae*, *H. influenzae*, and oral anaerobes. "Atypical" pneumonia is characterized by a more indolent onset of systemic symptoms such as headache, myalgias, nausea, and vomiting. Etiologic agents of atypical pneumonia are, more commonly, *M. pneumoniae*, *L. pneumophila*, and *C. pneumoniae* and, less commonly, the aforementioned viruses, fungi, and *C. psittaci*, *F. tularensis*, and *C. burnetii*. Other possible symptoms include sore throat/hoarseness with *C. pneumoniae* and altered mental status with *L. pneumophila*.

Patients may reveal vital sign abnormalities: fever/hypothermia, tachycardia, hypotension, increased respiratory rate, and decreased oxygen saturation. Such findings are particularly important in the decision of whether to treat in a hospitalized setting. Pulmonary exam findings may differ between typical and atypical presentations. Findings of typical pneumonia relate to the consolidation of lung parenchyma and include tactile fremitus, dullness to percussion, decreased breath sounds or rales, and egophony. Pulmonary findings of atypical pneumonia are usually underwhelming, with the exception of occasional rales. More common are the various associated findings, such as erythema multiforme, encephalitis/myelitis with *Mycoplasma*, or mental status changes with *Legionella*.

Diagnosis

The key diagnostic tools for CAP are the chest x-ray and microbiologic studies. Lobar pneumonia suggests more typical organisms, diffuse disease suggests more atypical organisms, and clear chest x-rays in an appropriate setting may suggest PCP. Noninfectious pulmonary syndromes in the differential diagnosis with suggestive radiologic features include CHF, vasculitis, atelectasis, and malignancy.

The microbiology studies to be obtained in patients with pneumonia include preantibiotic blood cultures and expectorated sputum Gram's stain and culture. Additionally, *Legionella* urine antigen should be obtained in those patients with suspected disease. Of note, sputum Gram's stain alone is believed to be sufficient for those cases that are appropriate for outpatient treatment (see Treatment below for clinical prediction rule). Other microbiologic studies available for the detection of pneumonia-causing organisms include induced sputum, antigen detection, and DNA probes/amplification. Induced sputum collections are used for the diagnosis of PCP and TB. Antigen detection tests are currently available for *S. pneumoniae*, *L. pneumophila*, and multiple viruses. DNA probes are being developed for the rapid detection of the atypical pneumonia agents.

Treatment

The Pneumonia Patient Outcome Research Team (PORT) has published methodology for the stratification of patients into *five severity classes* based on the variables of age, demographics, comorbid conditions, physical exam findings, and lab/radiographic findings. In step 1, patients are classified as risk class I (the lowest severity level) if they are aged <50 yrs, have none of five important comorbid conditions (neoplastic disease, liver disease, congestive heart failure, cerebrovascular disease, or renal disease), and have normal or only mildly deranged vital signs and normal mental status.

In step 2, all patients who are not assigned to risk class I on the basis of the initial history and physical exam findings alone are stratified into classes II–V, on the basis of points assigned for three demographic variables (age, sex, and nursing home residence), five comorbid conditions (listed above), five physical exam findings (altered mental status, tachypnea, tachycardia, systolic hypertension, hypothermia, or hyperthermia), and seven laboratory or radiographic findings (acidemia, elevated blood urea nitrogen, hyponatremia, hyperglycemia, anemia, hypoxemia, or pleural effusion). Point assignments correspond with the following classes: <70, class II; 71–90, class III; 91–130, class IV; and >130, class V. Mortality was low for risk classes I–III (0.1–2.8%), intermediate for class IV (8.2–9.3%), and high for class V (27.0–31.1%). Increases in risk class were also associated with subsequent hospitalization and delayed return to usual activities for outpatients and with rates of admission to the ICU and length of stay for inpatients in the Pneumonia PORT validation cohort. On the basis of these observations, Pneumonia PORT investigators suggest that patients in risk classes I or II generally are candidates for outpatient treatment, risk class III patients are potential candidates for outpatient treatment or brief inpatient observation, and patients in classes IV and V should be hospitalized. Subsequent studies have supported the use of the Pneumonia PORT prediction rule to help physicians identify low-risk patients who can be safely treated in the outpatient setting.

Current recommendations for treatment in the **outpatient setting** include a macrolide [e.g., azithromycin (Z-Pak), 500 mg PO × 1 day, then 250 mg PO qd × 4 days], doxycycline (100 mg PO bid), or a fluoroquinolone with enhanced activity against *S. pneumoniae* [e.g., gatifloxacin (Tequin), 400 mg PO qd]. Alternatively, some beta-lactams, such as amoxicillin-clavulanate (Augmentin), or a second-generation cephalosporin may be used. It has been suggested by some authorities that therapy with a macrolide or doxycycline should be reserved for the treatment of those patients <50 yrs without comorbid conditions, whereas the fluoroquinolones should be used in older patients and those with chronic disease.

Current recommendations for treatment in the **inpatient setting** include a regimen consisting of a beta-lactam plus a macrolide [e.g., ceftriaxone (Rocephin), 1 g IV qd, plus azithromycin, 250 mg PO qd] or a fluoroquinolone (e.g., gatifloxacin, 400 mg IV/PO qd). In those patients ill enough to require ICU placement, fluoroquinolone therapy should be combined with a beta-lactam. The preferred beta-lactams include ceftriaxone, cefotaxime (Claforan), or ampicillin/sulbactam (Unasyn). Parenteral PCN G remains the drug of choice for susceptible pneumococci and may be considered once the results of cultures/susceptibilities return. The preferred macrolides include azithromycin, clarithromycin (Biaxin), and erythromycin (E-Mycin). Of note, approximately 5% of PCN-resistant strains of *S. pneumoniae* are also resistant to macrolides *in vitro*. The preferred fluoroquinolones include those with enhanced activity against *S. pneumoniae*, such as levofloxacin (Levaquin), gatifloxacin, and moxifloxacin (Avelox). There is growing concern, however, that there is increasing resistance by *S. pneumoniae* to these agents. It should be remembered that the above recommendations apply to initial empiric treatment of CAP; therapy should be tapered to narrow-spectrum agents as microbiology test results become available.

Additional agents are sometimes used in the treatment of CAP in special circumstances. In those patients with comorbid conditions making them susceptible to *Pseudomonas* (COPD, cystic fibrosis), an appropriate beta-lactam with enhanced coverage [e.g., piperacillin-tazobactam (Zosyn)] with an aminoglycoside [e.g., tobramycin (Tobrex)] should be considered. In those patients at risk for aspiration pneumonia (neurologic disease, alcoholics) or those allergic to beta-lactams, a good regimen includes a fluoroquinolone plus clindamycin. Additionally, although vancomycin (Vancocin), linezolid (Zyvox), and quinupristin/dalfopristin (Synercid) have uniformly good activity against all *S. pneumoniae*, their use must be undertaken very carefully.

It is generally recommended that pneumococcal pneumonia should be treated until the patient has been afebrile for 72 hrs, whereas atypical pneumonias should be treated for approximately 2 wks. It is also believed to be reasonable to change from IV to PO therapy once a patient is hemodynamically stable and able to tolerate PO medications. Appropriate follow-up after antibiotic treatment includes repeat chest x-ray 6–12 wks after treatment to document resolution of the pneumonia and exclude any associated conditions, such as malignancy for a selected group of individuals (those >40 yrs and those who are smokers).

Prevention of CAP has been aided with the development of both the influenza and pneumococcal vaccines. The influenza vaccine is recommended to be given to those patients at risk for complications and health care workers. The pneumococcal vaccine is recommended to be given to those patients >50 yrs and those of any age with chronic medical illnesses.

LUNG ABSCESS

Lung abscess is defined as a collection of necrotic lung tissue contained within a cavity occurring as a result of progressive infection of the lung parenchyma. The reduction in the high incidence and mortality of lung abscess in the early part of the twentieth century may be attributed to two important discoveries: (a) that performance of tonsillectomy and oral surgery should be done in a supine, rather than seated, position; and (b) the discovery of PCN. Today, the incidence of lung abscess is approximately 5 in 10,000, and the overall mortality rate from lung abscess is in the range of 25%. Although the mortality rate from a primary abscess is estimated to be only 2%, that for a secondary abscess approaches as high as 75%.

Differential Diagnosis

Primary lung abscesses occur as a result of infection within the lung itself, whereas secondary lung abscesses occur in settings of extrapulmonary infection or sepsis, malignancy, or immunosuppression. Lung abscess may be seen as the end of a continuum from chronic aspiration pneumonitis, making it different from its purulent pulmonary counterparts of acute pyogenic pneumonia, necrotizing pneumonia, and empyema.

There are three important categories of bacteria responsible for the formation of primary lung abscess: (a) gram-positive anaerobic cocci (*Peptostreptococcus* species), (b) pigmented gram-negative bacilli (*Prevotella*, *Porphyromonas*, and *Bacteroides* species), and (c) *Fusobacterium* species. Additionally, most lung abscess material is polymicrobial. The prevalence of anaerobes and the polymicrobial nature of the lung abscess may be explained by the various virulence factors of the bacteria involved. Anaerobes possess different qualities or capabilities that may work synergistically to promote lung necrosis and cavitation. Aerobic bacteria (e.g., *S. aureus* and enteric gram-negative bacilli) are more common in cases of nosocomial noncavitary-acquired lung abscess. In contrast, the spectrum of organisms involved in the formation of cavitary lung lesions is more varied. Bacterial agents include *Pseudomonas* species, *Legionella* species, and *Nocardia*; fungal pathogens include *Histoplasma*, *Coccidioides*, *Blastomyces*, *Cryptococcus*, *Aspergillus*, and *Rhizopus*; parasitic organisms are rare but include *Paragonimus*, *Entamoeba*, and *Echinococcus*. Additionally, there are multiple noninfectious conditions that may promote the formation of cavitary lung lesions, including bronchogenic carcinoma, Wegener's granulomatosis, rheumatoid nodules, sarcoidosis, pulmonary infarction, and congenital pulmonary cysts.

Pathophysiology

The key etiologic factor in the formation of primary lung abscess is **aspiration.** Any condition that depresses consciousness, and thus the gag reflex, predisposes to aspiration (e.g., alcohol and sedative use, seizures, cerebrovascular accident, neuromuscular disease). Gingivitis may play an important role in that it may increase the infectious load of any aspiration material. Also, any condition that may impair local pulmonary host defenses (e.g., cough, mucociliary clearance, and alveolar macrophages) may be a contributing factor. Smoking, recent viral infections, diabetes, and chronic renal disease are examples.

With host defenses thus impaired, a state of indolent, chronic aspiration pneumonitis is established. With progressive necrosis, cavitation results. Lung abscesses may be multiple, but they are usually found as a single, dominant cavity. Air fluid levels may form when there is communication with the bronchial tree. Complications of lung abscess are progression to empyema, massive hemoptysis, and aspiration of abscess contents into the normal lung.

Clinical Manifestations

The clinical characteristics of lung abscess are both similar to and different from those of its purulent pulmonary counterparts. Fever, cough, sputum production, and chest pain are usual complaints, just as they are in patients with typical bacterial pneumonia. Weight loss, night sweats, hemoptysis, and anemia may also be described, just as they are in patients with necrotizing pneumonia. Putrid sputum and the indolent chronicity of symptoms may distinguish lung abscess from the other diagnoses. However, putrid sputum may be absent in as many as 40% of cases. Physical findings in a patient with lung abscess may involve those of chronic illness, such as wasting and signs of chronic anemia, as well as pulmonary cavitation, such as a limited area of hyperresonance on percussion and decreased breath sounds on auscultation. Additionally, the patient may exhibits signs of poor dentition, malodorous breath, and the ability to produce purulent sputum when requested.

Diagnosis

Chest x-ray is all that is usually necessary in the diagnosis of lung abscess. Lung abscesses usually involve the segments of lung that are dependent in a supine patient, namely the posterior segments of the upper lobes and the superior segments of the lower lobes. Additionally, they are more often found in the right-sided lung, presumably because the right main stem bronchus is less angulated with relation to the trachea in contrast to the left. Finally, lung abscesses are most often found in single lobes. Cavities are usually single and may vary in size. Air fluid levels may even be seen within the cavity. The most similar process of the differential diagnosis is necrotizing pneumonia; however, it is usually a more diffuse process of multiple smaller cavities on chest x-ray.

There is no evidence to suggest that CT scanning is essential to the diagnosis of lung abscess. It may be useful in detecting the pathogenic processes of early necrosis and cavitation before their appearance on chest x-ray. Additionally, because of better definition of pulmonary parenchyma, it may be useful in situations in which other diagnoses are being considered. Most important, CT may help to exclude the possibility of necrotic carcinoma or a cancerous mass causing a postobstructive process.

Because of the well-defined spectrum of pathogenic organisms involved, sputum culture is not necessary for treatment. Rather, methods such as fiberoptic bronchoscopy and percutaneous needle aspiration are used, like CT scanning, in excluding the possibility of carcinoma in those patients with risk factors for such disease who may present with lung abscess.

Treatment

PCN G (1.5–2.0 million units IV q4h) continues to be efficacious in the treatment of lung abscess, despite increasing resistance in a proportion of anaerobic bacterial isolates. However, there is evidence to support the use of clindamycin (Cleocin) (600 mg IV tid) over PCN. Two randomized trials comparing PCN and clindamycin revealed more rapid clinical response to treatment with clindamycin; defervescence and clearing of sputum were those markers used for response. Also, metronidazole (Flagyl) may be used in combination with PCN in those patients who cannot tolerate clindamycin. Another investigator has demonstrated that oral therapy is equivalent to parenteral therapy. Duration of therapy is believed to be determined on a case-by-case basis, with the end point being radiographic resolution; rarely is this resolution reached before 4–6 wks of antibiotic therapy. Thus, imaging should be obtained at intervals throughout the treatment period, with monitoring both for clinical signs of improvement and complications.

Drainage is well known to play a role in the treatment of abscesses. In terms of lung abscess, a drainage route is present through the bronchial airways if there is the presence of air within the abscess cavity. Thus, methods to promote expectoration are vital in the drainage process. Postural drainage and chest physiotherapy should be encouraged. Percutaneous catheter drainage or surgical drainage should be used in cases of severe and critical illness or in those resistant to medical therapy. Additional indications include massive hemoptysis or progression of lung abscess to empyema. Complications of such procedures include bronchopleural fistula and pneumothorax. Recurrent abscess may occur in a small minority of cases.

PULMONARY TB

TB is defined as a chronic infection caused by the bacterium *Mycobacterium tuberculosis* characterized by granuloma formation within infected tissues. The usual portal of entry and thus infection is the pulmonary system, but the disease may become widespread within an infected individual depending on both his or her immune and treatment status. Discussion in this section is limited to pulmonary TB.

TB is an epidemic of devastating proportions. It is estimated that one-third of the world population, or 1.7 billion people, is infected with the bacterium. Eight million new cases and 2 million deaths are reported each year. The distribution of TB is such that the third-world countries are burdened the most. According to the WHO in 1990, the rates of disease were 237 cases per 100,000 persons in Southeast Asia compared with 23 cases per 100,000 persons in Western Europe. The resurgence of TB in the United States in the late 1980s, which was considered secondary to the rise in HIV infection and immigration, has slowly declined due to major improvements in public health policy (e.g., reporting of disease, directly observed therapy, and treatment of both active and latent infections of TB).

Differential Diagnosis

The clinical characteristics and chest x-rays of TB may be similar to those with CAP. Occasionally, patients with TB may present with acute onset of disease and lobar pneumonia, as in typical pneumonia; however, more often they have a chronic indolent course, such as that of atypical pneumonias. Chronic fungal diseases (e.g., *Blastomyces* and *Histoplasma*), other mycobacterial diseases, and interstitial pulmonary diseases (e.g., hypersensitivity pneumonitis, eosinophilic granuloma, and sarcoidosis) must also be strongly considered. The keys to having a high index of suspicion for TB are history of exposure and predisposition to TB from immunosuppressive diseases (e.g., renal failure, diabetes, malnutrition, HIV).

Pathophysiology

The etiologic agent of TB is *M. tuberculosis*, an obligate aerobe, which is non–spore-forming and nonmotile. It is very slowly growing, with a doubling time of 15–20 hrs. Along with the other *Mycobacterium* species, it is distinguished by its ability to stain "acid fast"; surface lipids act to resist the destaining of carbolfuchsin with acid alcohol, and thus the bacteria retain a red color. These surface lipids and other protein and polysaccharide components of the cell wall are important immunoreactive structures that play important roles in the pathogenesis of and cell-mediated immunity to the disease.

The transmission cycle of TB has been well described. Beginning with a known tuberculous patient, infectious particles are generated with each activity involving forced expiration, including coughing, sneezing, breathing, and even singing. "Droplet nuclei" of respiratory secretions, with a size of 1–5 μm, each containing approximately 1–3 viable bacteria, are generated with the expirations. The droplet nuclei may remain suspended in air for up to several days; however, the bacilli are susceptible to environmental exposures, such as sun and ultraviolet light, and airborne droplets may be removed by highly efficient filtration systems. Successful transmission involves the inhalation of even just one infectious particle, which becomes deposited in the terminal alveoli of the new host. Other modes of transmission are less prevalent but include direct inoculation, such as through the skin, and vertical transmission, either transplacentally or directly by the birth canal.

Once infectious bacilli gain access to the pulmonary system, they come to lie in distal alveoli in the well-ventilated areas of the lower lung. Subsequently, nonspecific immune responses begin; macrophages ingest the infectious particles and spread to regional lymph nodes. Depending on host factors, the spread of the organism may be limited to the pulmonary system or may be great, entering the bloodstream, resulting in disseminated disease. Over the next several weeks, while the bacilli multiply within their intracellular environment, the macrophages present antigenic epitopes on their surface, allowing for generation of cell-mediated immunity through T cells by the host. Multiple cytokines, including chemotactic factors, interleukins, and interferons, are generated and released. In response to these activities, macrophages and monocytes are transformed into specialized histiocytic cells and organize to form granulomas. Over time, these granulomas may calcify, leading to lesions visible on chest x-ray. A **Ghon complex** is the combination of calcified lesions in the peripheral lung and hilar lymph node. Additionally, CD4$^+$ cells are subdivided into Th1 and Th2 cells whose balance is important in regulating the immune response.

The status of the infection is based on both the concentration of infecting bacilli and the extent of the generated immune response. In 95% of cases, the immune system successfully suppresses progression of disease, although it does not eradicate it. Patients in this state are said to have "latent infection"; they are asymptomatic and noninfectious. They will, however, have a positive cell-mediated immunity response to tuberculin skin testing. On the other hand, 5% of patients will not have the capability to contain their infection and will develop disease in 1–2 yrs. From those patients who develop latent disease, 95% of them never progress to active disease, whereas 5% of them have disruption of the balance of their immune system and clinically manifest TB. Patients at risk for progression to active disease include those with HIV infection, diabetes mellitus, chronic renal failure, head or neck cancer, organ transplantation, and silicosis.

Reactivation TB results when there is proliferation of organisms in an area of previously latent infection. Sites of reactivation involve those to which bacilli spread in the initial stages of infection, such as regional lymph nodes, apical portions of upper lungs, or even distant sites of disseminated disease. This form of TB is one of chronic, progressive wasting and constitutional symptoms.

Clinical Manifestations

The symptoms of a patient infected with TB may be subtle. Primary TB, or primary inoculation with infectious bacilli, is usually asymptomatic. In those patients who progress to pulmonary TB, the most prominent manifestation is cough. Mild forms of disease may have nonproductive cough, whereas advanced, often cavitary lesions may produce purulent, even bloody sputum. Dyspnea is less common but may be important in those patients in whom a pleural effusion is present. Chest pain may occur if there is extensive pleural inflammation. Constitutional symptoms appear more consistent, including fever, fatigue, night sweats, and weight loss. As previously mentioned, the symptoms of reactivation TB are those of generalized wasting, low-grade fevers, and drenching night sweats.

The key component to the history of TB is that of **exposure.** One should inquire as to the patient's history of TB and PPD status. Because the likelihood of transmission is highest in close quarters with poor ventilation, contact with persons with whom one lives is most important. Certain populations of people are more at risk for infection, including the homeless, IV drug users, prisoners, HIV-infected persons, and immigrants. Additionally, as mentioned previously, certain persons are more at risk for progression to disease after infection; it is important to remember these patients, as they too are candidates for tuberculin screening, as mentioned below.

The findings on the physical exam of patients with pulmonary disease are relatively unimpressive. Exceptions may be made for those patients with extensive disease. Crackles may be heard over areas of infiltration. Rales may be heard only posttussively, indicating apical disease. Amphoric breath sounds are those that are heard in cases of extensive cavitation. Wheezing may be heard in the presence of endobronchial lesions. Dullness to percussion may be noted in areas of disease, even in the area of the clavicles, indicating apical disease.

Amphoric Breath Sounds

Diagnosis

The diagnosis of TB involves identifying those patients who have disease and those patients who have latent infection.

Any patient who presents with symptoms, signs, and risk factors for TB should be assumed to have the disease, hospitalized, and isolated, and diagnostic testing should be initiated. Generally, TB isolation consists of airborne precautions in which the patient is placed in a negative-pressure room, and all visitors must wear an N95 mask when entering the room. It is important to be familiar with your health care facility's infection control policy as further guidelines (including when to discontinue isolation, transport policies, etc.) may vary. For sample isolation guidelines, refer to Chap. 30, Infection Control. Chest x-ray may be helpful in determining the level of suspicion of TB, although it cannot be used alone in the diagnosis. Findings indicative of TB include the Ghon complex, apical infiltrates, and cavitary lesions; findings such as local consolidation, diffuse disease, and pleural effusion are less specific but may be all that is present. Imperative in the diagnosis is culturing *M. tuberculosis*. Because of the slow-growing nature of the organism, presumptive diagnoses of active disease may be made using acid-fast smears or fluorochrome techniques. Samples for analysis are best obtained early in the morning on ≥3 separate days. Although positive AFB and fluorochrome results indicate that the patient has infectious mycobacterial disease, they do not specify the infecting organism as *M. tuberculosis*. Culturing the organism is necessary for exact identification and drug susceptibility testing; newer techniques have been developed to hasten these tasks during the culturing period, such as direct amplification testing. Drug susceptibility testing is indicated in the United States for all initial isolates and for subsequent isolates in persistently positive and relapsed cases of TB. Multiple techniques to obtain such information are currently available.

Identifying persons with **latent TB infection** is more difficult clinically than identifying those persons with active disease. This task has been made much easier with the development of the tuberculin skin test and guidelines for its use. Tuberculin skin testing uses a PPD, injected SC into the volar aspect of the forearm (Mantoux method), which, when given to a patient with latent infection, stimulates the cell-mediated immune response. Guidelines from the Infectious Diseases Society of America (IDSA) recommend performing tuberculin skin testing on all patients meeting one or more of the following criteria: HIV infection, injection drug use, homelessness, incarceration, or contact with a person with active pulmonary TB. Additional individuals who should be tested are immigrants from countries with high rates of TB, health care professionals, and persons living or working in long-term care facilities. The method of interpretation of the slightly imperfect PPD has been constructed to increase the predictive value of the test. Three different diameters of induration are significant for persons with different risks of infection. A 5-mm diameter reaction is considered positive for those persons with recent contact with known active TB, persons with HIV infection, other immunosuppressed persons, and persons with chest x-ray suggestive of old TB. A 10-mm diameter reaction is considered positive for those persons who have recently immigrated from countries with a high prevalence of TB, injection drug users, children <4 yrs, and persons who work or live in situations that may put them at risk for exposure to TB. A 15-mm diameter reaction is considered positive for all other persons. Any person who has a negative PPD but has a subsequent test within 2 yrs that reveals an increase of ≥10 mm is considered to have "converted," indicating recent infection and thus risk of progression to active disease. An additional note includes those immigrated persons who may have received the BCG vaccine. It is considered to be impossible to distinguish induration caused by TB versus BCG;

however, because the vaccine has proved to be ineffectual in preventing some cases of disease and because the prevalence of the disease is high in those countries where it is used, the history of receiving the vaccine should be ignored in interpretation of PPD testing.

Treatment

Guidelines for treatment of both active disease and latent infection have been described by the IDSA and the American Thoracic Society.

For those patients with suspected or confirmed **active tuberculous disease,** treatment should be initiated promptly, taking into consideration resistance patterns of the community. Therapy consists of the combination of isoniazid (Laniazid, Nydrazid) (INH) (300 mg PO qd), rifampin (Rifadin, Rimactane) (600 mg PO qd), pyrazinamide (pms-Pyrazinamide, Tebrazid) (2 g PO qd) ± ethambutol (15–25 mg/kg PO qd) or streptomycin. The IDSA recommends a threshold of 4%—meaning that if 4% of local isolates are resistant to INH, the four-drug regimen should be used. Because 84% of the population of the United States had >4% isolates resistant to INH, the four-drug regimen is the most recommended initial regimen for treatment of active TB; the fourth drug may be eliminated once drug resistance results have been reported. A full 6 mos of treatment are required for elimination of disease. INH, rifampin, and pyrazinamide must all be used daily for the first 2 mos; for the remaining 4 mos, INH and rifampin may be administered daily, twice weekly, or thrice weekly. Another approved regimen is to use the same initial drugs daily for 2 wks, then twice a week for 6 wks, and then taper to only INH and rifampin daily, twice weekly, or thrice weekly for the remaining 16 wks. Of note, slight variation of doses for these medications must be made for these alternative regimens (e.g., INH doses must be increased to 900 mg for both twice- and thrice-weekly dosing, whereas pyrazinamide must be increased to 4 g and 3 g, respectively). Finally, all of the drugs may be administered three times a week for the entire 6-mo period. A notable caveat is that rifampin must not be administered to those HIV-infected patients on nonnucleoside inhibitors or protease inhibitors secondary to drug interaction; rifabutin (Mycobutin) may be substituted. Adjuvant to the initiation of treatment, cases of TB should be reported to the public health authorities; such officials monitor the treatment of patients (i.e., directly observed therapy), locate and evaluate contacts, and study patterns of disease in the community.

For those patients with **latent TB infection,** treatment should be initiated with one of four regimens. Nine mos of INH (300 mg PO qd) is the preferred regimen for all adults. However, in those patients who are HIV negative, >18 yrs, and without fibrotic changes on chest x-ray, only 6 mos of INH is acceptable. Alternatively, 4 mos of rifampin (600 mg PO qd) alone may be used. Caveats to remember are that INH use in persons >35 yrs is associated with increased risk of toxicity and that rifampin use is not recommended in pregnant women; therefore, decisions regarding which regimen to use must be individualized.

In cases of active tuberculous disease, patients should be clinically monitored on a regular basis (e.g., once a month). Baseline tests to consider include hepatic enzymes, bilirubin, BUN/Cr and CBC, uric acid (if using pyrazinamide), and visual acuity (if using ethambutol). By 3 mos of therapy, both clinical improvement and negative smears/cultures should be obtained. If such goals have not been met, the possibilities of noncompliance and drug resistance need to be considered. **Directly observed therapy** has greatly aided in assuring compliance. Drug resistance testing is very helpful in confirming such cases; however, results may take up to 6 wks; therefore, decisions concerning the treatment regimen must be made without such information. The IDSA recommends that if drug resistance is suspected or confirmed, two drugs to which the organism is likely to be susceptible should be added to the regimen. Consultation with an infectious disease specialist is advised under these circumstances. Patients should then continue to be monitored with respect to their clinical symptoms and with smears and cultures for the duration of treatment.

In cases of latent TB infection, completion of therapy is less successful than in those cases of active TB. A performance indicator of 75% completion of therapy within 1 yr of initiation of treatment (vs. 100%) is what is expected under IDSA guidelines. **Monitoring**

of therapy should include periodic clinic visits. It is recommended that all patients with tuberculosis have counseling and testing for HIV infection, at least by the time that treatment is initiated, if not earlier. For patients with HIV infection, a CD4$^+$ lymphocyte count should be obtained. Patients with risk factors for hepatitis B or C viruses (e.g., injection drug use, birth in Asia or Africa, HIV infection) should have serologic tests for these viruses. For all adult patients, baseline measurements of serum amino transferases (AST and ALT), bilirubin, alkaline phosphatase, and serum creatinine and a platelet count should be obtained. Testing of visual acuity and red-green color discrimination should be obtained when ethambutol (EMB) is to be used. Routine measurements of hepatic and renal function and platelet count are not necessary during treatment unless patients have baseline abnormalities or are at increased risk of hepatotoxicity (e.g., hepatitis B or C virus infection, alcohol abuse). At each monthly visit, patients taking EMB should be questioned regarding possible visual disturbances, including blurred vision and scotomata; monthly testing of visual acuity and color discrimination is recommended for patients taking doses that, on a milligram per kilogram basis, are greater than 15–25 mg/kg and for patients receiving the drug for longer than 2 months.

NOSOCOMIAL PNEUMONIA

Nosocomial pneumonia (NP) is defined as the acquisition of a pulmonary infiltrate after 48–72 hrs of hospitalization. Included in this definition is the category of ventilator-associated pneumonia, which is those pneumonias that develop in patients who have been on mechanical ventilation for ≥48 hrs. Risk factors for the development of NP include mechanical ventilation, age, comorbid conditions, severity of illness, depressed level of consciousness, prior use of antibiotics, NG tubes, and the use of stress ulcer prophylaxis.

NP is the one of the most common of nosocomial infections. It has been documented to occur in 0.4–1.0% of hospitalized patients overall and in 25–58% of mechanically ventilated patients. NP results in extensions of hospital stays of 6–13 additional days and in approximately 25,000–100,000 deaths/yr. The overall mortality rate is calculated is 20–50%.

The spectrum of pathogens causing NP is less diverse than those responsible for CAP. Bacteria are implicated in >90% of cases, with viruses and fungi playing lesser roles. The most common bacteria are gram-negative rods, including *Pseudomonas aeruginosa*, *K. pneumoniae*, *Escherichia coli*, *Acinetobacter* species, *Serratia* species, and *Enterobacter* species, accounting for up to 70% of cases. *S. aureus* is the most important gram-positive cause, responsible for up to 30% of cases, with *Streptococcus* species and *H. influenzae* occasionally causing disease. *Legionella* causes NP in epidemics associated with contaminated hospital water supplies. Viral pathogens include influenza and RSV; fungal pathogens include *Candida albicans* and *Aspergillus* species. Important to recognize is the microbial spectrum in particular hospital institutions, as slight variations in the prevalence of disease-causing organisms may exist.

Differential Diagnosis

The differential diagnosis is limited primarily to airway colonization by the same organisms that are involved in the pathogenic process of NP. Differentiating between these two states is the key to successful treatment and is discussed within the sections below. Additionally, CHF, malignancy, atelectasis, and pulmonary hemorrhage may all mimic NP.

Pathophysiology

There are three important principles in the pathophysiology of NP: **disruption of host defenses, colonization, and aspiration.** The host defenses of specialized protective epithelium may be damaged by the placement of NG, endotracheal, and tracheostomy tubes; furthermore, once in place, these apparatuses bypass the upper respiratory tract defense systems. Two sites of colonization of the host important in the development of

NP are the airway and the GI tract. The airways of normal persons are colonized with gram-positive organisms such as *Streptococcus* species, *Staphylococcus* species, *H. influenzae*, *Moraxella*, and anaerobes; as a result, the proliferation of gram-negative bacilli is suppressed. However, it has been documented through convincing studies that those patients who are moderately to critically ill change their spectra of flora, becoming colonized with gram-negative rods within 4 days of hospitalization. The GI tract becomes an important source of nosocomial pathogens secondary to the use of medications for stress ulcer prophylaxis. Aspiration of newly colonized bacteria from both the airway and GI tracts is the likely mechanism for the institution of these pathogens into the lower respiratory tract. Evidence indicates that even 45% of normal persons microaspirate, whereas 70% of those with depressed mental status aspirate. Hematogenously spread NP involves other sites of infection, such as indwelling catheters, wounds, and even sinusitis. Contamination of various objects, including water supply, respiratory equipment, hands of health care workers, and enteral feeding solutions, have all been implicated as sources of organisms leading to NP.

Once obtaining access to the pulmonary tissue, the pathogenic organisms set up residence and incite the inflammatory response, resulting in interstitial infiltrate; most often, this inflammatory process progresses to a state of necrotizing pneumonia and cavitation. The two most common causes of NP, *Pseudomonas* and *S. aureus*, typically produce cavitation within 72 hrs, whereas *Klebsiella* and other gram-negative bacilli produce cavitation within 5–7 days.

Clinical Manifestations

Most important are the medical history and the history of the present medical course of those patients suspected of having NP. One should focus on comorbid conditions, such as cardiac, pulmonary, and rheumatologic disease; history of tobacco and alcohol use; and risk factors for pulmonary embolism and immunocompromised states. Increased duration of intubation, use of multiple antibiotics, use of steroids, or recent surgery may support the diagnosis of NP. Important features of the physical exam in the detection of NP include those that may favor the diagnosis and those that may favor any of the other diseases in the differential diagnosis. Particular attention should be paid to the vital signs, pulmonary exam, mental status, obvious sources of infection (catheters, wounds, purulent sinus drainage), signs of CHF, deep venous thrombosis, and even skin manifestation of rheumatologic disease.

Diagnosis

The task of diagnosing NP has proved itself to be more difficult than that of diagnosing its counterpart of CAP. Although chest x-ray, blood cultures, and expectorated sputum are the cornerstones of the diagnosis of CAP, they are less helpful in the determination of the presence of NP. The gold standard for the diagnosis of NP is histologic exam and culture of lung tissue. Because such information is rarely available, physicians have come to rely on clinical criteria and other types of respiratory samples in their decisions of diagnosis and treatment.

Obtaining respiratory samples and interpretation of their analysis have proved problematic, as it is difficult to distinguish between disease-causing organisms and colonizers. The use of sputum specimens from the upper respiratory tract is unquestionably limited given the high rate of colonization of the oropharynx, trachea, and ETTs. More invasive techniques of respiratory fluid collection have been developed to access and sample the lower respiratory tract, bypassing any contamination of the upper airway. **Fiberoptic bronchoscopy and blind bronchial sampling** are the means by which to obtain tissue by protected specimen brush and bronchoalveolar lavage. Once specimens are obtained, they may be used for Gram's stain and quantitative culture. Gram's staining of material from the distal airways, and in particular that obtained by bronchoalveolar lavage, has proved superior to that from proximal airways, with a positive predictive value of 92–95% and a negative predictive value of 57–95%. Quantitative culture allows for determination of pathogen versus colonizer depending on resultant growth; NP is defined as bacteria that are cultured at a concentration of 10^3 colony-forming units/mL by protected specimen brush and 10^4 colony-forming units/mL by bronchoalveolar lavage. Various other methods of analysis exist, including elastin fiber analysis and analysis of centrifuged lavage fluid. Elastin fiber analysis involves detection, with potassium hydroxide, of elastin fibers that are indicative of necrosis of lung tissue; centrifuged lavage fluid may be examined microscopically in an attempt to locate alveolar macrophages that may be harboring intracellular organisms.

Clinical characteristics and microbiologic data have been taken together in the formation of diagnostic criteria for NP, developed both by the CDC and individual investigators. The presence of NP is defined as presence of both clinical suspicion (fever, increased WBC count, purulent sputum) and histopathologic analysis of tissue consistent with pneumonia and at least one of the following: significant growth of pathogen on distal airway analysis, positive blood culture without other possible source, positive pleural fluid culture, chest x-ray with cavitation in the absence of malignancy, isolation of virus or *Legionella* from secretions, or serologic/antigen assay confirmation of infection with virus or *Legionella*.

Treatment

Treatment decisions rest on the determination of the severity of illness of the patient; severity of illness, in turn, parallels the risk that the causative organism is *P. aeruginosa*. Patients with mild to moderate illness, and thus lower risk for *Pseudomonas*, are usually those who were previously healthy without comorbid conditions who may have been on mechanical ventilation but received no prior antibiotic therapy. Organisms more likely to cause NP in these patients are *S. pneumoniae*, *H. influenzae*, and other less virulent gram-negative rods; appropriate treatment consists of monotherapy with beta-lactam plus inhibitor [e.g., ticarcillin/clavulanate (Timentin), 3.1 g IV q4h], second- or third-generation cephalosporin (e.g., ceftriaxone, 1–2 g IV qd), or fluoroquinolone (gatifloxacin, 400 mg IV qd). Patients with moderate to critical illness, and thus higher risk for *Pseudomonas*, are usually those patients with complicating medical problems who may have undergone prolonged mechanical ventilation and received multiple rounds of antibiotic therapy. Appropriate treatment may include monotherapy with agents such as piperacillin-tazobactam (Zosyn) (3.375 g IV q6h), imipenem-cilastatin (Primaxin IM, Primaxin IV) (0.5 g IV q6h), or cefepime (Maxipime) (1–2 g IV q12h). However, because such a regimen may have a failure rate as high as 60%, double coverage is most typically used. Combinations of beta-lactams with either an aminoglycoside (e.g., ticarcillin/clavulanate, 3.1 g IV q4h, plus tobramycin, 5 mg/kg IV qd) or fluoroquinolone are most typically used.

With regard to duration of therapy, no definitive studies have been performed. A treatment of 14–21 days is the general guideline. Necrotizing pneumonias may need treatment for up 28 days. Defervescence is the most used measure of response to treatment; resolution of leukocytosis, hypoxia, and chest x-ray are additional markers. Microbiologic studies reveal sterilization of distal airways secretion within 72 hrs of initiation of appropriate treatment. Once clinical improvement and adequate GI function are attained, there may be consideration to change from IV to PO mode of delivery of antibiotics. As with CAP, time to resolution of infiltrates on chest x-ray may take weeks; it may take even more prolonged periods of time in those patients with underlying pulmonary disease.

Numerous ideas have been formulated with regard to prevention of NP based on its principles of pathophysiology. Maintenance of gastric acidity with use of stress ulcer prophylaxis agents such as sucralfate (instead of antacids, H_2-blockers), use of antibiotic pastes on NG tubes, and acidification of enteral feeds are a few of those suggested to eliminate colonization of the GI tract. One large randomized trial showed that sucralfate at a dose of 1 g q48h reduced the risk of late-onset NP. Other prophylactic agents remain controversial. Semirecumbent positioning and jejunal feeding are believed to decrease the incidence of aspiration. Other strategies that have been studied are continuous lateral rotational therapy to assist in mobilizing secretions, chest physiotherapy and incentive spirometry to minimize atelectasis, and attention to proper hand washing and cleaning of respiratory equipment to reduce cross-contamination.

SEVERE ACUTE RESPIRATORY SYNDROME

Severe acute respiratory syndrome (SARS) is a viral respiratory illness that caused a global outbreak in 2003 with cases identified in more than two dozen countries in North America, South America, Europe, and Asia. It is caused by the SARS-associated coronavirus (SARS-CoV) and is primarily transmitted by close person-to-person contact. Droplets are spread when an infected person sneezes or coughs, and droplets are propelled up to 3 feet through the air and land on the mucous membranes (mouth, nose, eyes) of those nearby. The virus can also be spread when a person comes in contact with a surface containing infected droplets and then touches his or her nose, mouth, or eye(s). It is not yet clear whether airborne spread or other methods of transmission are possible. Through an immense international effort, the 2003 global outbreak was contained, but the disease may reemerge.

Clinical Manifestations

SARS may present with a high fever (temperature >100.4°F or 38°C) with chills and rigors or with mild respiratory symptoms. Other symptoms can include headache, an overall feeling of discomfort or malaise, diarrhea, and body aches. Within 2–7 days, patients may develop a dry cough, dyspnea, or hypoxemia. Many patients develop pneumonia. Some patients may recover, but some may decompensate rapidly. In 10–20% of cases, the respiratory illness is severe enough to require intubation and mechanical ventilation.

Laboratory Findings

Chest radiographs may remain normal throughout the course of the illness, but the respiratory phase is often characterized by early focal interstitial infiltrates that progress to more generalized, patchy, interstitial infiltrates. Areas of consolidation have been seen in the late stages of SARS. Absolute lymphocyte count is often decreased early in the illness. WBC counts are usually normal or decreased. At the peak of the respiratory illness, approximately 50% of patients have leukopenia and thrombocytopenia or low-normal platelet counts (50,000–150,000/mL). Early in the respiratory phase, elevated CPK levels (as high as 3,000 IU/L) and hepatic transaminases (two to six times the upper limits of normal) have been noted. Renal function is usually unaffected.

Treatment

To date, antimicrobials, antiviral agents, and steroids have been used in the treatment of SARS patients; however, the most efficacious treatment regimen for SARS is yet unknown. Current recommendations are to evaluate the patient for causes of CAP (cultures, viral antigen assays, and so forth) and treat for CAP as otherwise indicated.

Reporting of Severe Acute Respiratory Syndrome

Prompt identification is crucial, and all patients with these types of symptoms should be questioned about recent travel and potential contact with a SARS-infected individual. In the United States, clinicians who suspect cases of SARS should report cases to their state health department. The SARS Investigative Team can be reached at the CDC Emergency Operations Center (telephone, 770-488-7100). Outside the United States, clinicians who suspect cases of SARS are requested to report such cases to their local public health authorities. Additional information about SARS (e.g., infection control guidance and procedures for reporting suspected cases) is available at http://www.cdc.gov/ncidod/sars.

Contacts

Close contact is defined as having cared for or lived with someone with SARS or having direct contact with the respiratory secretions or body fluids of a SARS patient (e.g., kissing, hugging, sharing eating or drinking utensils, and touching or speaking with someone within 3 feet). Household contacts are at particular risk; the CDC has developed interim infection control recommendations for those with a suspected SARS patient in the household that should be followed for **10 days after the respiratory symptoms and fever resolve.** SARS patients should be advised to limit interactions outside of the home during this time. Health care workers are at increased risk and should follow the infection control recommendations outlined at http://www.cdc.gov/ncidod/sars/ic.htm#healthcare.

Travel

If an outbreak does recur, individuals should be advised to delay nonessential travel to areas where cases of SARS have been reported. Updated travel advisories and alerts can be found on the CDC Web site (http://www.cdc.gov/ncidod/sars/travel_advice.htm). If travel is necessary, individuals should be advised to wash their hands frequently, avoid close contact with large numbers of people, and consult a health care provider immediately if they develop any symptoms of SARS or have close contact with a SARS-infected individual.

References:

CDC Information for Clinicians: Severe Acute Respiratory Syndrome (SARS). http://www.cdc.gov/ncidod/sars/clinicians.htm. Last accessed 9/11/03.
CDC Information for Clinicians: Basic Information about SARS. http://www.cdc.gov/ncidod/sars/factsheet.htm. Last accessed 9/11/03.
CDC Preliminary Clinical Description for SARS. http://www.cdc.gov/mmwr/preview/mmwrhtml/mm5212a5.htm. Last accessed 9/11/03.

KEY POINTS TO REMEMBER

- The key to diagnosing acute bronchitis by physical exam is to distinguish it from URI and pneumonia.
- The most common etiology of CAP is *Pneumococcus*.
- Lung abscess holds fast to several principles: aspiration is causative, spectrum of organisms is limited, and chest x-ray is characteristic.
- Both active and latent forms of TB must be treated with one of the specific treatment regimens, and there must be close follow-up throughout the treatment course.
- The most common causes of NP are gram-negative bacilli.

REFERENCES AND SUGGESTED READINGS

Bartlett JG, Dowell SF, Mandell LA, et al. Practice guidelines for the management of community-acquired pneumonia in adults. *Clin Infect Dis* 2000;31:342–382.

Bartlett JG, Mundy L. Community-acquired pneumonia. *N Engl J Med* 1995;333:1618–1624.

Daniel TM. Tuberculosis. In: Isselbacher KJ, ed. *Harrison's principles of internal medicine*, 13th ed. New York: McGraw-Hill, 1994:710–718.

Davis B, Systrom DM. Lung abscess: pathogenesis, diagnosis, and treatment. *Curr Clin Top Infect Dis* 1998;18:252–273.

Fine MJ, Auble TE, Yealy DM, et al. A prediction rule to identify low-risk patients with community-acquired pneumonia. *N Engl J Med* 1997;336:243–250.

Gonzales R, Sande MA. Acute bronchitis in the healthy adult. *Curr Clin Top Infect Dis* 2000;20:158–173.

Horsburgh C Jr, Feldman RS, Ridzon R. Practice guidelines for the treatment of tuberculosis. *Clin Infect Dis* 2000;31:633–639.

Levinson ME. Pneumonia, including necrotizing pulmonary infections (lung abscess). In: Isselbacher KJ, ed. *Harrison's principles of internal medicine*, 13th ed. New York: McGraw-Hill, 1994:1184–1191.

Napolitano LA, Szekely LA, Thompson BT. Nosocomial pneumonia. In: Lee BW, Hsu SI, Stasior DS, eds. *Quick consult manual of evidence-based medicine*. Philadelphia: Lippincott–Raven, 1997:606–632.

Small PM, Fujiwara PI. Management of tuberculosis in the United States. *N Engl J Med* 2001;345:189–200.

Small PM, Selcer UM. Tuberculosis. In: Strickland GT, ed. *Hunter's tropical medicine and emerging infectious disease*. Philadelphia: WB Saunders, 2000:491–513.

Zaleznik DF. Evaluation and management of patients with hospital-acquired infections. In: Isselbacher KJ, ed. *Harrison's principles of internal medicine*, 13th ed. New York: McGraw-Hill, 1994:583–586.

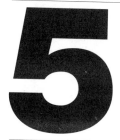

Cardiovascular Hardware Infections

Michele C. L. Cabellon

NATIVE VALVE INFECTIVE ENDOCARDITIS

Infection of the heart valves is a serious and possibly life-threatening disease. There are two main courses of presentation. **Acute bacterial endocarditis** usually has an onset within 3–10 days of initial infection and can be a fulminant course with the patient becoming critically ill quickly. **Subacute bacterial endocarditis (SBE)** has more of an indolent presentation with symptoms that may be present over several weeks, such as fatigue, weight loss, low-grade fevers, and signs of peripheral emboli. SBE usually affects previously damaged heart valves. Patients with prosthetic valves are at an exceptionally increased risk for infective endocarditis (IE) (see Prosthetic Valve Endocarditis). Here, native valve endocarditis is discussed.

Pathophysiology

It is not precisely clear why some individuals develop IE. The main theory is that a preexisting thrombus may exist at the site of damaged heart valves (classically, the mitral and aortic valves that have been involved in rheumatic fever) or at some congenital lesions, such as a ventricular septal defect. The clot gives a site for circulating bacteria to adhere. More clots can then form, resulting in a vegetation that consists of platelets, fibrin, microcolonies of bacteria, and inflammatory cells. It is believed that the bacteria are deep inside this mass of cells where they are protected from the environment, and they become relatively metabolically inactive, making it difficult for antibiotics to penetrate to the bacteria and be effective.

Risk factors for development of bacteremia and secondary IE include some dental and genitourinary procedures (see Prophylactic Recommendations for Infective Endocarditis) or other foci of infection, such as catheter-associated bacteremia. IV drug use is also a very common inciting factor for both acute bacterial endocarditis and SBE. Because of these usual routes of infection, *Streptococcus viridans* and *Staphylococcus aureus* are among the most common pathogens responsible for IE. Other organisms such as the HACEK group (*Haemophilus aphrophilus*, *Actinobacillus actinomycetemcomitans*, *Cardiobacterium hominis*, *Eikenella corrodens*, and *Kingella kingae*) and other gram-negative bacteria are also seen. Nosocomial infections can add a host of other less common bacteria.

Clinical Manifestations

The patient may become very ill quickly and experience high fevers (with acute IE) or may have low-grade temperatures with arthralgias, weight loss, and sweats (with SBE). Symptoms of CHF may be present. Pulmonary symptoms are significant with IV drug abuse because the lungs may be seeded from a right-heart vegetation. New rashes or hematuria may also be clues to the diagnosis.

Physical exam may be very helpful or may not be revealing at all. Cardiac murmurs are only useful if it is known whether the murmur is a new finding or if it has changed. Some cases of IE may not have an audible murmur at all. A full neurologic exam should be done. Neurologic changes may be a sign of septic emboli or mycotic aneurysms in the CNS. Clubbing is present in a small number of patients with SBE. An ophthalmologic exam also should be attempted to look for Roth's spots, although these are present in only 5% of patients. They are pale, centered, oval retinal hemorrhages, usually located proximally near the optic disc.

Classic skin findings are also very helpful but are most often not evident. Petechiae—nonblanching red lesions that turn brown—can appear and resolve in 2–3 days, cropping up in different patches later. Osler's nodes, seen in <25% of patients, are purple-red SC nodules, most often located on the pads of the fingers and toes. They are often preceded by severe focal pain or tingling in the area. Janeway lesions, seen in 2–11% of acute IE cases, are small hemorrhagic macules. These are usually located over the thenar and hypothenar eminences, palms, fingers, soles, and toes.

Diagnosis

The most important task in diagnosing IE is **obtaining adequate blood cultures before any antibiotics are given.** Three sets should be obtained initially (a set equals one aerobic and one anaerobic culture), each ≥1 hr apart and preferably from different locations. The microbiology lab should be advised that the diagnosis of suspicion is IE. If cultures remain negative after 48–72 hrs, they should be saved and incubated for 2–3 wks. In addition, a CBC for leukocytosis, a serum creatinine, and a UA looking for microscopic hematuria or casts (indicating immune complex deposition glomerulonephritis) should be obtained. A chest x-ray and an ECG (new heart block may be an indicator of intracardiac abscess) should be part of all workups. If there are any skin lesions present, a biopsy or aspirate can be sent for Gram's stain and culture.

The Duke Criteria, developed in 1994, have a high sensitivity and specificity in the diagnosis of IE (Table 5-1). These criteria were modified by Li et al. in 2000. These criteria added echocardiographic evidence and clinical findings as factors in the diagnosis of definite IE, whereas the previous Beth Israel Criteria relied on pathologic evaluation through surgery or autopsy as the only definitive way to diagnosis. The pieces of information are organized into major and minor criteria; to diagnose definite IE, two major, one major and three minor, or five minor criteria must be present. IE is rejected as a diagnosis if an alternate diagnosis is made, the symptoms resolve in ≤4 days of antibiotic therapy, or there is no evidence pathologically at surgery or autopsy after antibiotic therapy for ≤4 days. All other cases fall into the possible IE category.*

There has been debate over which type of echocardiogram is sufficient to help diagnose IE. TTE is a noninvasive study that is approximately 98% specific for vegetations but only <60% sensitive, especially for lesions <2 mm in size. In general, it can be used in low-risk patients to rule out IE, but if the patient is at high risk for IE or there is high clinical suspicion, a negative TTE does not help in ruling out vegetations. TEE has increased sensitivity and specificity for IE compared to TTE and should be used initially if there is an intermediate or high suspicion for IE, if the patient has a prosthetic valve, or if the patient is at high risk for complications associated with IE. A negative TTE and TEE have a negative predictive value of 95%. Still, if the clinical suspicion remains high or strengthens despite an initial negative TEE, the test should be repeated in 7–10 days to reassess the valves. A follow-up echocardiogram after treatment for IE is completed is not helpful because evidence for vegetations may persist for several years after the infection.

Treatment

In general, high serum concentrations of antibiotics are needed to diffuse into the vegetations, which are avascular and walled off with fibrin and other components. With the correct antibiotics, clinical improvement is usually seen within 5–7 days of therapy. If fever persists for >7 days on antibiotics, evaluation for an abscess or other complication should be considered. Blood cultures should be repeated daily until sterile. Additional blood cultures may be taken 4–6 wks after antibiotic therapy is completed to prove continued bacteremia resolution.

---

*Possible IE is defined by one major criterion and one minor criterion or three minor criteria in the 2000 modified Duke Criteria.

TABLE 5-1. DUKE CRITERIA FOR THE DIAGNOSIS OF INEFECTIVE ENDOCARDITIS (IE)

Major criteria

Positive blood culture

Typical microorganism for IE from two separate blood cultures

Streptococcus viridans, Streptococcus bovis, HACEK group **OR**

Community-acquired *Staphylococcus aureus* or enterococci in the absence of a primary focus

Persistently positive blood culture, from any organism, from

Blood cultures drawn >12 hrs apart **OR**

All of three or a majority of four or more separate blood cultures, with the first and last drawn ≥1 hr apart

Single positive blood culture for *Coxiella burnetii* or antiphase IgG antibody titer >1:800

Evidence of endocardial involvement through positive echocardiogram findings [transesophageal echocardiography recommended in patients with prosthetic valves, rated at least "possible IE" by clinical criteria, or complicated IE (paravalvular abscess); TTE as first test in other patients]

Oscillating intracardiac mass on valve or supporting structures, in the path of regurgitant jets, or on implanted materials, in the absence of alternative explanation **OR**

Abscess **OR**

New partial dehiscence of a prosthetic valve or new valvular regurgitation (not just an increase or change in a preexisting murmur)

Minor criteria

Predisposing heart condition or history of IV drug use

Documented fever ≥38°C (100.4°F)

Evidence of vascular phenomena: arterial embolism, septic pulmonary infarcts, mycotic aneurysm, intracranial hemorrhage, Janeway lesions

Immunologic phenomena: Osler's nodes, Roth's spots, glomerulonephritis, rheumatoid factor

Echocardiogram findings consistent with IE but not meeting major criteria (eliminated from modified Duke criteria)

Positive blood culture but not meeting major criteria or serologic evidence of active infection with a common IE organism

Adapted from Durack DT, Lukes AS, Bright DK. New criteria for diagnosis of infective endocarditis: utilization of specific echocardiographic findings. Duke Endocarditis Service. *Am J Med* 1994;96:200–209; and Li JS, Sexton DJ, Mick N, et al. Proposed modifications to the Duke Criteria for the Diagnosis of Infective Endocarditis. *Clin Infect Dis* 2000;30:633–638.

Empiric Therapy and Blood Culture–Negative Endocarditis

Antibiotics should be initiated empirically for acute IE after blood cultures are obtained. Coverage for *S. aureus* and gram-negatives is the target of therapy. Oxacillin (Bactocill, Prostaphlin), 2 g IV q4h, plus gentamicin (Garamycin), 1.5 mg/kg IV q8h, is the recommended regimen. Vancomycin (Vancocin) should be substituted for oxacillin if the patient is at high risk for resistance (e.g., nosocomial infections, nursing home residents, prosthetic valves, or IV drug use).

If no prior antibiotics have been given, blood cultures should be positive in >90% of patients with IE. Empiric therapy for SBE should be held if the patient is not toxic until initial culture results return. Cultures may remain negative for fastidious organisms such as the HACEK group, nutritionally variant streptococci (*Abiotrophia* species), or rare pathogens (e.g., *Bartonella*, *Coxiella*, or *Brucella*). If this is the case, empiric therapy to cover these can consist of ceftriaxone (Rocephin) or another third-generation cephalosporin plus gentamicin for 4–6 wks. Vancomycin can be added if there is a remaining suspicion for staphylococci.

Specific Therapies

- *S. viridans* and *Streptococcus bovis*: PCN G, 2 million units IV q4h for 4 wks, is used if the minimal inhibitory concentration (MIC) is <0.1 g/mL. If the MIC is ≥0.1 g/mL but is <0.5 g/mL, gentamicin, 1 mg/kg IV q8h, can be added for the first 2 wks of therapy. Vancomycin, 15 mg/kg IV q12h, is an alternative for those with PCN allergies.
- Group A beta-hemolytic *Streptococcus* and *Streptococcus pneumoniae*: PCN G, 2–4 million units IV q4h for 4–6 wks.
- Group B *Streptococcus*: *Streptococcus agalactiae* is the most common and can be present in the normal mouth, vaginal, and anterior urethral flora. Therapy is the same as for group A *Streptococcus*.
- Nutritionally variant *Streptococcus*: PCN G, 3–4 million units IV q4h, plus gentamicin, 1 mg/kg IV q8h, both for 4–6 wks.
- *Enterococcus*: Isolates must be evaluated for vancomycin and aminoglycoside resistance and MIC to PCN and vancomycin calculated. For PCN-sensitive *Enterococcus*, ampicillin, 2 g IV q4h, or PCN G, 3–5 million units IV q4h, plus gentamicin, 1.0–1.5 mg/kg IV q8h for 4–6 wks, is recommended. Vancomycin plus gentamicin can be substituted for those with PCN allergy or to treat beta-lactamase–producing strains.
- *S. aureus*: Oxacillin-sensitive organisms can be treated with oxacillin, 2 g IV q4h for 6 wks, with consideration of adding an aminoglycoside for the first 3–5 days of therapy to obtain a synergistic effect initially. Cefazolin may be a substitute for a nonimmediate PCN allergy. For cases of IV drug abusers with right-sided IE and no complications, a short 2-wk course of therapy consisting of both oxacillin and an aminoglycoside can be attempted, but it is suggested that if fever lasts for >5 days, standard therapy should be pursued. Oxacillin-resistant staphylococci should be treated with vancomycin, 1 g IV q12h for 4–6 wks.
- Coagulase-negative *Staphylococcus*: These infections are typically indolent and are more common after cardiac surgery. Therapy consists of vancomycin, 1 g IV 12h, and rifampin, 300 mg PO q8h for 4–6 wks, plus gentamicin, 1 mg/kg IV q8h for the initial 2 wks.
- HACEK group: These organisms are fastidious and slow-growing gram-negatives. The drug of choice is ceftriaxone, 2 g IV qd for 4 wks.
- *Escherichia coli* or *Proteus* species: These are uncommon pathogens but, if present, can be treated with ampicillin, 2 g IV q4h for 4 wks, or a broad-spectrum cephalosporin, plus gentamicin for the initial 2 wks.
- *Klebsiella* species: Similar to *E. coli* therapy, a third-generation cephalosporin with gentamicin for the initial 2 wks is adequate therapy.
- *Pseudomonas aeruginosa*: This pathogen appears most commonly with IV drug abusers. If the vegetations are right-sided, piperacillin (total of 18 g/day) or ceftazidime, plus tobramycin 5–8 mg/kg/day divided q8h, is required. Left-heart lesions almost always require surgery in addition to the above therapy.
- Anaerobes: IE secondary to anaerobic bacteria is rare. Treatment can consist of a combination of metronidazole (Flagyl) and a broad-spectrum PCN such as piperacillin, or imipenem.
- *Gonococcus* and *Meningococcus*: These are also rare causes of IE. PCN, 20 million units IV qd or a third-generation cephalosporin can be used for 4 wks.
- Fungal IE: Fungal IE is seen with IV drug abuse, with use of long-term IV catheters, in immunocompromised patients, and with prosthetic valves. It can present with negative blood cultures, bulky vegetations, and high frequency of emboli. Amphotericin B is the required medical therapy, and surgical intervention is almost always needed to fully eradicate the infection. Usually, 1–2 wks of amphotericin B is given before surgery, followed by 6–8 wks of postoperative treatment. Surgery should not be withheld to get adequate antibiotics on board, however, if the patient is decompensating.

Complications of Infective Endocarditis

CHF

The development of heart failure is the best predictor of prognosis, correlating with poor outcome for both surgery and medical treatment alone. A surgeon should be aware of the case early after diagnosis of IE. The decision to operate is based on the CHF class of the patient. It is better to take a patient with mild CHF to surgery earlier than to wait until full decompensation occurs.

Peripheral Emboli

The risk of developing emboli with IE is 22–50%, and it increases with larger size of vegetations, especially with streptococcal endocarditis. As many as 65% of cases involve the CNS, and a high mortality is involved if the middle cerebral artery is affected. Most emboli occur in the first 4 wks of antibiotic therapy.

Periannular Extension

Spread of infection from the valve can cause abscesses, fistulous tracts, shunts, or even heart block if extending from the aortic valve. The risk is greatest with prosthetic valves. TEE is needed to evaluate the area carefully if suspected. Almost all of these cases require surgery.

Splenic Abscess

Splenic abscesses are rare, with splenic infarction being much more common. Most often, *S. viridans* or *S. aureus* is the causative organism. Persistent bacteremia, fever, or outright sepsis may occur on antibiotics. If suspected, CT or MRI is the test of choice for evaluation. Splenectomy is the definitive therapy, and it should be done before valve replacement if needed.

Mycotic Aneurysms

Mycotic aneurysms are uncommon but are associated with high mortality, especially if located intracranially. Routine screening for these is not indicated unless symptoms are present, such as mental status changes, seizures, or headache. A contrast-enhanced head CT should be used for initial evaluation, and then angiogram of the cerebral arteries is the test of choice for further study (magnetic resonance angiography may also be considered). If the aneurysm is located distally to the first bifurcation of a major artery, the patient should be monitored with serial angiograms and taken to surgery if the aneurysm bleeds or enlarges. Multiple aneurysms and more proximal ones are managed in the same way. Some can resolve with antibiotics alone. Extracranial aneurysms often are asymptomatic until they rupture. Surgery is needed for cure. They should be suspected in any patient with suspicious signs (e.g., hematochezia, pulsatile mass).

PROSTHETIC VALVE ENDOCARDITIS

IE involving prosthetic valves is potentially more serious and has a greater risk for complications than native valve IE. The largest risk of developing prosthetic valve endocarditis (PVE) is in the initial 6- to 12-mo period postsurgery. The risk after this becomes approximately 0.4% per year, which is greater than that of the normal population.

There does not appear to be a difference in rates of PVE between aortic and mitral valve replacements. There also is no increased risk associated with the type of valve in place (mechanical or bioprosthesis). The development of PVE does appear to be greater for those valves replaced initially due to native valve endocarditis complications.

Pathophysiology

A newly replaced valve is not endothelialized, which puts it at greater risk for developing a sterile platelet fibrin thrombus. This gives bacteria a place to attach, as discussed in the section Native Valve Infective Endocarditis. Older valves become endothelialized, but the repetitive stress and aging of the valve also allow platelets to aggregate in the area.

PVE is classified into two categories. Early PVE, which occurs <2 mos from the initial valve replacement, is usually due to intraop contamination or nosocomial infections through catheters or other sources of bacteremia. Late PVE, which occurs >2 mos from cardiac surgery, is usually acquired in the community with more common endocarditis-causing organisms.

The most common organisms by far in early PVE are coagulase-negative staphylococci and *S. aureus* (with a high incidence of oxacillin resistance). Other pathogens, such as enterococci, gram-negative bacilli, diphtheroids, and fungi, including *Candida albicans*, are also seen but at a much lower frequency. As time passes from the initial cardiac surgery, more usual endocarditis organisms are most commonly seen in late PVE, including *S. viridans* and the HACEK group.

Infection of prosthetic valves often extends to the annulus and even the myocardium. Abscess, pericarditis, and functional obstruction of the valve with large vegetation are more common with PVE than native valve infection.

Clinical Manifestations

There must be a high index of suspicion for PVE in the post–valve replacement patient who continues to be febrile. The initial presentation may be indolent or fulminant to the point of sepsis or heart failure. The same physical findings found in native valve endocarditis may be present, including skin and autoimmune changes. A higher incidence of complications, such as peripheral emboli and mycotic aneurysms, may lead to one of these as the initial presenting symptom.

Diagnosis

The diagnostic evaluation is almost identical to the native valve workup (see Infective Endocarditis: Diagnosis). Blood cultures should be obtained initially and are positive in >90%. Anemia, leukocytosis, hematuria, and an elevated ESR may be present. New heart block or changes in the conduction system on ECG may indicate a septal abscess when dealing with aortic valve PVE.

The Duke Criteria (see Table 5-1) also apply to PVE and may be used in the diagnosis. TEE, rather than TTE, should be used as the initial study to evaluate the valve fully in all patients suspected of PVE. TEE is superior in defining pathology and dysfunction of prosthetic valves before surgery. If the initial study is nondiagnostic for vegetations and the suspicion for PVE is high, TEE should be repeated several days later for additional evaluation.

Treatment

All patients need to be hospitalized for initial treatment. If the symptomatology is mild and the patient does not appear toxic, antibiotics should be held until initial culture results are obtained because it is imperative to isolate the specific pathogen. Overall, IV antibiotic therapy is continued ≥6 wks for adequate treatment.

Empiric Therapy

Empiric treatment may be initiated after at least three sets of blood cultures have been obtained. The recommended short-term regimen consists of vancomycin and gentamicin, with the addition of a third-generation cephalosporin if other organisms such as the HACEK group are suspected. Culture results should be used to quickly tailor the regimen to the appropriate coverage.

Specific Therapies

- *Streptococcus*: PCN G, 18–24 million units IV/day divided into q4h for 6 wks, plus gentamicin, 1 mg/kg IV q8h for the initial 2 wks. If the MIC >0.1 μg/mL for PCN, gentamicin can be continued for 4–6 wks. Ceftriaxone, 2 g IV qd, or vancomycin, 15 mg/kg IV q12h, can be substituted for those with PCN allergy or high resistance to PCN.

- *Enterococcus*: Ampicillin, 2 g IV q4h, or vancomycin, 15 mg/kg IV q12h (for PCN resistance), plus gentamicin, 1 mg/kg IV q8h—all for 6 wks. If an aminoglycoside is contraindicated, the ampicillin or vancomycin should be extended for 8–12 wks.
- *Staphylococcus*: Associated with a very high mortality rate.
  - Oxacillin-sensitive *S. aureus*: Nafcillin (Nafcil) or oxacillin, 2 g IV q4h for 6–8 wks, plus gentamicin, 1 mg/kg IV q8h for 2 wks, plus rifampin, 300 mg PO q8h for 6–8 wks.
  - Oxacillin-resistant *S. aureus* or coagulase-negative *Staphylococcus*: Vancomycin, 15 mg/kg IV q12h for 6–8 wks, plus gentamicin, 1 mg/kg IV q8h for 2 wks, plus rifampin, 300 mg PO q8h for 6–8 wks.
  - Rifampin should be started only after two other agents have been initiated or one other antibiotic has been on board for ≥3–5 days due to the rapidity of selection for rifampin-resistant strains.
  - A fluoroquinolone may be substituted if an aminoglycoside is absolutely contraindicated.
- Diphtheroids: PCN G, 18–24 million units IV/day divided q4h, plus gentamicin, 1 mg/kg IV q8h for synergistic bactericidal effect—both for 6 wks. If the MIC for PCN is >4 μg/mL, vancomycin only should be used instead.
- HACEK group: ceftriaxone, 2 g IV qd for 6 wks, is the regimen of choice. If the organism does not produce beta-lactamase, ampicillin, 500 mg IV q4h, plus gentamicin, 1 mg/kg IV q8h, may be substituted. Most of these infections do not require valve surgery.
- *Pseudomonas* species: The preferred antibiotics are an antipseudomonal PCN [ticarcillin (Ticar) or piperacillin] plus tobramycin (total of 8 mg/kg/day). The peak serum concentration desired for tobramycin is 15 μg/mL.
- Fungal: More commonly seen now with more cardiac surgeries. The consensus is that all patients require surgery after initiating an antifungal agent, ideally for 1–2 wks prior. The drug of choice is amphotericin B, 0.7 mg/kg/day for candidal infections and up to 1 mg/kg/day for *Aspergillus* and *Mucor*. A total dose of 2 g of amphotericin is the goal. Because of the difficulty in eradicating fungal infections, some patients have been maintained on a prophylactic dose of fluconazole, 200–400 mg PO qd postoperatively for further protection.

Blood cultures should be obtained daily until bacteremia has cleared. Follow-up cultures should be taken 2–8 wks after completion of antibiotics. Serum concentrations of aminoglycosides and vancomycin need to be followed throughout treatment, along with serum creatinine. A weekly CBC should be obtained for patients on beta-lactams.

Indications for Surgery

There are a number of indications for surgical intervention with PVE, but in general, a surgeon should be aware of all patients so he or she is ready if the need for emergent surgery arises. Valve replacement should be pursued if (a) moderate or severe CHF is present; (b) the prosthetic valve is unstable or the infection has extended past the valve; (c) bacteremia persists despite antibiotics, or there is a relapse after treatment is completed; (d) vegetations are >10 mm; (e) blood cultures remain negative, but fever persists ≥10 days on antibiotics; or (f) the PVE is caused by any fungus, *Pseudomonas*, *S. aureus*, most *Enterococcus* species, or any other bacteria that normally require surgical repair with native valve IE. Surgery can usually be avoided if the patient is >12 mos out from initial valve replacement and the pathogen is documented as *S. viridans*, HACEK group, or enterococci. Postoperatively, antibiotics should be continued for a full 6-wk course in addition to preoperative treatment if the adjacent tissues to the valve are culture positive. If the infection seems to be confined to the prosthetic valve, the total preoperative and postoperative course of antibiotics is additive.

PROPHYLACTIC RECOMMENDATIONS FOR INFECTIVE ENDOCARDITIS

The American Heart Association published guidelines in 1997 for physicians to help protect patients with preexisting cardiac conditions from the risk of IE after potential bacteremia-causing procedures. There are no randomized, controlled trials involving humans to definitively support the guidelines, but the recommendations are based on evaluation from available data and are well accepted. In general, the patient's clinical condition should guide the approach to prophylaxis. The following is a summary of the guidelines.

Patients for Whom Prophylaxis Is Recommended

High-Risk Patients for Development of Infective Endocarditis

- Patients with prosthetic valves
- History of endocarditis
- Complex cyanotic congenital heart disease (e.g., tetralogy of Fallot, transposition of the great vessels)
- Surgically constructed systemic pulmonary shunts or conduits

Moderate-Risk Patients for Development of Infective Endocarditis

- Other uncorrected congenital malformations: patent ductus arteriosus, VSD, primum atrial septal defect, coarctation of the aorta, and bicuspid aortic valve
- Acquired valvular disease
- Hypertrophic cardiomyopathy
- Mitral valve prolapse only with valvular regurgitation or thickened leaflets (demonstrated by murmur of mitral regurgitation or echocardiographic evidence)

Procedures for Which Prophylaxis Is Recommended

In general, invasive surgical procedures or other procedures such as cardiac catheterizations or angioplasty in which aseptic technique is used do not need prior prophylactic antibiotics. This includes pacemaker or defibrillator placements, surgical biopsies, and cesarean section.

Dental Procedures

- Extractions
- Periodontal and endodontal (root canal) work
- Dental implants
- Initial placement of orthodontic bands
- Intraligamentary local anesthetic injections
- Prophylactic teeth cleaning

Respiratory Procedures

- Tonsillectomy/adenoidectomy
- Other surgical operations with the respiratory mucosa
- Bronchoscopy with a rigid bronchoscope (not flexible scopes; although if biopsy is to be taken, one may choose to give prophylaxis to high-risk patients)

GI Procedures

Prophylaxis is recommended for high-risk patients and is optional for moderate-risk patients.

- Sclerotherapy for esophageal varices
- Esophageal stricture dilation
- ERCP with biliary obstruction
- Biliary tract surgery
- Surgical operations involving intestinal mucosa
- High-risk patients: prophylaxis with TEE or endoscopy with biopsy

Genitourinary Procedures

- Prostatic surgery
- Cystoscopy
- Urethral dilation
- Vaginal hysterectomy and vaginal delivery considered only for high-risk patients

Prophylactic Regimens

Dental, Oral, Respiratory, or Esophageal Procedures

S. viridans (alpha-hemolytic *Streptococcus*) species are the most common organisms present as part of the oropharyngeal flora that cause IE. Prophylaxis is targeted at these. Amoxicillin, 2 g PO in adults and 50 mg/kg in children, is recommended 1 hr before the procedure. Clindamycin (Cleocin), 600 mg; azithromycin, 500 mg; or cephalexin, 2 g, are alternatives for PCN allergy. If the patient is unable to take oral medications, ampicillin, 2 g IV or IM, is recommended 30 mins before the procedure onset. No postprocedure dose of antibiotics is needed.

Genitourinary Procedures

Enterococcus faecalis is the most common organism after genitourinary manipulation to cause IE. Gram-negative bacilli are rare causes overall of endocarditis, making them less worrisome. Antibiotic prophylaxis is targeted at enterococci.

HIGH-RISK PATIENTS. Ampicillin, 2 g IV or IM, plus gentamicin, 1.5 mg/kg IV, given 30 mins before the start of the procedure and 6 hrs later; ampicillin, 1 g IV/IM, or amoxicillin, 1 g PO, is recommended for adults. If allergy to ampicillin exists, vancomycin, 1 g IV, plus gentamicin is an acceptable substitute. Children should be given ampicillin, 50 mg/kg, plus gentamicin, 1.5 mg/kg, initially and ampicillin, 25 mg/kg, or amoxicillin, 25 mg/kg PO, after the procedure.

MODERATE-RISK PATIENTS. Amoxicillin, 2 g PO 1 hr before the procedure, or ampicillin, 2 g IV/IM 30 mins before, for adults. Children receive amoxicillin, 50 mg/kg PO, or ampicillin, 50 mg/kg IV/IM, with the same time parameters. Again, vancomycin can be given for ampicillin allergies. No postprocedure doses are necessary with moderate-risk patients.

Cardiac Surgery

Periop antibiotics are recommended for prophylaxis against endocarditis, particularly with regard to staphylococci. First-generation cephalosporins or vancomycin, if a high rate of oxacillin resistance is present, are usually the antibiotics of choice. There is no evidence that coronary artery bypass graft surgery increases the risk for later endocarditis. Prosthetic valve surgery places patients in the high-risk category. Cardiac transplant patients are usually considered moderate risk.

MYOCARDITIS

Myocarditis is an acute infectious, autoimmune, or toxic process that affects the myocytes of the heart. The spectrum of illness ranges from asymptomatic cases to sudden death. In fact, myocarditis is one of the major causes of unexpected deaths in people <40 yrs. The diagnosis should be considered in anyone who has sudden onset of heart failure or arrhythmias in the setting of a febrile illness.

Pathophysiology

There are several different mechanisms by which the myocardium may be affected by inciting factors. The process may have a direct cytotoxic effect on the myocytes, there may be a secondary immune response, cytokines such as tumor necrosis factor may be expressed in the myocardium, or the causal agent may trigger abnormal apoptosis. Most causes of myocarditis are never identified. Most of these are likely viral in origin. Enteroviruses, especially coxsackie B virus, are the most widely seen viral cause, although there have been documented cases of almost any virus as the probable culprit. Bacterial myocarditis is rare and almost always is associated with extension of endocarditis. There have been some reports of chronic myocarditis being caused by *Chlamydia* species and *Mycoplasma*. Other noninfectious etiologies of myocarditis include pharmacologic drugs such as doxorubicin (Adriamycin), illicit drugs such as cocaine, autoimmune diseases, peripartum cardiomyopathy, and possible allergic origin with eosinophilic infiltration.

Classic Infectious Causes of Myocarditis

- Chagas' disease: This is the most common cause of myocarditis worldwide, endemic to Central and South America. The protozoan *Trypanosoma cruzi* can acutely be seen within the myocytes of infected patients. Only 1% of infections result in acute myocarditis, but 20% result in chronic heart failure from constrictive myopathy.

- Lyme disease: Up to 10% of acute infections with *Borrelia burgdorferi* can present with myocardial involvement. Classically, patients develop atrioventricular nodal abnormalities that may lead to syncope and left ventricular dysfunction. Most patients recover fully.
- Diphtheric myocarditis: This is the most common cause of death related to diphtheria infection. The myocardial inflammation is toxin mediated and not due to direct invasion by the organisms. Antitoxin must be initiated immediately to improve survival.

Clinical Manifestations

There is a broad spectrum of possible symptoms that may be associated with myocarditis, ranging from no symptoms to fulminant heart failure or death. A high index of suspicion is always necessary to make the diagnosis. Often, a history of upper respiratory symptoms or GI symptoms (e.g., cough, malaise, nausea, vomiting) a few weeks before onset is given, suggesting a possible viral cause. Fatigue, fever, and arthralgias may accompany heart failure symptoms or may be the only presenting features. Recent travel to Latin America or areas endemic for Lyme disease or a history of HIV may raise suspicion for this diagnosis.

Differential Diagnosis

In older adults with pulmonary edema, lower extremity edema, and orthopnea, heart failure due to other causes (e.g., coronary artery disease or valvular problems) is far more likely than myocarditis, but they all must be kept in the differential. It is easier to think of a myocarditis in younger patients with the same symptoms. Other causes of a generalized cardiomyopathy must also be ruled out, including alcohol use or other drug use and thyroid disease.

Diagnosis

Physical exam may show evidence of heart failure with crackles in the lung fields, jugular venous distention, or other signs of fluid overload. The ECG should give the tip-off that the myocardium is involved with supraventricular tachycardia, ectopy, ventricular arrhythmias, heart block, or myocardial infarction similarities. If myocarditis is suspected, a two-dimensional echocardiogram should be obtained in all patients to assess the extent of cardiac compromise. Chest x-rays may be normal or show evidence of cardiomegaly, pulmonary edema, or pleural effusions.

In the lab evaluation, a CBC may or may not show leukocytosis. The cardiac enzymes CK-MB and troponin I may be elevated as nonspecific indicators for myocyte necrosis. These are highest early on and may be normal at 1 wk into the course of the illness. An ANA titer, ESR, eosinophil count, and other rheumatologic tests may be indicated if the etiology is not obviously viral by the history. As far as making the exact viral diagnosis, serial antibody titers documenting a fall in the convalescent stage can be used, as well as viral serum PCR, but usually the exact virus is never isolated in this way. It is more helpful to culture from areas that may have been the initial site of the infection, such as the stool, throat, or nose.

The gold standard of making the diagnosis of myocarditis is by endomyocardial biopsy, but this procedure is rarely indicated today. In general, the Dallas Criteria, which classify histologic criteria, have low sensitivity and specificity when looking at only one small biopsied area of myocardium. Studies such as MRI and antimyosin scintigraphy are falling into favor now if the diagnosis is not obvious by two-dimensional echocardiography.

Treatment

Supportive care with bed rest is the first line of therapy. Diuretics, afterload-reducing medications, and possibly inotropes may be needed short term for heart failure management. Based on a few randomized clinical trials, there is no evidence to support routine use of corticosteroid therapy in patients with myocarditis, although it has been used with discretion when a high suspicion for an autoimmune cause is present. Antiviral drugs are also not helpful currently, with the exception of ganciclovir for CMV infection.

INFECTIOUS PERICARDITIS

Inflammation of the pericardium can be classified into several different types of clinical syndromes: acute, relapsing, tamponade, chronic, or constrictive. Most infectious etiologies have an acute presentation.

Pathophysiology

The possible causes of pericarditis are very broad. Idiopathic and viral etiologies are the most common, and they are usually the same enteroviruses that cause myocarditis. Bacterial sources are more common than with myocarditis but still are rare. They are usually extensions from head and neck infections, mediastinitis, and postoperative infections, or they can be hematogenously contracted. Meningococcemia can cause pericarditis either by direct bacterial invasion or through a reactive immune process. Primary pulmonary infection with *Mycobacterium tuberculosis* can progress to constrictive pericarditis in up to 1% of cases. Fungal causes are also rare but can result from disseminated histoplasmosis, coccidioidomycosis, or even candidiasis in the neutropenic patient. Often, the pericardial reaction is sterile in these cases and not the result of a direct seeding of the pericardium. The most common risk factor for fungal pericarditis is prior cardiothoracic surgery. HIV can cause pericarditis, but most often there is a secondary infection.

Clinical Manifestations

The classic symptom is **chest pain** that is *worsened by inspiration* and *relieved by leaning forward*. The patient may be short of breath if there is a large pericardial effusion present. Fever and tachycardia are usually evident. Specific symptoms, such as weight loss or night sweats, are important if the patient is at high risk for TB.

Differential Diagnosis

There are many alternative causes for pericarditis in addition to infectious etiologies. Neoplastic invasion or post-radiation or post-chemotherapy pericarditis are a consideration in the oncologic patient. Other infiltrative processes such as amyloidosis are common. Autoimmune disorders such as SLE can present with pericarditis and fever. Pneumonia, pulmonary embolism, and cardiac ischemia are nonpericardial problems in the differential.

Diagnosis

The physical exam may not be helpful unless there is a large effusion present in which signs of tamponade may be elicited (e.g., jugular venous distention, pulsus paradoxus). A friction rub on cardiac exam often waxes and wanes. The ECG may be most useful in making the diagnosis. Diffuse ST-segment elevation is the classic finding. A two-dimensional echocardiogram is usually indicated to rule out tamponade and to evaluate left ventricular function for associated myocarditis.

If a large effusion is present and drainage is required, *all* the fluid should be removed and sent for evaluation. AFB stain of the spun sediment should be ordered. PPDs are often negative in these patients. Viral isolation can be attempted through stool, nasal, or throat swabs, but as with myocarditis, antibody titers are often low yield.

Treatment

The main therapy for pericarditis is symptomatic with bed rest. NSAIDs can be used for pain. As with myocarditis, corticosteroid therapy should be avoided. The presence of a pericardial effusion is *not* an indication for drainage if the patient is hemodynamically stable. If hemodynamics become compromised or the effusion and symptoms remain present for >3 wks, drainage must be considered. In these situations, pericardiotomy with biopsy and drainage is much better than pericardiocentesis alone, with diagnosis rates of 55% and 20–25%, respectively. Because bacterial pericarditis is rare, empiric antibiotics are not necessary in all cases unless there is a clinical suspicion of bacterial seeding. If purulent pericarditis is suspected, in all cases surgical drainage should be pursued and a long course of appropriate antibiotics initiated.

MEDIASTINITIS: ACUTE AND SCLEROSING

The mediastinum is divided into four different compartments anatomically. Infection of any of these regions is most often acute and usually is a postoperative median sternotomy complication, although infection may also spread from the head and neck or may be secondary to esophageal perforation. A chronic form of mediastinitis also exists and is discussed later.

Acute Mediastinitis

Pathophysiology
Causes of **acute mediastinitis** include

- Anterior mediastinum: postoperative sternal infections
- Middle mediastinum: esophageal rupture, trachea or main bronchi rupture, extension of cervical infection, anthrax mediastinitis
- Posterior mediastinum: paravertebral abscess, tuberculous spondylitis

Cardiothoracic surgery by far promotes the most risk for mediastinitis, with an incidence of 0.4–2.4% postoperatively. The risk increases dramatically in post–cardiac transplant patients and those with an indwelling foreign body, such as a left ventricular assist device. The preoperative risk factors for mediastinitis are many and include diabetes mellitus, obesity, prior sternotomy, prolonged cardiopulmonary bypass, reexploration for bleeding, use of bilateral internal mammary arteries (it is believed that this decreases the blood supply to the sternum), and prolonged ICU stays.

For cases involving esophageal rupture, iatrogenic perforation during procedures is most common. Boerhaave's syndrome, esophageal malignancy, foreign bodies, or trauma may also result in tearing of the esophageal tissues. Extension from odontogenic or pharyngeal infections is rare. Ludwig's angina is mediastinitis resulting most often from an infection of the third mandibular molar tooth.

Postoperative infections are caused by gram-positive cocci >60% of the time, with *Staphylococcus epidermidis* the most common pathogen. Gram-negative bacilli and *Candida* are less common but are seen as well. The majority of head and neck infections and esophageal perforation–related mediastinitis cases are polymicrobial, usually with gram-negative bacilli and anaerobes. *S. viridans*, *Peptococcus*, *Peptostreptococcus*, *Bacteroides* species, and *Fusobacterium* species are the most common culprits.

Clinical Manifestations
Postoperatively, patients may complain of out-of-proportion chest pain that may be pleuritic or radiate to the neck. They also may describe dyspnea or dysphagia. All of these are usually accompanied by fever. Mediastinitis stemming from oral infections is usually self-evident, with severe throat pain, for instance, being the presenting symptom.

Differential Diagnosis
Any syndrome that may cause chest pain is in the differential diagnosis for mediastinitis, including gastroesophageal reflux disease and anginal pain, especially in those patients who are postoperative from cardiac surgery. Musculoskeletal pain such as costochondritis is also a possibility, but this is less likely, especially if there are fever and other signs of infection involved. Pericarditis, pneumonia, and osteomyelitis are other potential infections that may present like mediastinitis.

Diagnosis

Physical exam may reveal fever, tachycardia, crepitus, and edema over the sternal area. Hamman's sign is a crunching sound heard in synchrony with the cardiac rhythm. A chest x-ray is very helpful in looking for mediastinal widening, air–fluid levels, and subcutaneous emphysema. It is very important to look at a lateral film for superior mediastinal gas that may be missed on an anteroposterior film. If an esophageal perforation is suspected, a water-soluble contrast study should be ordered to look for extravasation into the surrounding tissues (**do not use barium**). Blood cultures should be drawn on all expected cases, preferably before antibiotics are given.

Postoperative mediastinitis is most often recognized by purulent drainage and erythema around the surgical wound. The sternum may become unstable. Plain films are less helpful here because there is often postoperative air evident that can be a normal finding. In these cases and all others in which the diagnosis is in question, a CT of the chest should be obtained.

Treatment

Postoperative mediastinitis most often requires sternal débridement, with rewiring and often surgical flaps to eradicate infection. Early closure of the surgical wounds is the key to decreasing morbidity and mortality in these patients. Antibiotics should cover staphylococci and gram-negatives empirically until cultures return. Vancomycin, 1 g IV q12h, and cefepime, 1 g IV q12h, or another extended-spectrum beta-lactam are good choices. The duration of therapy is debatable but at minimum should be 4–6 wks.

Esophageal perforations usually need surgical drainage and débridement. Antibiotic coverage should include anaerobic coverage in addition to gram-positives and aerobic gram-negatives, usually with metronidazole, clindamycin, imipenem, or a broad-spectrum beta-lactam (e.g., piperacillin). Anaerobic coverage should continue for the entire course of therapy even if cultures do not reveal any anaerobic organisms due to their difficulty to be grown in culture. *Candida* coverage (i.e., fluconazole) should also be strongly considered.

Complications of mediastinitis include pericardial effusions, tamponade, and sternal osteomyelitis. Delayed diagnosis leads to worsened outcomes, so always think of mediastinitis in your differential diagnosis of infection in the postoperative patient!

Sclerosing Mediastinitis

Chronic mediastinitis is known as *sclerosing* or *fibrosing,* and it is an invasive inflammatory infiltrate in the mediastinum, usually believed to be caused by granulomatous disease. *Histoplasma capsulatum* is the most common etiology, although TB, actinomyces, nocardia, blastomycosis, coccidioidomycosis, sarcoidosis, and silicosis have all been implicated. It is the most common cause of a nonmalignant mediastinal mass, usually found incidentally.

40% of patients are asymptomatic. Symptoms can range from chronic cough, dyspnea, wheezing, and hemoptysis to full pulmonary HTN and cor pulmonale. Fibrosing mediastinitis is also the most common cause of nonmalignant superior vena cava syndrome. The diagnosis is made by pathologic evaluation, usually by biopsy. Antibiotics, including antifungals, and corticosteroids are usually not indicated at the time of diagnosis because there is no active disease process present anymore. Surgery may be an option to clear scar tissue if the patient is extremely symptomatic.

CARDIAC PACEMAKER INFECTIONS

Infection may occur in the pocket around a pacemaker generator, which is the most common infection involving pacemakers. More rarely, infection may also involve the wires of the pacemaker. This is usually an extension from a pocket infection and often results in an endocarditis. Most of these present >6 wks out from pacemaker insertion. If the infection extends to the epicardial electrodes, pericarditis, mediastinitis, or even sepsis may occur.

Differential Diagnosis

The differential diagnosis is small, with infections of the cardiovascular system from an alternate source being the main discernment. Evidence of endocarditis, pericarditis, and mediastinitis should be ruled out. Bacteremia being shed from another part of the body may infect the pocket secondarily.

Pathophysiology

The pathogens most often responsible for pacemaker infections are *S. aureus* and coagulase-negative *Staphylococcus*. These are the usual skin organisms that infect the area at the time of insertion or shortly after while the wound is still healing. *S. aureus* usually presents within 2 wks of pacemaker insertion as a pocket infection. Other organisms, such as Enterobacteriaceae and even *Candida*, may also be seen but less often.

Clinical Manifestations

Fever and chills are the most common complaints. The patient may also notice redness, tenderness, swelling, or possibly drainage from the pocket area. Pulmonary symptoms, such as cough or purulent sputum suggesting a pneumonia or abscess, may occur in more advanced infections, particularly if the lung is seeded.

Diagnosis

Physical exam should include a careful inspection of the surgical wound site, looking for purulent drainage or fluctuance. Signs of endocarditis should be pursued. The majority of patients have a leukocytosis and an elevated ESR and CRP. Blood cultures should be obtained before antibiotics. If the patient continues to have persistent bacteremia or other signs of ongoing infection, a TEE should be pursued to rule out vegetations on the electrodes.

Treatment

In general, the two possible types of infections have different modes of treatment. Infection limited to the pocket can be treated by inserting a new pacemaker at an uninfected site while on appropriate antibiotics and then immediately removing the old generator. The infected pocket is left open for local wound management.

The consensus on pacemaker endocarditis is to remove the infected generator and electrodes and place the patient on a temporary pacing device while undergoing a minimum of 2 wks of appropriate endocarditis regimen antibiotics. Blood cultures after this time must be negative before a new pacemaker is inserted. It is then usually recommended that a full endocarditis regimen be completed starting when the new device is in place.

INFECTIONS OF IMPLANTABLE CARDIOVERTER-DEFIBRILLATORS

The incidence of infection with the transvenous implantable devices is small, approximately 0.8–1.5%. Most of these occur within 6 mos of the initial implantation.

Pathophysiology

Coagulase-negative *Staphylococcus* and *S. aureus* are the most common pathogens, likely from skin contamination around the time of the placement of the device. There are a good number of cases that are polymicrobial in origin as well, so a culture revealing more than one organism should be taken seriously.

Clinical Manifestations

Most commonly, patients describe pain and redness around the site of the device. Some may experience drainage from a poorly healed incision or possibly through a fistulous tract. If bacteremic from the infection, fever and chills may be part of the presenting symptoms.

Diagnosis

Confirmation of the infection can be done by culture of any of the fluid surrounding the area, usually obtained by fine-needle aspiration. Blood cultures should be drawn on all patients.

Treatment

Infection in the pocket of the implantable cardioverter-defibrillator usually requires complete removal of the device for total resolution. Antibiotics should cover coagulase-negative *Staphylococcus* and gram-negatives empirically and then should be tailored to the correct pathogens. Reimplantation of a new implantable cardioverter-defibrillator at an uninfected site should be done in ≥7 days or more, if possible, once blood cultures have cleared and the infection is under control.

INTRAVASCULAR GRAFT INFECTIONS

The incidence of infection involving synthetic surgical vascular grafts is <1–5%. Inguinal grafts (e.g., aortofemoral, femoropopliteal) are more prone to infection than aortic or other grafts, but aortic graft infection is associated with a higher mortality rate.

Differential Diagnosis

Wound infections that do not involve the graft must be differentiated from graft involvement. If only constitutional signs are present, other sources of infection must be ruled out before pursuit of the graft material is begun.

Pathophysiology

The most common method of infection is through intraop contamination. A graft may also become infected through contiguous spread from adjacent tissues (e.g., a wound infection) or through hematogenous seeding, even years after placement. *S. aureus* is the primary pathogen. Gram-negatives can be seen as well, especially with aortic grafts adjacent to the bowel. It is important to realize that coagulase-negative *Staphylococcus* infections may present months after the initial placing of the graft.

Clinical Manifestations

Fever and tachycardia are usually present to suggest infection. Abdominal pain or a mass may be evident. The patient may report weight loss, especially if the infection has been indolent for some time. There may be a leak in the skin around the surgical scar, suggesting a cutaneous fistula. All patients with a history of aortic graft who present with melena or rectal bleeding *must* be considered for possible aortoenteric fistula secondary to erosion of the graft into the bowel.

Diagnosis

The physical exam is the most important clue in suspecting an infected graft. A careful wound or scar inspection must be done. Look at the lower extremities for evidence of peripheral emboli.

Blood cultures before administering antibiotics should be obtained on all patients. A CT of the graft area is the test of choice to evaluate for false aneurysms, with U/S being less accurate. Sinography can be used to assess a possible tract if there appears to be a cutaneous fistula.

Treatment

Effective eradication of the infection involves complete resection of the synthetic materials and débridement of the surrounding tissues. A new graft should be inserted through a healthy site. Appropriate antibiotics based on culture evidence should be initiated postoperatively for a 4- to 6-wk course. The arterial stump at the anastomosis with the graft should be cultured as well, and if positive, it is recommended that antibiotics be continued for up to 6 mos.

KEY POINTS TO REMEMBER

- The diagnosis of IE includes blood culture and echocardiographic data.
- When IE is suspected, strongly consider TEE initially, as it has a higher sensitivity than TTE.
- If possible, hardware should be removed and blood cultures found negative before placement (however, this is not always possible).
- Generally, treatment of IE requires a minimum of 6 wks of IV antibiotics.
- Indefinite antibiotic suppression may be required when endovascular infections involve hardware that cannot be completely removed. ID consultation is strongly advised for these cases.
- Guidelines for antibiotic prophylaxis for the prevention of IE can be found at http://americanheart.org.

REFERENCES AND SUGGESTED READINGS

Bayer AS, Bolger AF, Taubert KA, et al. Diagnosis and management of infective endocarditis and its complications (AHA scientific statement). *Circulation* 1998;98:2936–2948.

Bayer AS, Scheld WM. Endocarditis and intravascular infections. In: Mandell GL, Bennett JE, Dolin R, eds. *Mandell, Douglas, and Bennett's principles and practice of infectious diseases*, 5th ed. Philadelphia: Churchill Livingstone, 2000:857–902.

Bone RC, Campbell GD Jr, Payne DK, eds. *Bone's atlas of pulmonary and critical care medicine*. Philadelphia: Lippincott Williams & Wilkins, 1998.

Chua JD, Wilkoff BL, Lee I, et al. Diagnosis and management of infections involving implantable electrophysiologic cardiac devices. *Ann Intern Med* 2000;133:604–608.

Dajani AS, Taubert KA, Wilson W, et al. Prevention of bacterial endocarditis. Recommendations by the American Heart Association. *JAMA* 1997;277:1794–1801.

Durack DT, Lukes AS, Bright DK. New criteria for diagnosis of infective endocarditis: utilization of specific echocardiographic findings. Duke Endocarditis Service. *Am J Med* 1994;96:200–209.

Feldman AM, McNamara D. Myocarditis. *N Engl J Med* 2000;343:1388–1398.

Kamath NV, Warner MR, Camisa C. Infective endocarditis: cutaneous cues to the diagnosis. *Consultant* 1999:3085–3097.

Karchmer AW. Infections of prosthetic valves and intravascular devices. In: Mandell GL, Bennett JE, Dolin R, eds. *Mandell, Douglas, and Bennett's principles and practice of infectious diseases*, 5th ed. Philadelphia: Churchill Livingstone, 2000:903–916.

Li JS, Sexton DJ, Mick N, et al. Proposed modifications to the Duke criteria for the diagnosis of infective endocarditis. *Clin Infect Dis* 2000;30:633–638.

Oakley CM. Myocarditis, pericarditis and other pericardial diseases. *Heart* 2000;84:449–454.

Rupp ME. Mediastinitis. In: Mandell GL, Bennett JE, Dolin R, eds. *Mandell, Douglas, and Bennett's principles and practice of infectious diseases*, 5th ed. Philadelphia: Churchill Livingstone, 1999:941–946.

Savoia MC, Oxman MN. Myocarditis and pericarditis. In: Mandell GL, Bennett JE, Dolin R, eds. *Mandell, Douglas, and Bennett's principles and practice of infectious diseases*, 5th ed. Philadelphia: Churchill Livingstone, 1999.

Wilson WR, Karchmer AW, Dajani AS, et al. Antibiotic treatment of adults with infective endocarditis due to streptococci, enterococci, staphylococci, and HACEK microorganisms: AHA. *JAMA* 1995;274:1706–1713.

Younes A, Johnson D. The spectrum of spontaneous and iatrogenic esophageal injury: perforations, Mallory-Weiss tears, and hematomas. *J Clin Gastroenterol* 1999;29:306–317.

Infections of the Gastrointestinal Tract

Melissa L. Norton

INFECTIONS OF ORAL MUCOSA

Acute Necrotizing Ulcerative Gingivitis

Pathophysiology

Acute necrotizing ulcerative gingivitis is a bacterial infection leading to ulcerative necrosis of the marginal gingivae, which may spread to other oral structures, including the tonsils and pharynx. The infection is believed to begin as aseptic necrosis secondary to mucosal capillary stasis. If untreated, it may cause necrosis of facial structures (cancrum oris, noma). Infections are polymicrobial, usually with anaerobic gram-negative bacteria, but can also have gram-positives and aerobes.

Clinical Manifestations

The infection begins as a painful, red lesion on the gingiva, which may be vesicular, or as the sudden onset of painful gums. There may be bleeding and involvement of the tonsils and pharynx, as well as high fevers, severe pain, and lymphadenopathy. As the infection spreads to deeper tissues, a necrotic ulcer forms with development of cellulitis of the lips and cheeks, which may progress to necrosis or sloughing.

Diagnosis

The diagnosis is made clinically, although cultures may direct therapy. Cultures need to be obtained from débrided materials to avoid contamination with normal oropharyngeal flora.

Differential Diagnosis

In the early stages of infection, the diagnosis may be confused with herpetic ulcers or aphthous ulcers. Behçet's syndrome is also in the differential.

Treatment

Initial therapy with broad-spectrum antibiotics is indicated. Antibiotics are usually given IV but may be given PO if the infection is caught early, before any necrosis develops. PCN, 250,000–400,000 U/kg/day divided PO q4–6h, and metronidazole (Flagyl), 500 mg PO q8h, are the antibiotics of choice for this infection, although a cephalosporin that covers aerobic gram-negatives may be needed as well. Débridement of necrotic tissues is also indicated. Reconstructive surgery may be necessary after the infection is treated.

Herpetic Gingivostomatitis

Herpetic gingivostomatitis infections are caused by HSV-1 and HSV-2, usually HSV-1. The disease can occur in infants, although it usually is a disease of children and adults.

Clinical Manifestations

The disease may be mild to severe, with symptoms that include fever, sore throat, malaise, and lymphadenopathy. Oral lesions consist of vesicles, usually <5 mm in diameter with an erythematous base, which appear 1–2 days after the onset of pain. These lesions are associated with painful red gingiva or palate. Symptoms persist for 2–3 days, although the vesicles may take 1–2 wks to resolve.

Diagnosis
The diagnosis may be made by direct immunofluorescence or viral culture of the ulcers.

Differential Diagnosis
The differential includes herpangina, VZV, and hand-foot-and-mouth disease in children. In adults, aphthous ulcers, Behçet's syndrome, cyclical neutropenia, and erythema multiforme are listed in the differential.

Treatment
Treatment is with acyclovir (Zovirax), 400 mg PO five times a day.

Herpangina

Herpangina is a viral infection caused by coxsackieviruses and echovirus, which produce oropharyngeal vesicles, generally at the junction of the hard and soft palate. The disease primarily affects children.

Clinical Manifestations
The disease is usually mild but can have fever, neck pain, sore throat, and headache. Lesions consist of multiple small white papules on an erythematous base, which usually spontaneously rupture in 2–3 days and seldom persist for >1 wk. Cervical lymphadenopathy is unusual.

Diagnosis
The diagnosis is made by culture of a sterile swab of the vesicles.

Differential Diagnosis
The differential includes HSV, hand-foot-and-mouth disease, and infectious mononucleosis.

Treatment
Therapy consists of symptomatic treatment only. The fever generally lasts up to 4 days, and the lesions generally resolve in 1–2 wks.

Hand-Foot-and-Mouth Disease

Hand-foot-and-mouth disease is a systemic infection by coxsackie A virus (usually serotype 16), which primarily affects children but can rarely affect teens and adults. Herpetic infections (including chickenpox), aphthous ulcers, and Behçet's syndrome) may be included in the differential diagnosis.

Clinical Manifestations
Vesicular eruptions on the hands, wrists, feet, and mouth are the classic presentation. Lesions are present on the hands and in the mouth >90% of time. Oral lesions may be present on the palate, tongue, or buccal mucosa. Associated symptoms may be mild to severe and may include fever, malaise, conjunctival injection, headache, and abdominal pain.

Diagnosis
The diagnosis is usually made clinically but is confirmed by culture of feces or swab of a vesicle.

Differential Diagnosis
The differential includes herpangina, HSV, aphthous stomatitis, Behçet's disease, and malignancy (lymphoma or acute leukemia).

Treatment
Treatment is symptomatic, with the clinical features resolving within 2–4 wks.

Syphilis

Syphilis is an infection by the organism *Treponema pallidum*, usually becoming clinically apparent 3 wks after exposure.

Clinical Manifestations
Primary infection consists of a painless ulcer with indurated margins at the site of exposure. Unilateral lymphadenopathy may occur. Untreated, the ulcer will spontaneously heal in 1–2 mos. Secondary syphilis of the oropharynx results in numerous maculopapular lesions with or without central ulceration. These lesions may be present on mucosal surfaces and on the skin. They may also be accompanied by fever and malaise.

Diagnosis
Primary syphilis is usually seronegative, so darkfield microscopy of the primary ulcer is necessary for diagnosis. Secondary syphilis may be diagnosed by serologic testing. The ulcers also may reveal spirochetes by darkfield microscopy.

Differential Diagnosis
Other diseases that may present with a genital ulcer include HSV, chancroid, lymphogranuloma venereum, granuloma inguinale, and Behçet's disease. However, the majority of these ulcers are painful. **Always** remember to check an HIV test in anyone suspected or proven to have syphilis.

Treatment
Benzathine PCN G, 2.4 million units IM in a single dose, is usually curative for primary or early secondary syphilis. Alternative treatments include doxycycline, 100 mg PO bid for 14 days, or erythromycin (E-Mycin), 500 mg PO qid for 14 days.

Oral Candidiasis

Candidiasis is caused by *Candida* species, usually *Candida albicans*. Oral candidiasis usually does not occur in immunocompetent individuals. Risk factors include advanced age, use of inhaled or oral steroids, recent use of broad-spectrum antimicrobials, denture use, and diabetes, HIV, or malignancy.

Clinical Manifestations
In patients using broad-spectrum antibiotics, lesions are often erythematous with a burning sensation of the tongue. Patients with cell-mediated immunity defects usually have thrush, a pseudomembranous form of disease, with a layer of white flecks of material that can be wiped off to reveal an erythematous surface, which may bleed.

Diagnosis
The diagnosis is usually made clinically. It can be made by microscopy of the exudate showing yeasts with hyphal forms. Culture is not as helpful, as *C. albicans* is present in the oral flora of 10% of the population.

Differential Diagnosis
The differential diagnosis includes oral hairy leukoplakia and pemphigus vulgaris.

Treatment
Treatment usually consists of modifying risk factors. This includes stopping antibiotics, advising the patient not to wear dentures at night, and stopping steroids if possible. Nystatin swish and swallow, 4–6 mL PO qid, or Mycelex troches, 5 times per day for 7–14 days, can be used. Immunocompromised individuals frequently require systemic therapy with fluconazole (Diflucan), 100–200 mg PO qd.

Other Infections

Patients with histoplasmosis or *Paracoccidioides brasiliensis* should be evaluated by an ID specialist.

Histoplasmosis
Generally, oral infections only occur with disseminated disease. Lesions tend to appear as erythematous areas that may ulcerate. A biopsy is needed to establish diagnosis. Treatment consists of amphotericin B or itraconazole (Sporanox).

Paracoccidioides Brasiliensis

Paracoccidioides brasiliensis is a major cause of systemic mycosis in Central America and South America, and it should be considered in any patient from these areas. Most patients have an oral mucosal ulcer with some surrounding edema. There may be perioral lesions that may be ulcerated or warty. Diagnosis is made by smear and culture, and treatment consists of oral imidazole [itraconazole (Sporanox)] compounds.

Salivary Gland Infections

Etiology

Salivary gland infections are usually viral in origin, including mumps virus, parainfluenza, coxsackievirus, echovirus, EBV, and HIV, although bacterial infections do occur. Risk factors for bacterial parotitis include advanced age, diabetes, dehydration, anticholinergic medication or diuretic use, and poor oral hygiene. Causative bacterial organisms include *Staphylococcus aureus*, *Streptococcus pyogenes*, *Streptococcus viridans*, and *Haemophilus influenzae*. Very rarely, mycobacterial infection may be the cause of salivary gland infection.

Clinical Manifestations

Viral infection usually begins with the gradual onset of painful swelling of parotid glands, either unilateral or bilateral. Mumps is also associated with orchitis, meningoencephalitis, fever, arthralgia, malaise, and headache.

Bacterial parotitis usually begins with rapid onset of pain, swelling, and induration. Manual palpation of gland is painful and can result in discharge of pus from the duct. There may be systemic features, with fever, rigors, and neutrophilia.

Diagnosis

The diagnosis is made through culture of secretions for viral and bacterial pathogens. The patient should also have a rise in convalescent antibodies for mumps virus. Fine-needle aspiration biopsy of the gland for cytology and culture may reveal nontuberculous mycobacterial infection.

Treatment

Bacterial infections need treatment with antibiotics, frequently with parenteral antibiotics such as nafcillin or oxacillin, 2 g IV q4h, if fever and neutrophilia are present. Surgical drainage is rarely necessary. Treatment of viral causes of parotitis usually consists of symptomatic therapy. Management of mycobacterial infection is conservative unless *Mycobacterium tuberculosis* is the cause, and treatment for this is with standard antituberculous therapy.

ESOPHAGEAL INFECTIONS

Pathophysiology

Infectious esophagitis is most commonly found in immunocompromised or immunosuppressed individuals. It is seen especially in the late stages of HIV infection. The most common esophageal infection is **candidiasis.** The candidal species is usually *C. albicans*, but other possibilities include *Candida tropicalis*, *Candida glabrata*, *Candida krusei*, *Candida parapsilosis*, or *Candida lusitaniae*. Esophageal candidiasis is usually associated with oral candidiasis. It is important to remember that even severe esophageal candidiasis may be asymptomatic. Viral causes of esophagitis include HSV and CMV infection, which are less often asymptomatic and less often present in the oropharynx as well. Each of these diseases may occur separately or may be present concurrently.

Clinical Manifestations

Infectious esophagitis usually presents with odynophagia or dysphagia. Symptoms may be present intermittently or may be associated with nausea if gastritis is also present, or the patient may be asymptomatic.

Diagnosis

Diagnosis is made almost exclusively by EGD, with biopsy, brush cytology, and cultures taken. Esophagogram may be used to identify esophagitis, but it is frequently normal or nonspecific. The endoscopic appearance of these infections is sometimes variable, but characteristically, HSV is associated with discrete ulcerations of the mucosa, particularly in the distal third of the esophagus; when severe, the ulcers may ooze blood. The diagnosis is best made by culture of the biopsy or brushings. Antibody staining is less sensitive and specific but faster than culture. There are four stages of severity of candidal esophagitis by EGD: diffuse mucosal hyperemia with or without edema; discrete white mucosal patches; mucosal ulceration, typically with a necrotic base; and bleeding or esophageal perforation. Biopsy specimens show typical hyphal elements. CMV is typically associated with extensive, large, shallow ulcers in the distal esophagus. The diagnosis is certain if typical cells are seen in the biopsy material (large cells with large, dense, intranuclear inclusions and small, dense intracytoplasmic inclusions are diagnostic, but they occur infrequently in the submucosa). Culture supports but does not establish the diagnosis.

Differential Diagnosis

Less common infectious causes of esophagitis include cryptococcosis, histoplasmosis, TB, and cryptosporidiosis. Noninfectious causes in the differential include lymphoma, Kaposi's sarcoma, squamous cell carcinoma, peptic esophagitis, aphthous ulcers, tablet mucositis, corrosive ingestion, and mucositis from chemotherapy.

Treatment

Treatment of candidal esophagitis is fluconazole, 100–200 mg PO qd. Itraconazole (Sporanox), 200 mg (20 mL) PO qd without food for 7 days, may also be used. In the past, patients who did not respond to fluconazole were often placed on parenteral amphotericin B. However, the newer antifungals caspofungin and voriconazole have been FDA approved for treatment of refractory candidiasis and have fewer side effects. Prophylaxis for candidal esophagitis is common but breeds resistance. HSV is treated with acyclovir, 400 mg PO five times a day; famciclovir (Famvir), 250 mg PO tid; or valacyclovir (Valtrex), 500 mg PO tid for 1 wk. For more severe infections, IV acyclovir is needed, usually at a dose of 5 mg/kg q8h. Relapses are common but may be prevented with therapy with acyclovir, 400 mg PO bid. CMV is treated with ganciclovir (Cytovene, Cytovene-IV) at an induction dose of 5 mg/kg IV q12h for 2–6 wks. This can be followed by a maintenance dose of 5 mg/kg IV qd, although there is no consensus regarding maintenance dosing for CMV esophagitis. An alternative maintenance dose is valganciclovir, 900 mg PO bid, which patients can take when able to take oral medications. Again, relapse is common.

INFECTIONS OF THE STOMACH

Helicobacter pylori infection causes chronic active gastritis, is the main cause of duodenal and gastric ulcers, and is a risk factor for gastric adenocarcinoma and lymphoma. Other infectious causes of gastritis are rare and usually are associated with immunocompromised states.

Pathophysiology

H. pylori is a spiral, gram-negative, urease-producing bacillus. Transmission occurs by either the fecal-oral or oral-oral route. *H. pylori* is primarily a gastric infection, although the bacteria may colonize areas of gastric metaplasia in the duodenum and esophagus. *H. pylori* infection has been associated with >90% of duodenal ulcers and 80% of gastric ulcers. Chronic infection is associated with a two- to sixfold increase in gastric cancer and MALT (*m*ucosa-*a*ssociated *l*ymphoid *t*issue) lymphoma.

Clinical Manifestations

Chronic infection in the majority of patients is asymptomatic. Patients may have chronic active gastritis, chronic persistent gastritis, or atrophic gastritis. Symptoms may include epigastric discomfort with a burning sensation, typically occurring when the stomach is empty. Less commonly, nausea, vomiting, and anorexia occur. Bleeding may occur, and signs and symptoms of anemia may be present.

Diagnosis

The diagnosis can be made by noninvasive tests or endoscopically. Endoscopy is performed to obtain mucosal biopsy specimens to perform urease testing and to send for histology and culture. Endoscopy is also used to document healing of gastric ulcers and to rule out malignancy. Noninvasive methods of identifying *H. pylori* infection include urea breath tests, which are easy and can also be used to document treatment success. Sensitivity and specificity range from 90 to 98%. Serology detecting IgG or IgA is reasonably sensitive (80–95%). A fall of >40% in IgG titers at 6 mos indicates treatment success, but quantifying titers is more expensive and difficult.

Treatment

There is a wide range of relapse rates recorded (approximately 20–40%). Treatment depends on acid suppression and eradication of *H. pylori* to prevent recurrence. A recent study suggests that due to an increase in clarithromycin- or metronidazole-resistant *H. pylori* isolates, treatment with either clarithromycin or metronidazole in the past may limit the effectiveness of the treatment regimen prescribed [1]. Appropriate use of antibiotics and avoidance of empiric treatment for *H. pylori* in the management of nonulcer dyspepsia are encouraged. In areas where drug-resistant strains are common, using a posttreatment test for cure (e.g., urea breath test) to confirm eradication may be a consideration. Multiple regimens exist for the eradication of *H. pylori* (Table 6-1).

INTESTINAL INFECTIONS

Infectious Diarrhea

Pathophysiology

The two major forms of infectious diarrhea include noninflammatory diarrhea and dysentery. Mechanisms leading to diarrhea include mucosal adherence, toxin production, and mucosal invasion. They are detailed below.

- Mucosal adherence leads to colonization and effacement of the intestinal mucosa, resulting in secretory diarrhea. Organisms such as enterotoxigenic *Escherichia coli* (ETEC) cause disease through this mechanism.
- Three forms of toxins can be produced. Enterotoxin causes fluid secretion without damaging the mucosa, resulting in watery, noninflammatory diarrhea. *Vibrio cholerae*, ETEC, *Salmonella*, *Campylobacter*, *Clostridium difficile* toxin A, and *Clostridium perfringens* toxin type A produce disease in this manner. Neurotoxin affects the autonomic nervous system, leading to enteric symptoms. *Staphylococcus* enterotoxin B, *Clostridium botulinum*, and *Bacillus cereus* produce disease through this means. Cytotoxin damages the mucosa, causing inflammatory colitis and dysentery. Examples of bacteria with cytotoxin production include *Shigella*, *E. coli* O157:H7, *C. difficile* toxin B, *Salmonella*, and *Campylobacter*.
- Mucosal invasion by the bacteria leads to penetration of the mucosa and destruction of the epithelial cells, resulting in dysenteric syndromes. *Shigella*, enteroinvasive *E. coli* (EIEC), *Campylobacter*, and *Yersinia* species all have this ability.

Clinical Manifestations

The diagnosis of infectious diarrhea is made by careful history and physical exam. Important points to consider include history of antibiotic use, history of recent or remote travel, duration of diarrhea, amount of weight loss, water supply, hobbies or occupation, pets, drugs, family exposure, and diet. It is important to distinguish between small and large bowel diarrhea. Large-volume, infrequent, or nocturnal diarrhea, gas, bloating, and periumbilical pain indicate the small bowel, whereas frequent

TABLE 6-1. TREATMENT MODALITIES FOR *HELICOBACTER PYLORI* INFECTION

Eradication rate (PrevPac), 86–92%
    Lansoprazole (Prevacid), 30 mg PO bid for 10–14 days
    Clarithromycin (Biaxin), 500 mg PO bid or tid for 10–14 days
    Amoxicillin (Amoxil), 1 g PO bid for 10–14 days

Eradication rate, 80–91%
    Omeprazole (Prilosec), 20 mg PO bid for 10 days
    Clarithromycin, 500 mg PO bid for 10 days
    Amoxicillin, 1 g PO bid for 10 days

Eradication rate, >80%
    Omeprazole, 20 mg PO bid for 14 days **OR** lansoprazole, 30 mg PO bid for 14 days
    Metronidazole (Flagyl), 500 mg PO bid for 14 days
    Amoxicillin, 1 g PO bid for 14 days

Eradication rate (Helidac), 86% (increased to 94–98% with addition of proton pump inhibitor[a])
    Bismuth subsalicylate (Pepto-Bismol), 525 mg qid for 2 wks
    Metronidazole, 250 mg PO qid for 2 wks
    Tetracycline, 500 mg PO qid for 2 wks
    H_2-receptor blocker for 4 wks

Eradication rate, 87–91%
    Omeprazole, 20 mg PO bid for 1 wk
    Metronidazole, 500 mg PO qid for 1 wk
    Clarithromycin, 500 mg PO bid for 1 wk

Eradication rate, 70–80%
    Omeprazole, 40 mg PO qd for 2 wks, then 20 mg PO qd for 2 wks
    Clarithromycin, 500 mg PO tid for 2 wks

[a]Clarithromycin may be substituted for metronidazole. Amoxicillin may be substituted for tetracycline.

small-volume stools with infraumbilical pain suggest the colon; tenesmus, incontinence, and urgency occur in colonic and anorectal inflammation.

- **Noninflammatory diarrhea** is confirmed by the absence of fecal leukocytes and blood in the stool. Associated symptoms may include nausea, vomiting, cramping, abdominal pain, arthralgias, myalgias, and chills but rarely fever.
- **Dysenteric syndrome,** or **acute dysentery,** is an inflammatory or invasive process that involves the colon and occasionally the distal small intestine. Symptoms include fever, low-volume stools with blood and mucus, chills, abdominal cramping, tenesmus, and vomiting.

Risk factors for death in diarrheal disease include malnutrition, immunosuppression, and complications such as dehydration, pneumonia, sepsis, and development of the HUS. Other risk factors include failure to receive rehydration or antimicrobial therapy when indicated, as well as infection with rotavirus (in children), invasive pathogens, and enterotoxigenic bacteria.

Diagnosis
In nonhospitalized patients with mild to moderate symptoms (<5 stools/day) and no fever, nausea, vomiting, or cramps, supportive therapy is indicated, and there is no need

for stool culture. All other patients must undergo testing, including exam for fecal leukocytes, stool culture, parasite exam, stool antigen testing, or stool toxin testing.

- An exam for **fecal leukocytes** is indicated in any patient with fever and moderate to severe diarrhea. Numerous leukocytes indicate an invasive enteric pathogen, such as *Shigella, Salmonella, Campylobacter, C. difficile, Yersinia enterocolitica, Aeromonas hydrophila, Vibrio parahaemolyticus*, EIEC, or enterohemorrhagic *E. coli* (EHEC). Mononuclear cells should lead to the suspicion of typhoid fever or amebic dysentery. If the exam for fecal leukocytes is positive, then the stool must be cultured.
- Exam for **ova and parasites** is indicated in all patients who have had diarrhea for >2 wks, have traveled to Russia or developing countries, are male homosexuals, or are HIV positive. Special stains are needed for amebic trophozoites, cryptosporidiosis, isosporiasis, and microsporidiosis, so one needs to specify which organisms one is looking for.
- **Stool antigens** now can lead to direct detection of *Isospora, Giardia, Cryptosporidium* species, and *Entamoeba histolytica* in feces. Stool toxin detection can lead to the isolation of *C. difficile* toxin and Shiga-like toxin.
- **Blood cultures** should be obtained in severely ill patients, when salmonellosis is suspected, or in any immunocompromised patient.
- **Endoscopy** is useful in identifying amebiasis and ruling out inflammatory bowel disease. It is also important in diagnosing patients when no pathogen can be identified by other means.

Treatment
Fluid and electrolyte replacement is the main therapy—first with volume resuscitation, then by matching output. Dietary alteration is helpful and includes a lactose-free diet, starches and cereals, crackers, and soup. Symptomatic therapy with antimotility agents, such as loperamide and bismuth sulfate, may reduce the number of stools. However, antimotility agents should be avoided if invasive forms of diarrhea are suspected, as they may worsen disease. Antimicrobial therapy is appropriate in patients living in industrialized regions with febrile dysentery, because such infections are usually invasive. Usually, a fluoroquinolone [ciprofloxacin (Cipro, Cipro XR), 500 mg PO bid for 3–7 days] is used in adults, although erythromycin, 500 mg PO qid for 5 days, and TMP-SMX (Bactrim DS), 1 DS tablet PO bid, also work.

Noninflammatory Diarrhea

The majority of cases of infectious diarrhea are noninflammatory, with no blood or fecal leukocytes, suggesting an enterotoxic bacterial, viral, or noninvasive parasitic process. Some organisms include *Salmonella typhimurium*, ETEC, *S. aureus, Cryptosporidium* species, *C. perfringens, B. cereus, Giardia lamblia, Rotavirus* species, and Norwalk agent.

Clinical Manifestations
See Infectious Diarrhea: Clinical Manifestations. Salmonellosis symptoms may range from watery diarrhea to acute dysentery. Patients may have moderate fever, and up to 5% have bacteremia. Severe intestinal hemorrhage may develop in up to 2% of cases, and perforation rarely occurs. *V. cholerae* infection presents with sudden onset of watery diarrhea and anorexia or abdominal discomfort followed by "rice water" stools. Diarrhea may be explosive and watery or dysenteric. The disease is usually self-limited, with symptoms resolving in 3–4 days, although death can occur from dehydration.

Diagnosis
See the section Infectious Diarrhea: Diagnosis.

Differential Diagnosis
Noninfectious causes of watery diarrhea include heavy metal poisoning (arsenic, tin, iron, cadmium, mercury, or lead), thyroid disease, VIPomas (vasoactive intestinal polypeptide tumors), hypoparathyroidism, adrenal insufficiency, sorbitol consump-

tion, lactase deficiency, and pancreatic insufficiency. Chronic noninflammatory diarrhea is usually related to giardiasis, tropical sprue, bacterial overgrowth syndromes, and *Cryptosporidium* or *Isospora belli* infection.

Treatment

Refer to the general treatment guidelines in the section Infectious Diarrhea: Treatment. Treatment of salmonellosis depends on the severity of illness and the patient's risk factors for more serious infection. Any symptoms suggesting bacteremia and any condition that places the patient in a high-risk group (age >65 yrs, malignancy, inflammatory bowel disease, renal dysfunction, post–renal transplant, presence of aortic aneurysm, HIV positive) indicate the need to be treated immediately.

Traveler's Diarrhea

Traveler's diarrhea is defined as three or more unformed stools per day in a person traveling in a developing nation. Infection is acquired through ingestion of fecally contaminated food or water. Infection may be severe and incapacitating, although it is rarely fatal. ETEC has been found to be the causative organism in approximately 50% of cases, with *Salmonella*, *Shigella*, *Vibrio*, and *Campylobacter* infection occurring less commonly. Protozoans and viruses also are uncommon causes of traveler's diarrhea.

Clinical Manifestations

Onset is usually 5–15 days after arrival, with malaise, anorexia, and cramping abdominal pain, followed by sudden-onset watery diarrhea. Nausea and vomiting occur in <25% of patients. Patients may have low-grade fever. The illness usually lasts 1–5 days.

Treatment

Traveler's diarrhea is almost always self-limited. Prevention includes avoiding raw fruits, vegetables, water, and ice cubes. All water should be heated, even bottled water. More information on preventive measures can be found at http://www.cdc.gov/travel/ or 1-877-FYI-TRIP (1-877-394-8747). Antibiotic prophylaxis breeds resistance, so it should only be given to patients with other medical conditions putting them at high risk for morbidity and mortality. For other treatments, see the section Infectious Diarrhea.

Bacterial Overgrowth Syndromes

Pathophysiology

Normal small bowel bacteria are lactobacilli, streptococci, and diphtheroids in few numbers. Organisms most commonly associated with overgrowth include aerobic enteric coliforms (Enterobacteriaceae) and anaerobic gram-negative fecal flora (bacteroides). Predisposing factors include achlorhydria, blind loop syndromes, cholangitis, impaired motility, surgery, diverticula, strictures, radiation damage, and episodes of acute infectious diarrhea (see the section Tropical Sprue). It can be caused by any condition that predisposes to intestinal stasis.

Clinical Manifestations

Bacterial overgrowth manifests as watery diarrhea in small bowel pattern, with large-volume, infrequent stools, bloating, gas, malabsorption, and periumbilical pain. Fevers, chills, and other systemic symptoms are not usually present.

Diagnosis

Diagnosis includes history, radiographic findings, and quantitative aerobic and anaerobic cultures of the upper small bowel contents by EGD. Serum cobalamin is often decreased, whereas serum folate is elevated.

Differential Diagnosis

The differential includes other infections (see earlier), food allergy, enzyme deficiency, endocrine disease (carcinoid tumor, Zollinger-Ellison syndrome, medullary carcinoma of the thyroid, thyrotoxicosis, and pancreatic insufficiency), as well as neoplasm, gluten enteropathy, and Wiskott-Aldrich syndrome.

Treatment

Patients with diarrhea and malabsorption should be treated, especially if they have a predisposing factor. Antimicrobial therapy needs to cover aerobes and anaerobes, such as amoxicillin-clavulanate (Augmentin), 250–500 mg PO tid; tetracycline, 250 mg PO qid; or ciprofloxacin, 250 mg PO bid, for intermittent 2-wk courses. Surgery and vitamin supplementation may be necessary.

Tropical Sprue

Tropical sprue is a disease characterized by a prolonged diarrheal illness and malabsorption of two or more substances in individuals in the tropics who have no other obvious reason to malabsorb. This disease is most readily identified in Asia and the Caribbean islands, and it is relatively common among the indigenous populations of Puerto Rico, Haiti, the Dominican Republic, Cuba, northern South America, Venezuela, Columbia, the Indian subcontinent, Myanmar, and the Philippines. It is mainly a disease of adults and generally does not develop until someone has lived in an endemic area for >6 mos. Rare cases have been documented in short-term travelers. The etiology is currently unknown.

Pathophysiology

There are some data supporting an infectious cause of sprue: Cases are often preceded by an episode of acute diarrheal disease, sprue appears to have an epidemic and seasonal nature, and it responds most often to antibiotic therapy. Small bowel bacterial overgrowth has been documented, but it is unclear if this is the cause of sprue. This may set off a cascade of events involving decreased intestinal motility, long-chain fatty acid consumption, and malabsorption. Intestinal abnormalities are present in both the small and large bowel. Partial villus atrophy is the hallmark histologic change in the small bowel. This is not specific for tropical sprue, however; it may be present in severe folate deficiency or with bacterial overgrowth.

Clinical Manifestations

The classic features are nonspecific and reflect malabsorption, including lactose intolerance, vitamin B_{12}- and folate-related anemia, iron-deficiency anemia, osteopenia, and fat malabsorption. Usually, the onset of sprue is abrupt, with most patients noting an acute episode of diarrhea. Prolonged diarrhea, abdominal cramping, anorexia, nausea, and weight loss are common. Patients describe crampy abdominal pain and multiple soft or loose stools daily, often with mucus. Symptoms are exacerbated by food consumption. Less commonly, peripheral edema, glossitis, stomatitis, and dermatitis may be present. Fever may occur at the onset of illness but rarely persists. Signs and symptoms of anemia may be present (pallor, fatigue, weakness). Late in the course, peripheral neuropathy, confusion, and high output CHF may develop. The disease may last months to years. Spontaneous recovery has been reported.

Diagnosis

The diagnosis should be considered in a patient presenting with chronic diarrhea, weight loss, and evidence of malabsorption. Travel history is important, as is exposure history, history of small bowel surgery, medications that alter motility, or any other risk factor for bacterial overgrowth. A social history to rule out risk factors for HIV should also be obtained. Blood work should include a CBC to screen for anemia, as well as vitamin B_{12}, folate, and iron levels if anemia is present. Stool studies should include a 72-hr collection for fecal fat, as well as a stool exam to rule out *Giardia*. Small bowel follow-through may show flattened mucosal folds, luminal dilatation, or flocculation.

Differential Diagnosis

The differential includes giardiasis, cryptosporidiosis, coccidiosis, capillariasis, celiac sprue, strongyloides infection, lymphoma, intestinal TB, blind loop syndrome, pancreatic tumor, Whipple's disease, and HIV.

Treatment

Combination therapy with tetracycline, 250 mg PO qid, and folate, 1 mg PO qd, for 1 mo for travelers, >6 mos for patients in endemic areas, is indicated. Relapses have been reported, but it is unclear if this is due to reexposure or reinfection.

Inflammatory Diarrhea

Acute dysentery is defined as frequent small bowel movements with blood, mucus, and tenesmus. It implies inflammatory invasion of the colonic mucosa from bacterial, cytotoxic, or parasitic infection. Fecal-oral spread is common, and outbreaks may be food- or water-borne.

Clinical Manifestations

Bacillary dysentery is most frequently caused by *Shigella* species and EIEC. EIEC infection is usually indistinguishable from *Shigella* infection. In childhood, cases may be complicated by the development of HUS. *Shigella dysenteriae* type 1 is associated with more serious disease and with an increased incidence of HUS. Intestinal obstruction occurs in 3% of patients and is a poor prognostic sign. Bacteremia and disseminated infection are rare. A Reiter's syndrome–like arthritis has been described in up to 10% of patients up to 6 wks postinfection.

EHEC infection may be sporadic or associated with food-borne outbreaks. Patients typically have no fever and no fecal leukocytes. Disease develops from the production of large amounts of Shiga-like toxin. The most commonly found subtype is *E. coli* O157:H7. This infection is associated with HUS in a larger proportion of patients than with shigellosis (8–10%).

Other organisms that commonly cause dysenteric syndromes include *V. parahaemolyticus*, *Salmonella enteritidis*, and *Campylobacter jejuni*.

Diagnosis

See the section Infectious Diarrhea: Diagnosis. Stool studies should show leukocytes even in the absence of blood. Stool culture may be used for *Shigella*. *Vibrio* species need special culture (thiosulfate citrate bile agar), as do *Yersinia* species (cold enrichment).

Flexible sigmoidoscopy to evaluate ulcers and to rule out pseudomembranous colitis may sometimes be helpful. Barium studies are unnecessary and may even be harmful.

Differential Diagnosis

The differential includes pseudomembranous colitis, necrotizing enterocolitis, and inflammatory bowel disease. Venereal exposure, especially among male homosexuals, may result in infection with gonorrhea, HSV, *Chlamydia trachomatis*, and *T. pallidum* as causes of proctitis, and *C. jejuni*, *C. trachomatis*, and *E. histolytica* as causes of colitis. Unusual causes of dysentery include spirillar dysentery, brucellosis, yersiniosis, adenovirus, schistosomiasis, *Trichinella spiralis*, and *Strongyloides stercoralis*.

Treatment

See the section Infectious Diarrhea: Treatment. All patients should have supportive therapy. When antimicrobial therapy is indicated, fluoroquinolones work very well. They have been shown to decrease fecal shedding and duration of illness with *C. jejuni*. Shigellosis should always be treated, as it is highly infective. Of note, EHEC should *not* be treated with antibiotics, as antibiotic therapy may predispose to development of HUS.

Chronic Inflammatory Diarrhea

Clinical Manifestations

Patients have a history of weeks to months of fever, abdominal pain, and weight loss in addition to diarrhea.

Diagnosis and Treatment

See the sections Inflammatory Diarrhea: Diagnosis and Inflammatory Diarrhea: Treatment, above.

Differential Diagnosis

The differential includes chronic *E. coli* infection, recurrent or relapsing *C. jejuni* or *Salmonella* infection, GI *M. tuberculosis* or syphilis, and parasitic infection, including coccidiosis, giardiasis, cryptosporidiosis, histoplasmosis, and blastomycosis (rare in North America).

Abdominal Pain with Fever

Several enteric infections are characterized by clinical syndromes of abdominal pain and fever, which are distinct from acute gastroenteritis. The portal of entry is usually the GI tract. Infection manifests as one of three syndromes: enteric fever; mesenteric adenitis, which can mimic appendicitis; or eosinophilia with abdominal cramps or diarrhea.

Enteric Fever

Pathophysiology

Enteric fever, also known as **typhoid fever,** is an acute systemic illness with fever, headache, and abdominal discomfort. The main organisms causing infection are *Salmonella typhi* and *Salmonella paratyphi*. Risk factors for *Salmonella* infection include postgastrectomy state, hypochlorhydria, altered intestinal motility, prior antibiotic therapy, sickle cell anemia, chronic liver disease, and CD4 cell deficiency. Organisms are ingested, multiply in intestinal lymphoid tissue, and disseminate systemically via a lymphatic or hematogenous route. Incubation lasts 5–21 days, infection may be food- or water-borne, and most cases are acquired abroad.

Clinical Manifestations

Symptoms include an insidious onset with fever, headache, and abdominal pain. Cough, conjunctivitis, and constipation or diarrhea may develop. Diarrhea occurs in 50% of patients. The physical exam may reveal abdominal tenderness, hepatosplenomegaly, rose spots on the upper abdomen or lower thorax, relative bradycardia, and mental status changes. Pharyngitis is infrequent. Rales may be present. Complications include pneumonia, endocarditis, osteomyelitis, arthritis, and meningitis.

Diagnosis

If diarrhea is present, exam of stool for leukocytes may reveal monocytes. Blood, stool, and urine cultures should be obtained for *Salmonella*. Urine and stool cultures are positive in <50% of patients. Multiple cultures should be obtained before beginning antibiotic therapy. Chest x-ray may reveal an infiltrate, although this is present in <10% of patients.

Lab values may reveal a variety of abnormalities. A CBC may reveal leukopenia; eosinophilia is rare. Mild DIC with elevation of the PT may be found. Liver function tests are often elevated, with alkaline phosphatase and transaminase levels being higher than bilirubin levels. A complement-mediated glomerulonephritis can be found, as can pyuria and proteinuria.

Differential Diagnosis

The differential includes *Y. enterocolitica*, *Yersinia pseudotuberculosis*, and *Campylobacter fetus* infection, as well as typhoidal tularemia. Also in the differential are intraabdominal abscess, infectious mononucleosis, amebiasis, pneumonia, rickettsial infections (typhus, Rocky Mountain spotted fever), acute hepatitis, influenza (especially B), *Legionella*, intestinal TB, and protozoan and helminth infections.

Rare causes include dengue fever, plague, intestinal anthrax, acute bartonellosis, acute brucellosis, malaria (with travel to tropics and endemic regions), rat-bite fever (*Streptobacillus moniliformis*), leptospirosis, relapsing fever (*Borrelia recurrentis*), abdominal actinomycosis, and psittacosis.

Noninfectious causes include eosinophilic gastroenteritis, malignancy involving the abdominal organs or lymph nodes, vasculitis, and granulomatous diseases.

Treatment

A fluoroquinolone is often used, such as ciprofloxacin, 500 mg PO bid for 10 days. A third-generation cephalosporin may also be used (e.g., ceftriaxone, 1–2 g IV qd). There is increasing resistance to chloramphenicol (Chloromycetin), TMP-SMX (Bactrim), and erythromycin, but all of these are still useful.

Mesenteric Adenitis

Pathophysiology
Infection is caused by *Y. enterocolitica* and *Y. pseudotuberculosis*, although beta-hemolytic *Streptococcus* may cause a few cases. The disease is caused when the organisms spread from the GI tract to the draining lymph nodes. The disease usually occurs in children and young adults, most often in winter and spring. Person-to-person spread and common-source infections have been documented, as has food-borne illness. *Y. enterocolitica* can also cause enterocolitis and terminal ileitis.

Clinical Manifestations
Symptoms and physical exam mimic acute appendicitis with fever; nausea and vomiting; abdominal pain, frequently with rebound tenderness; and diarrhea. A CBC may reveal leukocytosis.

Diagnosis
Stool cultures may grow *Yersinia* >50% of the time. Imaging by either U/S or contrast CT may help lead to an accurate diagnosis.

Differential Diagnosis
Acute appendicitis, actinomycosis, infectious mononucleosis, and parvovirus B19 infection (pseudoappendicitis) are included in the differential. Disseminated *Mycobacterium avium* complex should be considered in AIDS patients.

Treatment
The majority of cases are self-limited. In patients who are severely ill, antibiotics are needed. If possible, antibiotic choice should be based on sensitivity testing. If no sensitivity testing is available, consider a third-generation cephalosporin, a fluoroquinolone, tetracycline, chloramphenicol, or TMP-SMX (Bactrim). Because of the difficulty in distinguishing mesenteric adenitis from acute appendicitis, many cases still undergo exploratory surgery.

Abdominal Pain or Diarrhea with Eosinophilia

Pathophysiology
Eosinophilic gastroenteritis is characterized by infiltration of the GI tract with eosinophils. This may be due to a variety of infectious causes. Infectious causes include bacterial overgrowth, Whipple's disease, and parasitic infection, including *S. stercoralis*, *Ascaris lumbricoides*, *Toxocara* infection (visceral larva migrans), *T. spiralis*, various nematodes, and *I. belli*.

Clinical Manifestations
Patients usually present with diarrhea as well as abdominal pain, nausea, vomiting, and weight loss. Steatorrhea and protein-losing enteropathy may occur. These patients may develop edema or anasarca. GI bleeding, malabsorption, and gastric outlet obstruction may develop. Peripheral eosinophilia is present in up to 75% of patients.

Diagnosis
Stool should be cultured and examined for leukocytes and parasites. Charcot-Leyden crystals may be found in the stool. Definitive diagnosis is made by EGD, which shows patchy involvement, so multiple biopsies are needed.

Differential Diagnosis
Noninfectious causes include vasculitis, regional enteritis, ulcerative colitis, food allergy, and SLE. Also, solid tumors and lymphomas may cause abdominal pain, diarrhea, and eosinophilia.

Treatment

Treatment of the underlying infection is usually curative, but corticosteroids may be helpful.

FOOD-BORNE ILLNESSES

Food-borne illnesses result from the ingestion of foods contaminated with pathogenic organisms, toxins, or chemicals. The estimated incidence of food-borne disease ranges from 6.5 million to 80 million cases/yr worldwide. The diagnosis of food-borne disease should be considered when an acute illness with GI or neurologic manifestations affects two or more persons who have shared a meal during the previous 72 hrs. Over 50% of reported food-borne disease outbreaks in the United States are of unknown cause.

Clinical Manifestations

Clinical syndromes generally involve noninflammatory diarrhea, dysentery, or gastroenteritis (see the sections Noninflammatory Diarrhea: Clinical Manifestations and Inflammatory Diarrhea: Clinical Manifestations). The **time course** of symptoms is often the major clue to the organism causing the symptoms (Table 6-2).

- Nausea and vomiting within **1–6 hrs** of ingestion suggest a preformed toxin (*S. aureus* and *B. cereus*), whereas abdominal cramps and diarrhea within 8–16 hrs of ingestion are usually caused by toxins produced *in vivo* (*B. cereus* and *C. perfringens*).
- Fever, abdominal cramps, and diarrhea within **1–3 days** of ingestion imply tissue invasion (*Salmonella, Shigella, C. jejuni, V. parahaemolyticus*, and EIEC). *V. cholerae* non-01 infection may cause bloody diarrhea with fever. *Y. enterocolitica* is common in the United States and is becoming more common in Canada and Europe. Some strains produce heat-stable enterotoxin, but illness is usually caused by direct invasion.
- Abdominal cramps and watery diarrhea within **1–3 days** are usually caused by ETEC, *V. parahaemolyticus, V. cholerae* non-01, and *V. cholerae*. *C. jejuni, Salmonella*, and *Shigella* can also cause disease. Usually, the disease is enterotoxin or cytotoxin mediated. Symptoms usually resolve in 76–92 hrs but may last >1 wk.
- Bloody diarrhea without fever within **3–5 days:** *E. coli* O157:H7 produces this distinct syndrome of hemorrhagic colitis. The bacteria are noninvasive. Infection is characterized by severe abdominal cramping and diarrhea, which is initially watery but subsequently grossly bloody. The mean incubation is 4–8 days, and uncomplicated illness lasts 1–12 days. Fever and leukocytosis may herald the development of thrombotic thrombocytopenic purpura or HUS.

TABLE 6-2. COMMON ORGANISMS CAUSING FOOD-BORNE ILLNESS

Staphylococcus aureus: ham, poultry, egg salad, pastries

Bacillus cereus: fried rice, meats, vegetables

Clostridium perfringens: beef, poultry, gravy, Mexican food

Escherichia coli O157:H7: undercooked beef, raw milk

Salmonella: poultry, beef, egg, dairy products

Shigella: egg salads, potato salads, lettuce

Campylobacter jejuni: raw milk, poultry (spring, summer)

Vibrio cholerae: shellfish

Yersinia enterocolitica: milk, tofu, pork

Enteroinvasive *E. coli*: cheese

Enterotoxigenic *E. coli*: salad, cheese, sausage, seafood, cheese, hamburger

Clostridium botulinum: vegetables, fruits (especially home-canned), fish

- The classic presentation of botulism is nausea, vomiting, diarrhea, and paralysis within **18–36 hrs**. Paralysis and weakness are descending and can last for weeks to months. Nausea and vomiting occur in 50%; diarrhea occurs in 25% of patients. The differential includes Guillain-Barré syndrome, which can develop 1–3 wks after *Campylobacter* infection. Guillain-Barré syndrome is usually an ascending weakness/paralysis with sensory findings and abnormal nerve conduction studies.

Diagnosis

Diagnosis is made by appropriate specimens from patients (see the section Infectious Diarrhea: Diagnosis). Also, any leftover food should be cultured, as well as the food preparation environment and food handlers, where applicable.

Differential Diagnosis

Noninfectious causes of food-borne illness include heavy metal poisoning (copper, zinc, tin, cadmium). Symptoms usually resolve 2–3 hrs after removal of the offending agent. Abdominal cramps and diarrhea can be caused by poisonous mushroom ingestion. Symptoms begin within 6–24 hrs of ingestion and usually resolve in 24 hrs but can be followed 1–2 days later by hepatorenal failure. Paresthesias within 1 hr of ingestion usually result from niacin consumption or shellfish poisoning.

Treatment

In general, supportive therapy is indicated. Treatment is instituted where appropriate, as noted in the section Infectious Diarrhea: Treatment. Prevention is based on proper storage and preparation of food. Cold food must be refrigerated to <40°F (4°C), and food must be cooked to >140°F (60°C). Cases must be reported to the public health service.

Other Food-Borne Diseases

Listeriosis (pregnant women, immunocompromised patients) causes fever, myalgia, meningitis, and bacteremia. Sources include cole slaw, dairy products, and cold processed meats. Incubation is 2–6 wks, with a case fatality rate of 25%. *Vibrio vulnificus* from raw oysters can lead to myonecrosis or bacteremia and is usually seen in patients with liver disease. Group A beta-hemolytic *Streptococcus*, *Bacillus anthracis*, *Francisella tularensis*, *Brucella* species, parasites, HAV, and Norwalk virus are all associated with food-borne outbreaks as well.

Water-Borne Diseases

Giardia, E. coli O157:H7, HAV, *Shigella, S. typhi*, other *Salmonella* species, ETEC, *C. jejuni, Cryptosporidium, Cyclospora, Isospora*, and Norwalk agent can be (but are not always) water-borne diseases. *E. histolytica* and *Balantidium coli* resist chlorination and are therefore associated with water-borne outbreaks as well.

ANTIBIOTIC-ASSOCIATED DIARRHEA/COLITIS

Antibiotics are the most important predisposing factor to the development of *C. difficile* colitis, but *C. difficile* colitis *can* happen without antibiotic exposure. Other risk factors include abdominal surgery and chemotherapy. Classically, *C. difficile* causes pseudomembranous colitis, but many patients do not develop pseudomembranes. An important fact to remember is that the most common type of antibiotic-associated diarrhea is related to the antibiotic itself and resolves with removal of the antibiotic therapy.

Pathophysiology

C. difficile is a spore-forming, gram-positive obligate anaerobe that is present in the normal flora of 3% of healthy adults. However, colonization rates are 10–30% of hospitalized patients. *C. difficile* infection results in acute inflammation of the colonic mucosa. Disease results from spore germination, colonization, overgrowth, and then toxin production. At least two toxins are produced: Toxin A is an enterotoxin, and toxin B is a cytotoxin. Different strains of *C. difficile* may have one, the other, both, or no toxins.

During infection, usually only the epithelium and superficial lamina propria are affected, although in more severe cases, deeper tissues are involved. Pseudomembranes may be found throughout the colon but are worst in the rectosigmoid region. The ileum is rarely involved unless a previous colostomy/ileostomy is present. A far less likely cause of antibiotic-associated diarrhea may be *S. aureus*.

Clinical Manifestations

Infection results in profuse watery or green mucoid, foul-smelling diarrhea with cramping abdominal pain usually beginning 4–10 days after starting antibiotic therapy. However, the diarrhea can start within 24 hrs of initiation of antibiotic therapy. The diarrhea may be Hemoccult positive. Patients may develop toxic megacolon, perforation, and peritonitis. Disease develops most frequently in middle-aged to elderly patients. Higher-risk patients include women, cancer or burn patients, patients undergoing abdominal surgery, intensive care patients, and anyone exposed to even short courses of antibiotics. Most antibiotics have been associated with the development of *C. difficile* diarrhea. High fever, abdominal tenderness, and leukocytosis point to a diagnosis of colitis rather than benign diarrhea.

Diagnosis

Diagnosis is based on isolation of *C. difficile* toxin. Culture of the organism is not as helpful, as 25% of *C. difficile* strains cannot make toxins and are therefore not able to cause colitis. Also, a percentage of people have *C. difficile* as normal flora. Endoscopy may be useful in distinguishing *C. difficile* colitis from other forms of colitis when the diagnosis is in doubt.

Differential Diagnosis

Diarrhea from antibiotic use is number one in the differential. Withdrawal of the antibiotic results in resolution of the diarrhea. In patients with nonspecific colitis associated with antibiotic usage, consider Crohn's disease, ulcerative colitis, ischemic colitis, or infection with other intestinal pathogens, such as EIEC, *Salmonella*, *E. histolytica*, *S. aureus*, *Campylobacter*, *Yersinia*, or *Strongyloides*.

Treatment

Antimicrobial therapy consists of metronidazole, 500 mg PO tid for 7–14 days, or vancomycin (Vancocin), 125 mg PO qid for 7–14 days. Patients may be treated with IV metronidazole, 500 mg tid for 10–14 days or until signs and symptoms have resolved, if they are too sick to take PO. Antidiarrheal agents should be avoided, because they may promote toxin accumulation in the gut lumen and may make the patient symptomatically worse.

Relapses should be retreated with a single antibiotic for 3–4 wks. If relapse again occurs, treat with vancomycin and metronidazole PO combination therapy.

Prevention is aimed at effective antibiotic therapy of the infected patient; contact precautions, vinyl gloves, and careful hand washing are required. Disinfectants that kill spores include sodium hypochlorite and possibly iodine disinfectants. Alcohol foams do *not* kill *C. difficile* spores. Prophylaxis is *not* recommended.

WHIPPLE'S DISEASE

Whipple's disease was originally described by George Whipple in 1907. This disease is rare; most patients are white men with a mean age in their 40s at diagnosis. The disease is characterized by infiltrates of macrophages that stain intensely with periodic acid-Schiff (PAS) stain in almost all organ systems.

Pathophysiology

Whipple's disease is a multisystem disorder that commonly affects the small intestine and its lymphatic drainage, but pathologic features are present in most organs of the body. There may be a subtle cell-mediated immune deficit in these patients, but it is unclear whether this predisposes to the disease or is a result of the disease. There is a positive association with HLA B27. The areas of greatest involvement are the lamina propria of the small intestine and its lymphatic drainage, the heart, the valves, and the CNS. The causative organism is a rod-shaped bacillus with a cell wall consisting of a trilaminar membrane, which stains PAS-positive. The organism has *never* been cultured, but it has been seen by light and electron microscopy and has been identified using molecular genetic techniques. It is now known as *Tropheryma whippelii*. The organism may actually be intracellular and has been found in a variety of cells, including epithelial cells, immune cells, and smooth muscle cells.

Clinical Manifestations

The onset of disease is usually insidious, and migratory arthralgias involving the proximal joints usually precede diarrhea by years. Symptoms include weight loss, diarrhea, arthralgia, abdominal pain, GI bleeding, and CNS complaints. Diarrhea may be watery or steatorrheic. Signs include weight loss, hypotension, lymphadenopathy, skin pigmentation, fever, edema, glossitis, abdominal mass or tenderness, ascites, splenomegaly, and an abnormal neurologic exam. Neurologic signs are a late finding and can involve personality changes, hyperreflexia, paresis, dementia, ataxia, and myoclonus. Cardiac involvement is rare at presentation, but CHF is a common terminal event in untreated disease. Sudden cardiac death, atrial fibrillation, and other arrhythmias have also been reported.

Diagnosis

The diagnosis should be considered in anyone with arthralgias, diarrhea, abdominal pain, and weight loss, *especially* if the arthralgias preceded the other symptoms. Small bowel biopsy is the initial investigation of choice, usually by endoscopy. Pathology must be sent for PAS staining, and electron microscopy for *T. whippelii* is diagnostic.

Differential Diagnosis

These patients initially frequently undergo rheumatologic workup to rule out rheumatoid arthritis and seronegative spondyloarthropathy. Also, SLE, sarcoidosis, Addison's disease, celiac disease, inflammatory bowel disease, and giardiasis are considered in the differential.

Treatment

If CNS symptoms are present, then ceftriaxone (Rocephin), 2 g IV bid, plus streptomycin, 1 g IV qd for 2 wks, should be given. After this, the patient should receive TMP-SMX DS PO bid for 1 yr. If the patient has no CNS involvement at presentation, then benzyl PCN may be substituted for ceftriaxone. CNS relapses have been treated with chloramphenicol, 2 g PO qd for 1 yr, although there are no studies supporting this treatment. Some patients have been treated with PCN V, 250 mg PO qid for 1 yr, whereas others have been treated with Bactrim DS PO bid for 1 yr alone. However, these regimens are not recommended. Symptomatic treatment of specific organ systems should be undertaken as well. One cannot follow the presence of PAS-stained macrophages to monitor response, as these may never go away. Many patients develop clinical relapse years after treatment.

APPENDICITIS

Acute appendicitis may occur at any age but most commonly occurs between the second and third decades of life. The mortality rate from appendicitis has decreased dramatically over the last 60 yrs and is currently <1/100,000 cases. The incidence of the disease is much lower in underdeveloped countries and in lower socioeconomic groups for unclear reasons.

Pathophysiology

Obstruction of the appendiceal lumen leads to inflammation, gangrene, and rupture if no intervention is taken. The rupture may get walled off, forming a local process. If not, the infection may spread to diffuse peritonitis. The two most common sites for loculation are the pelvic recess and the right subhepatic space. Organisms are predominantly colonic microflora, consisting of anaerobes, gram-positive cocci, and Enterobacteriaceae.

Clinical Manifestations

Patients frequently present with vague pain in the upper abdomen or periumbilical area, followed by migration of the pain to the right lower quadrant with development of anorexia, nausea, and vomiting. The patient may have tenderness at McBurney's point, fever, rebound, guarding, and abdominal rigidity. The patient may have the psoas or obturator signs, depending on the location of the appendix and surrounding inflammation. A CBC may reveal leukocytosis.

Diagnosis

The diagnosis is made by history and physical exam and should be considered in any case of lower quadrant abdominal pain. Imaging modalities (e.g., chest x-ray to rule out pneumonia, obstructive series to rule out perforation, and abdominal CT or U/S to visualize the appendix) are useful.

Differential Diagnosis

The differential includes PID, inflammatory bowel disease, mesenteric adenitis, diverticulitis, acute cholecystitis, hepatitis, right lower lobe pneumonia, pyelonephritis, Meckel's diverticulum, tubo-ovarian conditions, and intestinal obstruction.

Treatment

The primary therapy is surgical intervention. Antimicrobial therapy is indicated if rupture is suspected. A variety of regimens are effective. Antibiotics must cover gram-negative aerobic *and* anaerobic bacteria. Ampicillin-sulbactam (Unasyn), 3 g IV q6h, or an equivalent antimicrobial may be used.

DIVERTICULITIS

Pathophysiology

Diverticulitis refers to infection of the diverticula, including extension into adjacent tissues. Obstruction from a fecalith results in inflammation or micropuncture of diverticula, which may lead to confined perforation with epicolic abscess formation, fistula formation, or, less commonly, free perforation with peritonitis. Organisms usually include anaerobes and gram-negative bacilli.

Clinical Manifestations

The patient typically presents with left lower quadrant pain and a change in bowel habits. The patient can have fevers, chills, nausea, and vomiting. Microscopic rectal bleeding occurs in up to 25% of cases. Occasionally, patients can present with signs of perforation, including shock and peritonitis. Lab tests often reveal a leukocytosis.

Diagnosis

The diagnosis is frequently made on clinical grounds. Barium studies should be deferred until the inflammatory process has abated somewhat. Plain films may be helpful to rule out perforation. CT scanning is helpful to evaluate for abscess formation.

Treatment

Diverticulitis is primarily a medical, not surgical, disease. Nonoperative management should be tried for the first few attacks of acute, uncomplicated diverticulitis, including NPO status, IV fluids, and IV antimicrobial therapy. The patient may need percutaneous drainage of any abscess. Antibiotics should be broad spectrum as in peritonitis and appendicitis (see Infections of the Peritoneum: Treatment and Appendicitis: Treatment). Patients who are less ill can be treated with TMP-SMX DS, 1 pill PO bid for 10 days, *and* metronidazole, 500 mg PO bid for 10 days. Ciprofloxacin, 500 mg PO bid, may also be used with metronidazole. Surgical intervention is indicated if the patient does not respond to conservative management in 48–72 hrs or has recurrent attacks at the same location, if there is fistula formation, if obstruction or perforation develops, or if carcinoma is suspected.

PERITONEAL INFECTIONS

Primary Peritonitis

Also known as **spontaneous bacterial peritonitis,** primary peritonitis is almost exclusively found in patients with liver disease and ascites, although it can occur in patients with other causes of ascites, such as CHF and malignancy.

Pathophysiology

The route of infection is usually not apparent but could be from hematogenous spread, transmural migration through the intact GI tract wall from the intestinal lumen, or ascending infection from the female genitourinary tract through the fallopian tubes. Typical organisms include *E. coli, Streptococcus pneumoniae, Klebsiella pneumoniae,* other streptococci, and Enterobacteriaceae. Anaerobes are found in ≤5% of cases. Rare causes include *S. aureus, Chlamydia pneumoniae, Neisseria gonorrhoeae,* and *M. tuberculosis.*

Clinical Manifestations

Manifestations include fever in the majority of patients. Other symptoms may include abdominal pain, nausea, vomiting, diarrhea, encephalopathy, and hepatorenal syndrome.

Diagnosis

Any cirrhotic patient with ascites and fever needs to have spontaneous bacterial peritonitis ruled out. Diagnosis is made by paracentesis, with fluid sent for culture (in blood culture bottles), cell count, and differential. Blood cultures also need to be obtained, as bacteremia may be present in up to 75% of patients with peritonitis from aerobes. The diagnosis is supported if the neutrophil count in the peritoneal fluid is >250. Cases in which the ascites fluid culture is negative do occur frequently. CBC may reveal leukocytosis, but this is not reliable.

Treatment

Treatment is successful in most cirrhotic patients, especially if gram-positive organisms are found and treatment is instituted early in the disease course. Poorer prognosis is associated with renal failure, hyperbilirubinemia, hypoalbuminemia, and encephalopathy. In patients with ascites caused by nephrotic syndrome, the survival rate is >90%. Initial therapy usually consists of a third-generation cephalosporin, such as ceftriaxone, 2 g IV qd, or a broad-spectrum PCN or carbapenem until culture results are back, and then therapy can be tailored to the specific bacteria if one is found. Treatment should continue for 7 days if blood cultures are negative or 2 wks if blood cultures are positive. Alternative antibiotic treatments include the quinolones (e.g., ciprofloxacin, 500 mg PO bid).

Secondary Peritonitis

Pathophysiology

Infection results either from a perforation of the GI tract, resulting in spillage of the intestinal contents into the peritoneum, or from contiguous spread from a visceral infection or abscess (i.e., pancreatitis with infection). Organisms usually include *E. coli,*

Enterobacteriaceae, anaerobes, and *Enterococcus* and, less likely, *Staphylococcus* species, *M. tuberculosis*, and *Pseudomonas aeruginosa*. If the large intestine perforates, *E. coli*, enterococci, *Bacteroides fragilis*, anaerobic gram-positive cocci, and *Clostridium* species are the main bacteria causing infection. In animal models, *E. coli* is responsible for early sepsis, whereas *B. fragilis* is responsible for late abscess formation.

Clinical Manifestations
Manifestations include severe abdominal pain, nausea, vomiting, anorexia, fevers, chills, and abdominal distention. Patients may have abdominal tenderness, hypoactive or absent bowel sounds, rebound, guarding, and abdominal rigidity. Bacteremia is present in 20–30% of cases. CBC usually reveals leukocytosis with a predominance of neutrophils.

Diagnosis
Abdominal series is necessary to rule out free air and obstruction. A chest x-ray to rule out a pulmonary problem is helpful. An abdominal CT or U/S to evaluate for the source of the infection may be required.

Differential Diagnosis
The differential includes any abdominal infection, pelvic infection, inflammatory bowel disease, pneumonia, sickle cell crisis, diabetic ketoacidosis, tabes dorsalis, porphyria, SLE, and uremia.

Treatment
Antimicrobial therapy should be broad spectrum while awaiting culture results and organism identification. Multiple different regimens are effective but must cover *both* gram-negative aerobic and anaerobic organisms, and treatment should continue for ≥5–7 days. Ampicillin-sulbactam, 3 g IV q6h, or a third-generation cephalosporin with metronidazole works well (e.g., ceftriaxone, 1–2 g IV qd, plus metronidazole, 500 mg IV q8h). Surgical management of the source of infection needs to be undertaken with repair of any perforations and removal of necrotic or infected material. Prognosis depends on the patient's age, duration of peritoneal contamination, presence of foreign material (e.g., bile or pancreatic secretions), the primary intraabdominal process, and the microorganisms involved in infection.

Peritonitis Secondary to Indwelling Peritoneal Dialysis Catheters

Peritonitis secondary to indwelling peritoneal dialysis catheters is very common at an average rate of one infection per person undergoing peritoneal dialysis per year. Recurrent peritonitis is a main reason to discontinue continuous ambulatory peritoneal dialysis.

Pathophysiology
Infections usually originate from contamination of the catheter by skin organisms. Infections also occur due to exit site infections, subcutaneous tunnel catheter infections, transient bacteremia, and contamination of the dialysate delivery system during bag exchanges. Organisms are usually *S. aureus*, *Staphylococcus epidermidis*, *Streptococcus* species, *E. coli*, *Klebsiella*, *Enterobacter*, *Proteus*, and *P. aeruginosa*. Less commonly, *M. tuberculosis*, *Aspergillus*, *Nocardia*, and *Candida* species can lead to peritonitis. Gram-positive bacteria account for 60–80% of all isolates.

Clinical Manifestations and Diagnosis
Patients describe abdominal pain, tenderness, nausea, vomiting, fever, and diarrhea. The diagnosis is usually made by analysis and culture of the dialysate. The dialysate is almost always cloudy, and microscopic exam reveals a leukocyte count >10 with a predominance of neutrophils. Gram's stain reveals the organism <50% of the time. Blood cultures are rarely positive. Negative cultures of the dialysate occur in 5–10% of cases.

Treatment
Patients can be treated with intraperitoneal antibiotics, such as vancomycin, and an aminoglycoside or third-generation cephalosporin. (Intraperitoneal dialysis dosages: vanco-

mycin, 1.0 g/L dialysate loading dose, then 25 mg/L dialysate maintenance dose; gentamicin, 0.6 mg/kg body weight in only one dialysate exchange qd; ceftazidime, 250 mg/L dialysate loading dose, then 125 mg/L dialysate maintenance dose.) Most patients show clinical improvement in 2–4 days. If symptoms persist past 96 hrs, reevaluation for the source of the infection should be undertaken to rule out a GI source. If patients are severely ill or blood cultures are positive, then antibiotics can be given parenterally. Depending on the organism and the severity of the illness, patients may need their catheters removed. This is especially true if the infection is due to fungi or multiple organisms; if the patient has persistent skin or tunnel infections, recurrent peritonitis with the same organism, or *P. aeruginosa* peritonitis; or if there is concern for bowel perforation. Prognosis is generally favorable.

INTRAABDOMINAL ABSCESS

Pathophysiology

Intraabdominal abscess is usually a complication of primary or secondary peritonitis, including appendicitis, diverticulitis, biliary tract infection, pancreatitis, perforated peptic ulcers, inflammatory bowel disease, trauma, and abdominal surgery. The location of the abscess generally depends on the site of the primary disease and the direction of dependent peritoneal drainage. Organisms are usually polymicrobial and involve normal gut flora. Frequently, *E. coli* and *B. fragilis* are the dominant aerobe and anaerobe, respectively. Several studies have shown the cause of intraabdominal abscesses to be anaerobes in >50% of all cases. Other organisms found include *Klebsiella*, *Proteus*, *P. aeruginosa*, *S. aureus*, and *Enterococcus*.

Clinical Manifestations

The abscesses may be intraperitoneal, retroperitoneal, or visceral. Characteristically, there is an acute course with high fever, shaking chills, abdominal pain, and localized tenderness. Occasionally, this can be a chronic, indolent disease. Subphrenic abscesses usually accompany chest findings, including costal tenderness and pleural and pulmonary involvement. A CBC may reveal leukocytosis.

Diagnosis

Diagnosis is typically made with U/S or CT scan. CT scan is most accurate and also may allow guidance for drainage. U/S also allows guidance for drainage but with a lower success rate, and it is most suitable for right upper quadrant, retroperitoneal, and pelvic abscesses. Gallium scanning has low sensitivity and is not routinely used.

Treatment

Treatment is dependent on adequate drainage, either surgical or percutaneous, with appropriate antibiotic coverage active against both aerobic and anaerobic bacteria, as in secondary peritonitis (see the section Secondary Peritonitis: Treatment).

Pancreatic Abscess

Pathophysiology

Pancreatic abscesses usually develop as a complication of pancreatitis of any cause. Abscess formation occurs in 1–9% of patients after acute pancreatitis. Organisms are usually *E. coli*, Enterobacteriaceae, enterococci, anaerobes, *S. viridans*, and occasionally *S. aureus*.

Clinical Manifestations

Manifestations are varied. The patient may simply not respond to conservative management or may acutely decompensate after a period of improvement. Usually, patients are febrile with symptoms of pancreatitis. With abscess rupture, there may be signs of peritonitis.

Diagnosis
The diagnosis is usually made with CT scan, as this can image the pancreas more clearly than can U/S. Radionuclide scans may be helpful in differentiating pseudocyst formation from abscess formation.

Treatment
Early drainage is most important, and percutaneous drainage alone is frequently inadequate. Prophylactic antibiotic use early in the course of pancreatitis is ineffective at preventing abscess formation. Antimicrobial therapy is the same as for secondary peritonitis (see Secondary Peritonitis: Treatment) and may be tailored if specific organisms are identified.

Splenic Abscess

Pathophysiology
Splenic abscess is an uncommon lesion, usually developing during the course of bacterial endocarditis due to *S. aureus* or *Streptococcus*. Enterobacteriaceae and anaerobes have also been recovered. Candidal infection also occurs but is rare. Usually, the abscess develops as a metastatic process with hematologic seeding. However, some splenic abscesses do develop from contiguous spread.

Clinical Manifestations
Frequently, the patient describes left upper quadrant abdominal pain, although referred pain to the left shoulder does occur. Splenomegaly, tenderness to palpation, fevers, chills, nausea, and vomiting also occur.

Diagnosis
The diagnosis is made with U/S, CT, or MRI of the spleen.

Treatment
Initial antibiotic therapy should have a broad spectrum of activity and should cover *Staphylococcus*, *Streptococcus*, anaerobes, and gram-negative bacilli. Percutaneous drainage and splenectomy may be necessary.

Pancreatic Infection

Pathophysiology
Usually, infections of the pancreas are complications of pancreatitis and include abscess formation (see the section Pancreatic Abscess), infected necrosis, and cholangitis (see Chap. 7, Infections of the Hepatobiliary System). Infection of necrotizing pancreatitis is common, and the risk is related to the duration and extent of necrosis. Acute pancreatitis is rarely caused by infection, however. Organisms causing infection include *E. coli*, Enterobacteriaceae, enterococci, *S. aureus*, *S. epidermidis*, anaerobes, *Candida* species, *Klebsiella*, *Proteus*, and *Pseudomonas*. Anaerobic bacteria have been reported in 6–16% of cases.

Clinical Manifestations
Infected necrotizing pancreatitis clinically appears no different from sterile pancreatitis. In the patient with severe pancreatitis and fever that are not responding to conservative measures, pancreatic infection needs to be ruled out.

Diagnosis
The diagnosis is made with U/S or CT scan of pancreas. If the presence of infection is uncertain, then CT-guided biopsy (sensitivity, 96%; specificity, 99%) may need to be performed. Blood cultures are usually not positive but should be drawn.

Treatment
Treatment is accomplished by drainage of any infected pseudocyst. Laparotomy with débridement of necrotic pancreatic tissue and purulent material with infected necrosis is indicated. These patients must also receive broad-spectrum antibiotics as in peritonitis (see Primary Peritonitis: Treatment).

KEY POINTS TO REMEMBER

- Bacterial infections of the oropharynx and salivary glands need prompt antibiotic therapy.
- The majority of viral infections are treated symptomatically.
- Patients with suspected esophageal or gastric infections usually need endoscopy.
- Duodenal ulcers = *H. pylori* infection.
- If you think a patient has a food-borne illness, report it.
- The majority of cases of infectious diarrhea are self-limited. Always work up prolonged diarrhea, bloody diarrhea, and profuse diarrhea.
- Do not give antibiotics if the diarrhea is bloody and has no WBCs.
- Do not give antimotility agents if the diarrhea has WBCs or is from *C. difficile*.
- If a patient has diarrhea associated with an antibiotic, stop the antibiotic, then check for *C. difficile*.
- Alcohol foams do not kill *C. difficile* spores.
- Only high-risk patients receive prophylactic antibiotics for traveler's diarrhea.
- Always cover gram-negatives and anaerobes.
- If a patient with cirrhosis and ascites has a fever, then tap him or her to rule out spontaneous bacterial peritonitis.
- Peritonitis from peritoneal dialysis catheters can be treated with intraperitoneal antibiotics if the case is mild. Some infections require removal of the peritoneal dialysis catheter.
- Peritonitis in patients without peritoneal dialysis catheters means that there is likely a leak somewhere; find it and fix it if possible.
- Pancreatic infection is hard to identify, so think about it early and if suspicious, get tissue.
- Intraabdominal abscesses require drainage and antibiotics (cover gram-negatives and anaerobes).
- Most abscesses develop from another infection; always find and fix the source.

SUGGESTED READING

Cohen J, Powderly WG. *Infectious diseases*, 2nd ed. Edinburgh: Mosby, 2004:457–467, 469–475, 477–496, 497–502, 517–528.

Connor DH, et al. *Pathology of infectious diseases*. Stamford, CT: Appleton & Lange, 1997:572–575.

Gorbach SL, et al. *Infectious diseases,* 2nd ed. Philadelphia: WB Saunders, 1998:514–515.

Mandell GL, et al. *Mandell, Douglas and Bennett's principles and practice of infectious diseases,* 4th ed. New York: Churchill Livingstone, 1995:945–1029, 1030–1031, 1934–1955, 1964–1979, 2013–2038, 2070–2077.

Suerbaum S, Michetti P. Medical progress: *Helicobacter pylori* infection. *N Engl J Med* 2002;347:1175–1186.

Walsh JH, Peterson WL. Drug therapy: the treatment of *H. pylori* infection in the management of peptic ulcer disease. *N Engl J Med* 1995;333:984–991.

Wong CS, et al. The risk of the hemolytic-uremic syndrome after antibiotic treatment of *Escherichia coli* O157:H7 infections. *N Engl J Med* 2000;342:1930–1936.

REFERENCES

1. McMahon BJ, Hennessy TW, Bensler JM, et al. The relationship among previous antimicrobial use, antimicrobial resistance, and treatment outcomes for *Helicobacter pylori* infections. *Ann Intern Med* 2003;139(6):463–469.

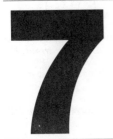

Infections of the Hepatobiliary System

Melissa L. Norton

CHOLECYSTITIS

Pathophysiology

In >90% of cases, cholecystitis is caused by the impaction of gallstones in the cystic duct. Causative organisms usually consist of normal intestinal flora: *Escherichia coli*, *Klebsiella*, *Enterobacter*, *Proteus*, and enterococci, as well as anaerobes. The source of infection is believed to be ascending infection from the intestines.

Clinical Manifestations

Initial obstruction of the cystic duct may be accompanied by epigastric pain, nausea, and vomiting. With persistent obstruction, pain shifts to the right upper quadrant and becomes increasingly severe. Pain may radiate to the right shoulder and scapula. Fever may occur. Repeated chills and fever, jaundice, and hypotension suggest the development of cholangitis. Some patients can present with sepsis or altered mental status (especially in the elderly). The CBC reveals leukocytosis, and patients may have hyperbilirubinemia, mild transaminase elevation, and alkaline phosphatase elevation. Complications of cholecystitis may include empyema, gangrene of the gallbladder, emphysematous cholecystitis, pericholecystic abscess, intraperitoneal abscess, cholangitis, peritonitis, liver abscess, and bacteremia.

Diagnosis

Imaging with either U/S or technetium hepatoiminodiacetic acid scan is diagnostic. U/S may reveal stones, a thickened gallbladder wall, a dilated lumen, and pericholecystic fluid. Technetium hepatoiminodiacetic acid scan may reveal that the cystic duct is occluded and the gallbladder is not visualized. CT scan may pick up some of these findings but should not be used for initial screening. Abdominal MRI is sensitive in detecting gallbladder disease, but it is expensive.

Differential Diagnosis

The differential includes myocardial infarction, perforated ulcer, right lower lobe pneumonia, intestinal obstruction, hepatitis, and right kidney disease.

Treatment

Treatment consists of IV fluid resuscitation and broad-spectrum antibiotic therapy [e.g., ampicillin/sulbactam (Unasyn), 3 g IV q6h, or piperacillin/tazobactam, 3.375 g IV q6h]. The role for antibiotics in uncomplicated cholecystitis remains unclear. Available evidence suggests that periop antibiotics are a helpful adjunct to prevent postop infectious complications. Antibiotic therapy should definitely be given in severely ill patients, patients with any complications, and the elderly. Immediate surgery is indicated for emphysematous cholecystitis, perforation, and suspected pericholecystic abscess. The timing of surgery in uncomplicated cholecystitis is controversial; surgery is usually performed within 6 days of onset of symptoms, although if the patient stabilizes and responds to medical management, the surgery can be delayed for 6 wks.

CHOLANGITIS

Cholangitis is a disease characterized by varying degrees of inflammation or infection involving the hepatic and common bile ducts. Infection can be acute, recurrent, idiopathic, or secondary to pancreatitis or cholecystitis.

Pathophysiology

Obstruction of the common bile duct results in congestion and necrosis of the walls of the biliary tree followed by proliferation of bacteria within the biliary tree. Often, the common bile duct obstruction is due to gallstones. However, it may also be due to tumor, chronic calcific pancreatitis, parasitic infection, or a complication of ERCP. Organisms are similar to those pathogens associated with cholecystitis (see Cholecystitis: Pathophysiology).

Clinical Manifestations

Patients usually have a history of gallbladder disease. The onset is usually acute, with fevers, chills, right upper quadrant pain, tenderness over the liver, and prominent jaundice. The classic presentation of Charcot's triad is fever, right upper quadrant pain, and jaundice. There often is marked leukocytosis, hyperbilirubinemia, elevated alkaline phosphatase, and elevated transaminases. The patient may have lab evidence of DIC. Blood cultures may be positive in >50% of all patients. Complications of cholangitis include bacteremia, shock, gallbladder perforation, hepatic abscess, and pancreatitis.

Diagnosis

U/S can be used to evaluate gallbladder size, the presence of stones, and the degree of bile duct dilatation. ERCP is valuable in evaluating bile duct obstruction, but this is seldom feasible in acutely ill patients.

Differential Diagnosis

The differential includes cholecystitis, hepatic abscess, perforating ulcer, pancreatitis, intestinal obstruction, right lower lobe pneumonia, and myocardial infarction.

Treatment

Treatment consists of IV fluid resuscitation and broad-spectrum antibiotics. Antibiotic therapy consists of a third-generation cephalosporin such as ceftriaxone (Rocephin), 2 g IV q24h, and metronidazole (Flagyl), 500 mg IV q8h, or ampicillin/sulbactam (Unasyn), 3 g IV q6h. Clindamycin (Cleocin), 600–900 mg IV q8h, can be substituted for metronidazole. Antibiotic therapy is mandatory but alone does not sterilize the biliary tree in the face of obstruction. Therefore, prompt decompression of the common bile duct is mandatory, either surgically or percutaneously. The patient may require ERCP for sphincterotomy.

ACUTE HEPATITIS

Acute viral hepatitis is a common disease. HBV, HCV, and HDV can also progress from an acute to a chronic infection, leading to chronic liver disease, cirrhosis, and hepatocellular carcinoma as well as extrahepatic disease, such as polyarteritis nodosa, cryoglobulinemia, and glomerulonephritis.

Clinical Manifestations

Symptoms range from asymptomatic illness to fulminant hepatic failure. The four stages of acute hepatitis include the incubation period, the preicteric phase, the icteric phase, and convalescence. The incubation period varies in presentation, the initial symptoms are nonspecific, and the onset of symptoms may be sudden or insidious.

Malaise and weakness, with anorexia, nausea, vomiting, and vague, dull right upper quadrant pain, are common. This preicteric phase usually lasts 3–10 days. Fever rarely persists into the icteric phase. A minority of patients present with a serum sickness–like illness. This involves fever, rash, and migratory, nondeforming arthritis and is most commonly associated with HBV, although it also occurs with HCV infection. The onset of jaundice and dark urine marks the icteric phase; pruritus is common. Fulminant hepatic failure may develop within 8–12 wks of the onset of symptoms. 30–60% of cases of fulminant hepatic failure are due to HBV. Symptoms include lethargy, fatigue, somnolence, and personality changes, followed by stupor and coma.

There are very few specific physical findings in the preicteric phase. Urticaria may be present if a serum sickness–like syndrome develops. In the icteric phase, jaundice and a slightly enlarged and tender liver may be present. A minority of patients may have a palpable spleen tip. Excoriations on the skin are frequently present. Signs of hepatic encephalopathy and asterixis may be present if fulminant hepatic failure develops.

Large elevations of AST and ALT (>eightfold normal) may occur. The AST is usually higher than the ALT. A mild to large elevation in bilirubin and a mild elevation in alkaline phosphatase and LDH (one to three times normal) are common. The WBC count is normal or slightly low, although a mild lymphocytosis may occur. Platelet count abnormalities are worrisome for the development of DIC with fulminant hepatic failure. The PT is generally normal; any elevation is a serious sign and worrisome for the development of fulminant hepatic failure.

Specific viral types are covered below; please see continued discussion in Diagnosis, Differential Diagnosis, Treatment, and Prevention.

Viral Types

HAV

HAV is an acute, self-limited disease that rarely causes death. There is an incubation period of 15–50 days, with an average of 3–4 wks.

CLINICAL MANIFESTATIONS. The prodromal stage frequently begins as an influenza-like illness with myalgia, headache, fever, and malaise. The incidence of jaundice increases with age, so that <10% of patients <6 yrs old develop jaundice, whereas >80% of patients >15 yrs old develop jaundice. Infection is usually not as severe or long lasting as HBV. The average mortality is 0.4% (4/1000), but the elderly are at higher risk of death. A prolonged cholestasis appearing late in the acute phase and lasting several months may be seen, but acute HAV infection never leads to chronic hepatitis. HAV is spread via the fecal-oral route, although transmission through contaminated food and water has been reported. Fecal shedding is found during both the incubation period and the early symptomatic phase of illness.

DIAGNOSIS. Anti-HAV antibody is detectable in the serum by the resolution of clinical disease. IgM is detectable up to 6 mos after exposure, and IgG conveys protective immunity.

HBV

HBV infection causes more serious disease than does HAV, with a propensity to development of chronic hepatitis.

CLINICAL MANIFESTATIONS. The incubation period is usually 45–180 days, averaging 2–3 mos. Usually, HBV has a more insidious onset and a more prolonged course than does HAV. The occurrence of the serum sickness–like syndrome favors the diagnosis of HBV infection. Jaundice is present in approximately 50% of patients. The average acute case fatality rate is 0.5–1.0%. Transaminase levels may be 20–50 times baseline levels. HBV is spread by parenteral transmission, sexual contact, and perinatal exposure, although in 30–50% of cases, no exposure can be found.

DIAGNOSIS. The diagnosis rests on serologic testing. In acute infection with recovery, HBsAg appears during the incubation period and persists throughout the clinical illness. HBsAb usually becomes detectable 8–9 mos after exposure. In <5% of cases, HBsAg is rapidly cleared, in which case HBsAg will be present in the convalescent period. HBcAb usually appears during the symptomatic period. HBeAg is also present into the symptomatic period, with development of HBeAb several months after exposure. However, 5–10% of patients do not clear HBsAg and become chronically infected.

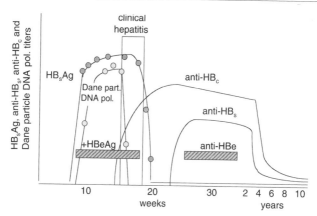

FIG. 7-1. Time after HBV infection. A schematic representation of the typical course of self-limited primary HBV infection. HB_C, hepatitis B core; HB_SAg, hepatitis B surface antigen; part., particle. (Courtesy of Dr. Bradley Stoner, Washington University School of Medicine, St. Louis, Missouri.)

In these patients, HBsAg may be detected for years. HBeAb or HBeAg may be detected, as HBeAg will be present during times of high replication, but HBeAb will be present during periods of low replication. HBcAb will be present (Fig. 7-1).

HDV

HDV, also known as *delta agent*, absolutely requires the presence of HBV for infection and replication. HDV is endemic to the Mediterranean basin, the Middle East, and portions of South America. Outside of these areas, infection occurs most commonly in IV drug abusers and in patients with a history of multiple blood transfusions. This is an uncommon infection in health care workers and male homosexuals.

CLINICAL MANIFESTATIONS. There are two forms of infection: acute HBV and HDV coinfection or, more commonly, acute HDV infection superimposed on chronic HBV infection. Clinically, HDV tends to be a severe illness with a high mortality rate (2–20%). HDV often has a protracted course and frequently leads to cirrhosis. In one series of patients, >50% of patients with chronic HDV developed cirrhosis.

DIAGNOSIS. Many patients test negative for HDV in the acute phase, as antibodies rise in the convalescent stage. Most patients with acute coinfection clear both infections, but superinfection frequently results in chronic HDV infection on top of chronic HBV infection. High titers of HDV antibody indicate ongoing infection.

HCV

Acute HCV infection does occur, but most commonly HCV infection presents as a chronic hepatitis. The primary route of transmission is blood exposure, such as transfusion or IV drug use, but up to 20% of patients have no identifiable exposure. Needle-stick transmission is estimated to be up to 10%. HCV may also be transmitted sexually but at a lower rate than HBV. Perinatal transmission is rare but does occur. The incubation period is 2–26 wks, with an average of 6–8 wks.

CLINICAL MANIFESTATIONS. 20–25% of HCV infections have an acute presentation with icterus, and acute HCV infection has a mortality rate of <1%. The vast majority of patients have no signs or symptoms. Acute HCV has a more insidious onset and a more indolent course than does acute HBV. Transaminase levels may reach 10–20 times normal. Patients with chronic HCV may report generalized fatigue or vague abdominal pain as their only symptom.

DIAGNOSIS. The diagnostic screening test is HCV antibody. The presence of HCVAb suggests prior exposure to HCV but does not convey immunity. Seroconversion may not occur early in illness; only 40% of patients with acute HCV infection have HCVAb. HCVAb is present in >95% of patients with chronic infection.

HEV

Epidemiologically, HEV resembles HAV, with fecal-oral transmission and occurrence as both epidemic and sporadic cases. Most cases occur in developing parts of the world, including India, Southeast Asia, Africa, and Mexico, in association with contaminated drinking water. Outbreaks largely affect young adults and have unusually high mortality rates in pregnant women. Secondary cases in families are uncommon. U.S. cases are usually associated with a history of travel to endemic areas.

CLINICAL MANIFESTATIONS.   Clinical manifestations of HEV are similar to those of HAV. HEV has an incubation period of 2–8 wks, averaging approximately 6 wks. HEV is an acute, self-limited disease, often with a cholestatic picture. The serum alkaline phosphatase tends to be somewhat higher and transaminases tend to be somewhat lower than in other acute hepatitides. Prolonged jaundice can occur, but HEV infection does not lead to chronic hepatitis. The case fatality rate is estimated to be 1–3%, although among pregnant women, it is 5–15%. Illness severity is known to increase with age.

DIAGNOSIS.   Anti-HEV antibodies may be detected, but in the United States, serologic testing is currently only available through the CDC. IgM is usually detectable by the onset of symptoms.

Non-A, Non-B Hepatitis

Non-A, non-B hepatitis is the category used when serologic tests for other viruses are negative. These cases occur sporadically and are transmitted via blood exposure. Previously, HCV accounted for most of these cases before reliable serologic tests were available.

Diagnosis

Patients in whom acute hepatitis is suspected should be tested for anti-HAV IgM, HBsAg, anti-HBc IgM, and anti-HCV antibody. Anti-HAV IgM makes a diagnosis of acute HAV infection. HBsAg makes the diagnosis of HBV but does not distinguish between acute and chronic disease, whereas anti-HBc IgM confirms the diagnosis of acute HBV. If patients have tested positive for HBsAg, the test should be repeated q2mos until HBsAg disappears. If HBsAg is present 4–6 mos after acute infection, the patient is chronically infected. Anti-HDV should be sought only when evidence of HBV infection is found. The presence of anti-HDV suggests coinfection. Titers can help to separate acute from chronic hepatitis. HCV can be diagnosed by anti-HCV antibody but, again, does not distinguish between acute and chronic infection. Anti-HEV testing is rarely necessary in the United States or Western Europe. If all initial serologies are negative, anti-HCV should be rechecked in 6 mos; if positive, the patient should be followed for development of chronic hepatitis.

Differential Diagnosis

The differential includes infectious causes such as EBV, CMV, rubella, rubeola, mumps virus, and coxsackie B virus. These viruses can cause mild liver enzyme abnormalities but are rarely accompanied by jaundice. In immunocompromised hosts, EBV, CMV, HSV, and VZV can cause disseminated infection with hepatic involvement. Yellow fever is a cause of acute hepatitis in Central America, South America, and Africa but only in the United States after recent travel to endemic areas. Bacterial sepsis, mycobacterial disease, rickettsial disease, fungal disease, brucellosis, tularemia, and *Legionella* may all cause hepatitis. Early syphilis can be accompanied by significant serum transaminase elevation (3–8 times normal), although jaundice is rare. Leptospirosis is unusual in the United States; Q fever is associated with prominent constitutional symptoms, and jaundice occurs in only 5% of patients. Noninfectious causes may include many drugs that can cause hepatitis, including acetaminophen, INH, and alcohol. Usually, the AST is elevated out of proportion to the ALT in acute alcohol-related hepatitis. Anoxic liver injury can occur from hypotension, heart failure, or cardiopulmonary arrest. Finally, cholestatic liver disease and other diseases (e.g., Wilson's disease, sickle cell disease, acute Budd-Chiari syndrome, tumor infiltration of the liver, and Gilbert and Dubin-Johnson syndromes) can lead to acute hepatitis–like syndromes.

Treatment

Treatment of acute viral hepatitis is primarily supportive. Most patients do not require hospitalization and can be managed at home with rest, avoidance of alcohol, and avoidance of most medications. Symptomatic therapy for nausea, vomiting, and pruritus may be needed. Patients should be hospitalized if there is evidence of severe dehydration, bilirubin level >15–20 mg/dL, PT prolongation, or any other evidence of hepatic failure. Monitoring should be 1–2 times/wk of transaminases, alkaline phosphatase, bilirubin, and PT for 1–2 wks, and then every other week until all return to normal. Corticosteroids have not been shown to shorten disease course or lessen symptoms; in fact, they may predispose to longer illness and more relapses. Liver biopsy is indicated when the diagnosis of viral hepatitis is in doubt, more than one explanation of acute liver injury exists, if drug-related hepatitis is a possibility, or when specific therapy is being considered. Management of fulminant hepatic failure includes hospitalization, hepatology consultation, vitamin supplementation, FFP and blood products if a GI bleed is evident, and treatment of encephalopathy with lactulose. Transplantation should be considered. If stage IV hepatic coma is present, mortality exceeds 80%, usually from progressive liver failure, GI bleeding, sepsis, or cerebral edema.

Prevention

There is no immunization for HCV, HDV, or HEV. An HAV vaccine has been developed, which is 85–100% effective in preventing disease. Patients at high risk should be vaccinated (e.g., homosexual men, travelers, patients with chronic liver disease, military personnel), and communities with high rates of infection (e.g., American Indian) should routinely vaccinate children. Vaccination doses should be given at 0 and 6–18 mos. HAV Ig can be given to travelers to intermediate- and high-risk areas and to exposed individuals and close contacts of those individuals within 2 wks postexposure. HAV Ig is not indicated for casual contacts. Anti-HAV IgG is present in vaccinated individuals.

Immunization against HBV should be given to patients with multiple anticipated transfusions, IV drug abusers, homosexual men, and family members or sexual contacts of all HBsAg carriers, as well as to health care workers. The CDC recommends vaccination of all infants and sexually active adolescents. High-risk individuals should be screened before immunization to avoid vaccinating patients who are chronic carriers or have already recovered from infection. Anti-HBs IgG is present in vaccinated individuals.

CHRONIC HEPATITIS

Chronic viral hepatitis is defined as the presence of liver inflammation persisting for ≥6 mos and associated with HBV, HCV, HDV, or non-A, non-B infection. Information on diagnosis and treatment is discussed separately under Viral Types. Please see Acute Hepatitis: Prevention for information on prevention. Early referral to a hepatologist for evaluation is recommended.

Clinical Manifestations

Signs and symptoms span a wide spectrum, from asymptomatic patients who are discovered by lab test abnormalities to patients with mild nonspecific symptoms to patients with reactivation and severe or fulminant disease. Occasionally, patients may initially present with polyarteritis nodosa (HBV), glomerulonephritis (HBV, HCV), mixed cryoglobulinemia (HCV), or porphyria cutanea tarda (HCV).

Physical exam findings may include spider angiomata, hepatomegaly, splenomegaly, ascites, jaundice, gynecomastia, testicular atrophy, asterixis, and loss of body hair. Lab data for HBsAg, anti-HBs, anti-HBc, HBeAg, anti-HBe, anti-HCV, HDV antigen, and anti-HDV should be assessed. Histologic confirmation is necessary to document the presence and severity of disease. Histologic severity of disease is an important prognostic indicator for survival. Transaminases, bilirubin, and alkaline phosphatase levels should all be ascertained. A PT and albumin level should be checked to monitor synthetic function.

Viral Types

Chronic HBV

Chronicity occurs in 5–10% of adults with acute HBV. Susceptibility to chronicity is increased in the immunosuppressed and coincidental infection with HCV or HDV. Treatment of chronic HBV infection is interferon alfa, 5 million units SC qd for 16 wks or, alternatively, 8–10 million units SC three times/wk for 16–24 wks. Approximately one-third of patients respond with sustained loss of replication and with histologic remission. 10% of patients have loss of HBsAg. Use of interferon alfa is restricted to patients with normal synthetic function and elevated transaminases without evidence of decompensated liver disease (no GI bleeding, ascites, or encephalopathy). CBC and liver function tests need to be monitored q2–4wks during therapy. Patients who are HIV negative and those with higher transaminase levels and lower levels of HBV DNA are more likely to respond to therapy. Several nucleoside analogs have an inhibitory effect on HBV replication and are currently being studied. Lamivudine (Epivir, Epivir-HBV) has been shown to decrease HBV DNA levels in both posttransplant reactivation HBV and in chronic HBV. Some patients develop resistance to lamivudine therapy. Combination therapy is currently being studied. Liver transplantation is a possibility, but infection posttransplant does occur.

Chronic HCV

Patients are frequently asymptomatic and are identified by giving blood or at the time of abdominal surgery. Patients also present with end-stage liver disease. Treatment consists of interferon alfa, 3 million units SC three times/wk for 12–18 mos, but results may be short lived. The response to interferon alfa therapy is variable, but results in a short-term study showed a response rate of 30–50%. Predictors of poor response include cirrhosis, male gender, advanced age, and the presence of HCV genotype 1a or 1b. PO ribavirin has been shown to reduce transaminase and HCV DNA levels, but these were not sustained. Studies have shown an improved response to combination therapy than to monotherapy alone. Combination therapy is currently being used as standard treatment. Pegylated interferon alfa has a longer half-life and duration of therapeutic activity than interferon alfa and has been approved by the U.S. FDA for the treatment of chronic HCV. Treatment results in a higher rate of response than with interferon alfa alone. If disease progresses with no response to treatment, liver transplantation is the only treatment option, but the HCV may reinfect the graft.

Chronic HDV

Chronic HDV occurs only in the presence of chronic HBV. Diagnosis is made by persistence of HDV antigen in the liver or anti-HDV titers. The incidence of chronicity is <5% in coinfection but >50% in superinfection. Therapeutic trials have not uncovered a treatment for chronic HDV infection. The success of interferon alfa is limited, and years of treatment may be required for any response. Persistence of virus after transplantation is also a problem.

Differential Diagnosis

The differential diagnosis includes autoimmune hepatitis, alpha$_1$-antitrypsin deficiency, hemochromatosis, Wilson's disease, primary biliary cirrhosis, primary sclerosing cholangitis, granulomatous hepatitis, SLE, and drug-induced chronic hepatitis. Alcoholic liver disease is in the differential as well.

GRANULOMATOUS HEPATITIS

Granulomas in the liver are a manifestation of a broad range of disease processes. Usually, they reflect a systemic granulomatous disease (approximately 75%). Patients can present with abnormal liver tests but remain asymptomatic, or they may present with nonspecific symptoms such as fever, malaise, anorexia, or even jaundice.

Diagnosis

Diagnosis is based on liver biopsy.

Differential Diagnosis

The differential includes mycobacterial disease (tuberculous and nontuberculous), lepromatous leprosy, brucellosis, tularemia, granuloma inguinale, melioidosis, listeriosis, cat-scratch disease, Q fever, syphilis, histoplasmosis, coccidioidomycosis, candidiasis, CMV, EBV, viral hepatitis, schistosomiasis, visceral larva migrans, fascioliasis, *Capillaria hepatica*, and several noninfectious causes. The noninfectious causes include sarcoidosis, hypersensitivity diseases (erythema nodosum, drug reactions), primary liver disease (primary biliary cirrhosis), neoplasms (Hodgkin's disease), host defense defects (hypogammaglobulinemia), temporal arteritis, idiopathic granulomatous hepatitis, ulcerative colitis, Crohn's disease, and allergic granulomatosis.

Treatment

Treatment is directed at the underlying cause, if known. If no cause can be identified, consider treatment with antituberculous drugs. If there is no clinical response to antituberculous drugs after 2 mos of treatment, discontinue and consider corticosteroid treatment.

HEPATIC ABSCESS

Bacterial abscesses of the liver are relatively uncommon and are usually associated with biliary tree obstruction or GI tract infection. Pyogenic abscesses may also occur in patients with chronic granulomatous disease and sickle cell anemia.

Pathophysiology

Infections are frequently polymicrobial. The majority of abscesses have enteric gram-negatives, including *E. coli* and Enterobacteriaceae, as well as anaerobes, such as *Bacteroides* species. *Staphylococcus aureus* occasionally causes abscess formation, and *Yersinia enterocolitica* and *Candida* species rarely do.

Clinical Manifestations

Fevers and chills of days' to weeks' duration occur with right upper quadrant pain and possibly pleuritic symptoms, depending on the location of abscess. Over half of all patients have tender hepatomegaly. Jaundice is not present unless ascending cholangitis is the cause of the abscess or unless there is extensive involvement with multiple hepatic abscesses. Blood cultures may be positive in up to half of patients. The alkaline phosphates level is usually elevated.

Diagnosis

U/S, CT, and MRI are all highly sensitive techniques. Technetium sulfur colloid liver scans are capable of detecting 85% of lesions ≥ 2 cm. Lab tests usually reveal an elevated alkaline phosphatase, mild elevations in the transaminase levels, and leukocytosis.

Treatment

Drainage of the abscess is important and may need to be repeated several times, particularly if there are multiple lesions. Drainage can frequently be done percutaneously. Broad-spectrum antibiotics are indicated. Traditionally, ampicillin (Principen, Totacillin), 2 g IV q6h; metronidazole (Flagyl), 500 mg IV q8h; and an aminoglycoside are used, although ampicillin-resistant gram-negative bacilli are increasing; thus, metronidazole, 500 mg IV q8h, and a third-generation cephalosporin such as ceftriaxone, 2 g IV q24h, may be substituted. Some case reports have demonstrated that antibiotics alone may work without drainage, but this is not currently recommended. Antimicrobial therapy should last ≥ 4 wks. If the patient's fever does not abate after 2 wks of percutaneous drainage and antibiotics, then surgical drainage should be undertaken. Surgery is required for loculated or highly viscous abscesses, as these cannot be drained percutaneously.

AMEBIC ABSCESS

Amebic abscesses complicate approximately 3–9% of cases of amebic colitis and may occur months to years after a case of amebic colitis. Over 90% of cases occur in men.

Pathophysiology

Infection is caused by *Entamoeba histolytica*.

Clinical Manifestations

Clinical differentiation between amebic and pyogenic liver abscess is difficult. Often, patients with amebic abscess have a history of diarrhea and may lack spiking fevers. Frequently, amebic abscesses are solitary and occur in the right lobe of the liver.

Diagnosis

The workup is the same as with pyogenic abscess, but because this is not a purulent lesion, gadolinium scans do not show increased uptake. Percutaneous aspiration is recommended to rule out pyogenic abscess (typically amebic abscess yields a brown fluid that is sterile without foul odor). The diagnosis is typically made by finding *E. histolytica* by microscopy or aspirate of the wall of the abscess.

Treatment

Treatment consists of metronidazole, 750 mg IV or PO q8h for ≥10 days. Therapeutic aspiration has been debated and is usually reserved for patients with extremely large abscesses to decrease the risk of rupture (12–30% mortality with rupture). Paromomycin (Humatin), 500 mg PO tid for 7 days, or diloxanide, 500 mg PO tid for 10 days, may also be needed to remove luminal amebic cysts from the GI tract.

KEY POINTS TO REMEMBER

- Uncomplicated acute cholecystitis should be treated with surgery ± antibiotics.
- Ascending cholangitis needs antibiotics *and* drainage. Always cover gram-negative and anaerobic bacteria.
- Treatment for acute hepatitis is supportive.
- The major complications of acute hepatitis are chronic hepatitis and fulminant hepatic failure.
- Vaccines are available for HAV and HBV.
- There is not a lot of treatment available for chronic hepatitis, so refer your patients to a hepatologist for evaluation early.
- Pyogenic abscesses need to be drained, but amebic abscesses do not (unless they are big).

REFERENCES AND SUGGESTED READINGS

Cohen J, Powderly W, eds. *Infectious diseases*, 2nd ed. Edinburgh: Mosby, 2004:529–553.

Connor DH, et al., eds. *Pathology of infectious diseases*. Stanford, CT: Appleton & Lange, 1997:365–382, 1131–1132.

Fauci AS, et al., eds. *Harrison's principles of internal medicine*. New York: McGraw-Hill, 1998:1677–1692, 1696–1704, 1176–1179, 1725–1736.

Gorbach SL, et al., eds. *Infectious diseases*, 2nd ed. Philadelphia: WB Saunders, 1998:834–883, 884–890.

National Institutes of Health. NIH consensus statement on hepatitis C: 2002. *NIH Consensus and State-of-the-Science Statements* 2002;19(3).

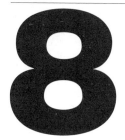

Urinary Tract Infections

Michele C. L. Cabellon

ASYMPTOMATIC BACTERIURIA

The screening and treatment of asymptomatic bacteriuria have been topics of debate among physicians. Overall, it is generally believed that screening is of little value except for two particularly high-risk groups. The first group is pregnant women, who should be screened during the first trimester and then every month after that if the initial culture is positive. The second group is patients undergoing urologic surgery, who have a high chance of becoming bacteremic after instrumentation. Many of the studies surrounding this issue have been done on elderly institutionalized patients who are the population with the greatest incidence of bacteriuria.

Bacteriuria may be as high as 25–50% and 15–35% in institutionalized women and men, respectively. The incidence increases with increased disability in patients. Although it may be difficult to ascertain symptoms from some of these patients, some studies have suggested that GU symptoms often do not correlate with episodes of bacteriuria. Also, despite some conflicting studies, there have been no good data to support that asymptomatic bacteriuria has any negative effects on long-term morbidity and mortality.

Overall, it is not recommended to treat these elderly institutionalized patients with antibiotics. Clinical judgment should prevail in deciding treatment when GU symptoms are present or when systemic symptoms of infection are prevalent, such as fever or mental status changes. A negative urine culture helps in pinpointing a source of infection, but a positive urine culture may or may not be helpful in distinguishing the cause. If antibiotics are used, a posttreatment urine culture is not needed, because the chance of recurrent bacteriuria is high. More studies need to be done in ambulatory populations to extrapolate these findings to other patients.

ACUTE UNCOMPLICATED BACTERIAL CYSTITIS IN WOMEN

UTIs are the second most common infectious cause of physician visits and use of prescription antibiotics. Most are limited to the lower urinary tract but may lead to pyelonephritis and bacteremia. The definition of uncomplicated cystitis according to the guidelines by the Infectious Diseases Society of America (IDSA) is the presence of urinary symptoms, including dysuria, frequency, or urgency, in the setting of bacteriuria in adult nonpregnant women. Diabetic patients are not included in this classification. Male patients are more likely to have UTI in the first 3 mos of life, but thereafter female patients have a much higher incidence.

Pathophysiology

Cystitis is almost always an ascending infection. Colonization of the periurethral area precedes infection and may persist between episodes. The colonizing bacteria ascend into the bladder along the mucosal sheath after either mechanical introduction or sexual activity. Fimbriae play a key role in bacterial adherence to the bladder mucosa.

There is actually a very narrow spectrum of common bacteria as the cause for uncomplicated UTIs. *Escherichia coli* accounts for approximately 80%, with *Staphylo-*

coccus saprophyticus as the second most common at 5–15%, occurring mostly in younger sexually active women. The remainder of infections are usually due to other gram-negative enterics, such as *Klebsiella* or *Proteus* species. Other bacterial causes are rare and usually should only be considered if the patient has recurrent UTIs or does not respond to first-line therapy.

Many of the most common risk factors associated with increased UTI are related to sexual intercourse, especially in younger women. Sexual intercourse in itself is a risk, due to the ease of introducing vaginal organisms into the urinary tract. Other factors include delayed postcoital micturition and the use of contraceptive devices such as diaphragms and spermicides, which may irritate the mucosa around the urethra. A history of a recent UTI puts women at a higher risk, and this is usually due to reintroduction of bacteria into the urinary system rather than a recurrence from the previous infection.

Clinical Manifestations

The usual symptoms of acute cystitis are dysuria, urgency, and frequency. A patient may have one or all of these. Other, less common symptoms may be nausea, vomiting, and suprapubic discomfort. These may also be the presenting symptoms of urethritis secondary to gonorrhea or *Chlamydia* infection or vaginitis due to yeast or *Trichomonas*. Thorough questioning about sexual history and vaginal discharge is warranted to help distinguish the appropriate diagnosis in these patients. Low-grade fever may occur but is usually absent. The patient may have suprapubic tenderness on physical exam.

Diagnosis

Every evaluation starts with a general physical exam, and a pelvic exam with a wet prep and vaginal cultures should be strongly considered if the history gives any question to the diagnosis. Usually, a urine dipstick is the initial and may be the only urine exam needed to make the diagnosis. Depending on the dipsticks used and the existing literature, leukocyte esterase has anywhere from 75 to 96% sensitivity for detection of pyuria. With the narrow spectrum of bacterial causes, you can be fairly confident in treating an uncomplicated UTI with a positive dipstick and no further studies. No urine culture is necessary in this instance.

If there are symptoms suggestive of a UTI but the urine dipstick is negative for leukocytes, a UA with microscopic analysis may be sent. Vaginal abnormalities are then a bigger possibility and must be ruled out. A urine culture may be considered if there are still strong suspicions for a UTI. A culture with growth of >100,000 colony-forming units per HPF is very specific (>99%) for UTI; however, sensitivity is quite low (approximately 50%). Suggestions have been made that as few as 1000 organisms in the setting of pyuria may be a reasonable standard for presumptive treatment.

Suprapubic aspiration of urine is another means of diagnosing UTI. Although this procedure is rarely performed, any bacteria identified by this method should be considered significant and treated.

Differential Diagnosis

Dysuria caused by bacterial cystitis should be distinguished from dysuria due to vulvovaginitis. The dysuria in vulvovaginitis tends to be external in nature and may be accompanied by a vaginal discharge. Urethritis due to chlamydial, gonococcal, or HSV infection needs to be considered as well in sexually active patients.

Treatment

The goal of treatment is to eradicate infection and limit morbidity with minimal toxicity. According to the IDSA guidelines, TMP-SMX (Bactrim), 160 mg/800 mg PO bid, as **3-day therapy** is the current standard of treatment. This was derived from available evidence through randomized, controlled trials. A metaanalysis of two studies comparing 3-day vs 7-day therapy with TMP-SMX revealed the same bacteriuria eradication rates in both groups. Although the 3-day group had a slightly higher recurrence rate of bacteriuria, the 7-day group had greater adverse effects from the treatment, such as rash or yeast infections.

Trimethoprim alone (100 mg PO bid) and the fluoroquinolones (ciprofloxacin, 500 mg PO bid) are believed to be equivalent therapies for alternative 3-day treatment if there is a reason sulfa cannot be used (e.g., allergy). Trials looking at ciprofloxacin (Cipro) and norfloxacin have shown excellent eradication rates with the 3-day regimen. It is recommended that fluoroquinolones not be used for first-line therapy to help protect against bacterial resistance to the drugs and also due to their expense.

Other possible alternative therapies include beta-lactams and nitrofurantoin (Macrodantin). Beta-lactams have been shown to be less effective therapy as 3-day regimens and are not recommended unless the bacteria has known susceptibility to the drug. Nitrofurantoin has been shown to have decreased eradication rates when compared to TMP-SMX on a 3-day regimen. It is suggested that a 7-day course is given if this drug is chosen as therapy, although there are few studies to support this.

Follow-Up

No follow-up visit or posttreatment urine culture is recommended unless the patient is still experiencing symptoms during treatment or the symptoms recur. It can be expected that >90% of cases of bacteriuria will be eradicated with initial treatment. There is a low risk of recurrence if treated by the above guidelines.

UTIs IN MEN

Young Men

UTIs in young men are rare, but they do not all indicate an anatomic abnormality, as was once believed. There are definite risk factors that increase the chances of men developing acute cystitis. Lack of circumcision increases the area of possible colonization with organisms. Insertive anal intercourse in both homosexual and heterosexual men increases exposure to *E. coli*. A female sexual partner with vaginal colonization of uropathogenic organisms may also increase the man's chances of developing a UTI.

Pathophysiology

Pathogens are generally the same as those responsible for UTI in women. *E. coli* causes >50% of all cases, with *Proteus, Providencia, Klebsiella*, and other gram-negative enterics causing the rest. Gram-positive cocci, particularly *Enterococcus* and *Staphylococcus* species, may also be uncovered as pathogens in up to one-fifth of infections.

Clinical Manifestations

Symptoms are generally the same as in women, with dysuria, urgency, and frequency being the most common. The patient may present with suprapubic or flank pain. A penile discharge is more suggestive of urethritis, but this may be associated with cystitis.

Diagnosis

A UA and urine culture are recommended before treatment in all male patients with urinary symptoms. If the patient is presenting for the first time with these symptoms, no further evaluation is needed to examine the patient's urinary tract. It is generally accepted that imaging studies can be saved for patients with recurrent UTI or for those who do not respond to treatment. Male patients who appear to have pyelonephritis also may be considered for imaging.

Differential Diagnosis

The differential diagnosis includes urethritis, nephrolithiasis, and prostatitis as the most common. STDs should be screened for if appropriate. Pyelonephritis can be a complication of simple cystitis. Other infections of the genitalia, such as epididymitis, usually do not present like cystitis, but they also must be remotely considered.

Treatment

Most male patients can be treated with a 7-day course of antibiotics. Three-day shortened courses are not recommended, as they have not been shown to be as effective as in women. Antibiotic choice is the same as for women: TMP-SMX, 160 mg/800 mg PO bid, as the first-line agent. Trimethoprim alone, 100 mg PO bid, or a fluoroquinolone (e.g., ciprofloxacin, 500 mg PO bid) can be used if unable to use sulfa drugs due to allergy. No follow-up culture is recommended unless there is a recurrence of symptoms.

Elderly Men

Elderly men have a much higher incidence of anatomic abnormalities, with benign prostatic hypertrophy being the most common. This makes them somewhat more susceptible to UTI, but the initial evaluation for an elderly patient is no different from that for younger men, as stated in the section Young Men. The causal organisms are similar and treatment identical. The threshold for assessment of urinary outflow tract obstruction should be low for an elderly man presenting with recurrent symptomatic bacteriuria.

COMPLICATED UTIs

When talking about complicated UTIs, a wide range of clinical syndromes are encompassed, including urosepsis. This definition involves patients with anatomic or functional abnormalities, metabolic problems, or immunocompromised states, and also unusual pathogens.

Pathophysiology

The pathogens responsible for UTIs in these types of patients are often more broad than those seen in normal patients with simple cystitis. Many of these infections are polymicrobial. If the patient has been hospitalized many times or has been exposed to antibiotics, resistant organisms are more likely.

Clinical Manifestations

Patients generally describe the typical urinary symptoms seen in uncomplicated infections, such as dysuria, urgency, and frequency. In addition, these types of patients are more likely to have generalized symptoms, such as fatigue, nausea, vomiting, or headache, and these may be present without the urinary clues. A high suspicion must be kept in order not to miss the UTI.

Diagnosis

A pretreatment urine culture and Gram's stain must be obtained in all of these patients due to the broad range of possible organisms. The culture may show polymicrobial involvement, and it is important to cover all organisms identified, even if one is predominant. If the patient presents with pyuria and all urine cultures are negative, fastidious organisms would be a consideration, and the lab should be notified to test AFB stains and hold cultures for longer periods.

Differential Diagnosis

The differential is identical to that for uncomplicated UTI, including vaginitis and other gynecologic problems in women and prostatitis in men. Also, more serious processes must be considered, including renal stones and abscesses. Again, any intraabdominal process may present in a similar fashion as a complicated UTI, especially if nausea and vomiting are involved.

Treatment

A 10- to 14-day course of antibiotics is recommended as initial therapy. The important thing to remember is that broad coverage is needed, pending pathogen identification. Fluoroquinolones are an excellent choice if the patient is well enough to be treated as an outpatient. For hospitalized patients who need IV antibiotics, there are several choices: ampicillin, 1 g IV q6h, plus gentamicin, 1 mg/kg IV q8h, imipenem/cilastatin, 0.5–1 g IV q6–8h, piperacillin/tazobactam (Zosyn), 3.375 g IV q6h, or cefepime (Maxipime), 1 g IV q12h, are all appropriate to provide broad gram-negative coverage, including for *Pseudomonas* species. Staphylococcal infection is also a concern, so vancomycin, 1 g IV q12h, is the likely agent of choice for empiric coverage until culture results are available. If *Enterococcus* or *Pseudomonas* species are recovered from culture, longer courses of antibiotics (14 days) are preferred. Any foreign body, such as stents that are in place, must be removed for complete resolution of the infection. A follow-up urine culture 1–2 wks posttherapy is recommended.

RECURRENT UTIs IN WOMEN

Many women experience a recurrence of a UTI within several months despite adequate treatment initially. At least 90% of the time, these are instances of reinfection rather than recurrence. Very few patients have urinary tract abnormalities. Most often, recurrent UTIs are associated with sexual intercourse.

Pathophysiology

Sexual intercourse in itself is a risk, and urinary symptoms usually occur 12–48 hrs postcoital. Spermicide use, diaphragm use, and lack of hormone replacement therapy in postmenopausal women all put the patient at risk by allowing alteration of the vaginal flora, increasing *E. coli* colonization. Other risk factors include urinary and fecal incontinence, excessive bowel movements, incomplete bladder emptying, diabetes mellitus, any GU abnormality including post-childbirth changes (e.g., cystocele), age >65 yrs, and immunocompromised state.

Clinical Manifestations

Symptoms are the same as in simple cystitis, such as dysuria and frequency. If symptoms are identical to prior episodes of UTI in a particular patient, more confidence can be made in the diagnosis of recurrent UTI.

Diagnosis

All patients should undergo pelvic exam to look for vaginal irritation and to assess for prolapse of any organs. Rectal tone and perineal sensation should also be assessed. Costovertebral angle tenderness should be ruled out. Checking a postvoid residual should be considered if indicated from the history in older patients.

UA should reveal pyuria, which is 80–90% sensitive and 50–75% specific for infection. Microscopic hematuria may also be seen. A urine culture should be obtained the first few times the UTI recurs to document pathogens. If the cultures show a different organism each time or if they are polymicrobial, vesicovaginal fistula should be considered, along with possible self-injection if all other diagnoses are excluded. Negative urine cultures with negative nitrites on dipstick suggest an alternate diagnosis from UTI.

Differential Diagnosis

The differential diagnosis for recurrent UTI is broad but includes vaginitis, vulvovaginitis (possibly due to excess washing), detrusor muscle instability, pelvic muscle dysfunction, interstitial cystitis, or even superficial carcinoma *in situ*. The physical exam should help to distinguish some of these conditions from each other.

Treatment

Most of these infections can be treated like an uncomplicated UTI with a 3-day course of therapy. Longer 7-day courses of antibiotics are recommended for diabetic patients and the elderly. Long-term treatment can consist of three different methods. In patients in whom recurrence is obviously related to sexual intercourse, treatment can consist of postcoital self-administration of an oral antibiotic, usually TMP-SMX, 80 mg/400 mg, in a single-strength dose. If recurrence is very frequent, daily or every-other-day prophylaxis with single-strength TMP-SMX can be used. The third method is for very reliable patients who can monitor their own symptoms and direct their own treatment. These patients are given urine dipsticks and can self-administer a 3-day course of antibiotics. If the symptoms do not resolve in 2 days, they can then alert their physicians for further management.

Other possible therapies for relief from recurrent UTI include changing the form of contraception the patient is using and more frequent voiding, especially during the immediate postcoital period. For postmenopausal women, estrogen cream for the vaginal mucosal areas is very helpful for restoring lactobacilli to the flora, even if the woman is already on oral hormone replacement. Cranberry juice ingestion has also been shown in a randomized, controlled trial to help prevent infection by producing hippuric acid, a bactericidal agent that concentrates in the bladder.

A urology referral should be made for any suspected anatomic abnormality, especially if the patient is experiencing gross hematuria. Urinary stones, continued dysuria despite negative cultures, or any other unexplainable symptom should also be considered for referral.

ACUTE PYELONEPHRITIS IN WOMEN

The definition of acute pyelonephritis according to the IDSA guidelines is the presence of flank pain or fever with urinary symptoms in young, nonpregnant women with normal urinary tract anatomy.

Pathophysiology

Pyelonephritis most frequently results from an ascending infection from the lower GU tract. The pathogens responsible for acute pyelonephritis are very similar to those for acute cystitis. *E. coli* is the cause in >80% of cases, but these may be particularly "uropathogenic" strains that have adaptations such as pili and enzymes that help them adhere to the uroepithelium, allowing them to ascend. Other gram-negative enteric pathogens are also common, and gram-positives, such as *Enterococcus*, may also be involved.

Clinical Manifestations

The main symptoms patients may describe that differentiate pyelonephritis from cystitis are flank pain and fever. They may also have or have had dysuria, frequency, or urgency. Nausea and vomiting may be present. If the infection is advanced, signs of sepsis may be evident with hypotension and tachycardia. Physical exam should look for costovertebral angle tenderness in addition to pain along the flank or anywhere throughout the abdomen.

Diagnosis

All patients should have a urine Gram's stain and culture obtained. The Gram's stain provides an early clue for treatment direction, although approximately 20% is negative. The UA should show pyuria, and usually RBCs are also evident. There may be leukocytosis with a left shift. No other tests are recommended for initial workup if this is the patient's first episode of pyelonephritis.

Differential Diagnosis

Despite what might be an obvious-looking clinical picture for pyelonephritis, a complete differential diagnosis should be considered. This should include nephrolithiasis, appendicitis, cholecystitis, pancreatitis, diverticulitis, or even a lower lobe pneumonia. Appropriate tests should be ordered if any of these is a possibility. An incidental lower UTI may be found in addition to one of the above, which may complicate the picture.

Treatment

The consensus by IDSA recommends treatment for 14 days for all cases of pyelonephritis. Analysis of all available randomized, controlled trials concludes that 2 wks of therapy is adequate, and longer treatment shows no benefit. Shorter lengths of therapy (5–7 days) have been postulated and even used by some physicians, but there are no good trials to support this.

There are basically two treatment groups for acute pyelonephritis. For **mild cases** in which patients may have a low-grade fever, may have a normal or mildly elevated WBC count, and are able to tolerate PO intake, treatment may be initiated in the outpatient setting. The recommended first-line antibiotic is a PO fluoroquinolone, usually ciprofloxacin, 500 mg PO bid. TMP-SMX, 160 mg/800 mg PO bid, may also be used if the bacteria are susceptible. One dose of an IV antibiotic is sometimes used as the initiation of treatment—often a third-generation cephalosporin or an aminoglycoside. There are no available data on any benefit of this.

For **severe cases** of pyelonephritis in which the patient has a high fever, leukocytosis, and signs of dehydration or sepsis, or if the patient is pregnant, hospitalization is recommended for IV hydration and antibiotics. In such clinical scenarios, an IV fluoroquinolone alone, a third-generation cephalosporin with or without an aminoglycoside, or an aminoglycoside with or without ampicillin is recommended as first-line therapy. If an *Enterococcus* species is suspected, ampicillin, 1 g IV q6h, with or without gentamicin, 1 mg/kg IV q8h, should be considered. Regimens may be switched to equivalent PO forms when the patient's fever has abated and he or she is able to tolerate PO intake.

If fever or pain continues after 72 hrs on appropriate antibiotics, a repeat urine culture should be obtained to be sure the causal bacteria is being covered, and imaging should be considered. An abdominal CT or renal sonogram should be obtained if perinephric abscess, renal stones, other forms of obstruction, or urinary tract abnormalities are suspected. There is no benefit to imaging all women during the initial evaluation, as the majority of cases are uncomplicated and resolve with initial antibiotics.

Follow-Up

A follow-up urine culture is generally recommended 2 wks after treatment completion to ensure clearing of the bacteriuria. This is for all cases, despite resolution of symptoms.

PROSTATITIS

Prostatitis is a group of syndromes that affects >50% of men in their lifetime. The diagnosis should be considered in any man who reports urinary symptoms, pelvic pain, or sexual dysfunction. There are four main classifications of prostatitis: acute and chronic bacterial (5–10%), nonbacterial (60%), and chronic pelvic pain syndrome (30%). Symptoms and treatment are similar for each group, and it can be a challenge to diagnose which type of prostatitis is present.

Acute Bacterial Prostatitis

Pathophysiology

Acute prostatic infections usually affect young men, aged 20–30 yrs. It can also present in older men who have had their GU tracts recently manipulated. Risk factors are Foley catheter insertion, urinary procedural instrumentation, and unprotected insertive anal intercourse, although there are cases of acute prostatitis without any of these prior circumstances.

The usual causative organisms are similar to those causing UTIs in women. *E. coli* is the most common, accounting for >80% of cases. Other common organisms are *Proteus* and *Providencia* species, with *Klebsiella* and other gram-negatives comprising the remainder. Gram-positives such as staphylococci can also be seen, but they are rare. STDs such as *Chlamydia trachomatis* may also present as prostatitis but are less common.

Clinical Manifestations

Patients describe urinary symptoms, such as dysuria, frequency, and urgency, and may have trouble with obstruction and problems initiating micturition. Low back, rectal, or perineal pain may also be the presenting symptoms. Fever, chills, and myalgias are often present.

Diagnosis

Physical exam reveals a boggy and possibly enlarged prostate that is very tender to the touch. Prostatic massage should not be attempted in this case due to pain and to a possibility of resultant bacteremia. A Gram's stain and urine culture are usually all that is needed to make the diagnosis. These, along with a CBC and blood cultures if the patient has a septic appearance, should be sent on every patient.

Differential Diagnosis

Prostatitis must be discerned from cystitis because the length of treatment is very different. Epididymitis and orchitis may be associated with acute prostatitis or may be seen alone. Noninfectious processes, such as nephrolithiasis, may present in a similar way. Once a rectal exam is performed, it should help make the diagnosis more obvious.

Treatment

A fluoroquinolone, usually ciprofloxacin, 500 mg PO bid, is the antibiotic of choice in treating prostatic infections. Fluoroquinolones have small molecular size, low protein binding, and high lipid solubility, which allow the drugs good penetration into the prostate for the most common pathogens as well as coverage for *Chlamydia* (overall, PCNs and cephalosporins have poor penetration into the prostate). An alternative, if needed for a fluoroquinolone allergy, is TMP-SMX, 160 mg/800 mg PO bid. An IV form of a fluoroquinolone or a third-generation cephalosporin may be used if the patient is unable to tolerate PO intake. The antibiotic may then be altered after culture results are received. Treatment should continue for 2–4 wks. Any GU instrumentation should be avoided, so if the patient is experiencing extreme retention symptoms, a suprapubic catheter may be warranted.

Prognosis is generally good with these patients, and a quick response to antibiotics should be expected. If the infection is left untreated, it may progress to epididymitis or orchitis. Prostatic abscess is a rare complication and needs surgical drainage if present. It may be considered with an extremely high fever and severe acute urinary retention.

Chronic Bacterial Prostatitis

Pathophysiology

Chronic bacterial prostatitis is generally seen in the middle-aged to older population of men. The risk factors are the same as for acute prostatitis. Prostatic calculi are seen in the majority of patients at this age, and one theory is they account for the chronic infection due to microcolonies of bacteria that exist inside the stones.

The same organisms in acute bacterial prostatitis are generally the culprit here as well. *E. coli* is the most common, followed by other gram-negative enteric pathogens.

Clinical Manifestations

The most common presentation is recurrent UTIs with the same organism on urine culture each time. During episodes, patients may describe low back pain, perineal, or testicular pain. They also may have dysuria, ejaculatory pain or hematospermia, or prostatic obstructive symptoms to help with the diagnosis.

Diagnosis

The physical exam is usually not helpful, as the prostate is most often normal in size and texture, and it is not particularly painful. Transrectal U/S of the prostate is also not helpful unless another problem is suspected, such as an abscess. History is the best clue to making this diagnosis.

Traditionally, the four-cup prostatic localization test has been used to attempt to isolate bacteria in the prostate. This entails collecting four urine specimens for analysis: Initial urine stream is collected in the first cup; then mid-urine stream is collected in the second cup; then a prostatic massage is performed, and prostatic secretions are collected in the third cup; and then urine after the massage is collected in the fourth cup. This test was meant to help distinguish urethritis, cystitis, and prostatitis. The initial two cultures must be negative to diagnose prostatitis. There are no good data to support that this test is superior to other methods in diagnosis, despite the fact that the test is uncomfortable and time consuming for both the patient and the examiner. One preliminary study has suggested that a pre– and post–prostatic massage test is just as effective as the four-cup test, with only two samples to collect. Many physicians have now adopted this as their method of diagnosis.

Differential Diagnosis

When encountering multiple recurrent UTIs, one must worry about reinfection, although it would be more common to have several different pathogens in this case. Some other focus of infection higher in the urinary tract must be ruled out, such as chronic pyelonephritis, nephrolithiasis, or a renal abscess. Anomalies of the GU tract or another type of obstructing lesion are also possibilities.

Treatment

Long courses of antibiotics are warranted in chronic bacterial prostatitis. Again, oral fluoroquinolones are the antibiotic of choice (ciprofloxacin, 500 mg PO bid). Alternatives are TMP-SMX or doxycycline. A 6-wk treatment course is recommended initially. If the patient relapses, 3 mos of therapy should be tried. Patients who continue to have symptoms may fare better on chronic low-dose antibiotic suppression. Transurethral prostatectomy is only effective in approximately 30% of cases.

Nonbacterial Prostatitis

Nonbacterial prostatitis is a classification for patients who have the signs and symptoms of chronic bacterial prostatitis, leukocytes in the prostatic fluid, and repeatedly negative urine cultures. Evaluation is the same as for bacterial prostatitis. Many hypotheses have been made regarding the etiology of the prostatic inflammation, and one is that the cause is still infectious but due to agents not detected on typical urine culture, such as *C. trachomatis*, *Mycoplasma* species, *Ureaplasma urealyticum*, *Trichomonas vaginalis*, or a viral cause. This is supported by the fact that many of these cases are in young, sexually active men who have had a history of untreated urethritis, but there is still no good evidence to support this idea.

To treat this condition, a single trial of 4 wks of a fluoroquinolone (ciprofloxacin, 500 mg PO bid) is usually recommended to cover the typical pathogens, but there is no evidence that this is beneficial. Other therapies that have been used are NSAIDs, finasteride (Propecia, Proscar), and alpha-blockers in conjunction with antibiotics. Again, there are no randomized, controlled trials to support this, but there are case reports that some relief may be provided to patients with this regimen.

Chronic Pelvic Pain Syndrome

Pain of the pelvis or perineum is the most prominent symptom of this syndrome. Patients rarely have urinary or prostatic symptoms. Prostate exam is usually normal. Urine cultures are negative, and prostatic secretions do not contain leukocytes. Antibiotics are not indicated here. Reassurance, stress management, analgesics, and muscle relaxants are often used as therapy. Little is known otherwise about the etiology or mechanisms of this syndrome.

EPIDIDYMITIS AND ORCHITIS

Epididymitis

Infection of the epididymis is the result of extension of a more distal infection in the urethra that has spread retrograde. It is most common in young, sexually active men, but it can also be seen in older men who have had Foley catheters inserted or other GU procedures performed.

Pathophysiology

In sexually active patients, the most common causative organisms are sexually transmitted *C. trachomatis* and *Neisseria gonorrhoeae*. In patients >35 yrs or in children, *E. coli* is the most common bacteria responsible. Other gram-negative enteric pathogens are also possible causes if the GU tract has been manipulated.

Clinical Manifestations

Patients describe dull pain and ache in the unilateral affected scrotum. The pain may radiate to the flank. Patients may also report urinary symptoms if they have a concurrent urethritis. They may have a history of a recent urethral discharge.

Diagnosis

The epididymis is swollen and very tender on exam, and lifting the ipsilateral testicle is extremely painful. The epididymis may eventually become a hard mass if untreated. A UA and urine culture should be obtained to identify pyuria and bacteriuria.

Differential Diagnosis

The other main worrisome diagnosis in the differential is testicular torsion. If this is suspected, a testicular U/S should be obtained immediately. Testicular neoplasms usually do not present with pain, but they must still be considered.

Treatment

Treatment for epididymitis depends on how it was suspected to be contracted. In sexually active men, the antibiotic of choice is doxycycline, 100 mg PO or IV q12h, usually for 2 wks. Other types of infections should be treated with a fluoroquinolone. Initial bed rest and scrotal elevation are also recommended.

Orchitis

Acute orchitis is almost always an extension of epididymitis, and the evaluation and treatment are essentially the same. A rare cause of orchitis is the mumps virus. Treatment is symptomatic relief with analgesics. Usually, the problem resolves spontaneously in 7–10 days without residual effects. If the orchitis is bilateral, the patient is at risk for sterility later in life.

UTIs IN DIABETIC PATIENTS

An increased incidence of bacteriuria is seen in patients with diabetes mellitus. In addition, there is also an increased incidence of upper UTIs, some being very severe. It is believed that a major contributing factor is neuropathy of the bladder, which causes decreased sensation of the bladder mucosa and resultant decreased emptying.

Pathogens are generally the same as with nondiabetic patients, with gram-negatives such as *E. coli* and *Klebsiella* species being the dominant organisms. Patients with simple cystitis and no other complicating factors can be treated as outpatients with a 7- to 10-day course of TMP-SMX, 160 mg/800 mg PO bid, with care for patients on PO antihypoglycemics because the antibiotic can rarely potentiate hypoglycemia. Another good alternative is the fluoroquinolones, especially if there is concern for *Pseudomonas*. Any diabetic patient with signs of an upper UTI should be hospitalized and treated initially with appropriate IV antibiotics—usually an extended-spectrum beta-lactam (e.g., cefepime, 1 g IV q12h, or piperacillin/tazobactam, 3.375 g IV q6h) and coverage for *Enterococcus* species with vancomycin, 1 g IV q12h.

Diabetic patients are at greater risk of developing **severe complications** with upper UTIs, such as perinephric abscess, renal papillary necrosis, renal cortical abscess, and emphysematous pyelonephritis and cystitis. If a diabetic patient has signs of pyelonephritis, a plain abdominal film should be considered to evaluate for air in the urinary tract. If any suspicion is present, a CT of the abdomen, which is the test of choice, should be obtained. If emphysematous pyelonephritis is present, immediate surgical attention is needed for emergent nephrectomy. Emphysematous cystitis can be treated adequately with systemic antibiotics.

UTIs IN PREGNANT WOMEN

Pregnant women have increased susceptibility to upper UTIs, which is believed to be secondary to relaxation of the ureters by progesterone. Pyelonephritis increases the chance of premature delivery and low birth weight of the fetus.

All pregnant women with asymptomatic bacteriuria should be treated with antibiotics. Patients should be screened in their first trimester and treated if bacteriuria is present. They should then be screened every month until the delivery for further episodes of infection. Three days of antibiotics are recommended, with amoxicillin, 500 mg PO q8h, nitrofurantoin, 100 mg PO qid, or a PO cephalosporin being an appropriate choice. Any pregnant woman with pyelonephritis should be hospitalized.

URINARY CANDIDIASIS

The treatment of *Candida* species in the urine has been a debated topic. It is generally believed that most cases are due to colonization after urinary tract instrumentation. The IDSA published practice guidelines in 2000 for the treatment of candidiasis, which are summarized here.

Pathophysiology

Three major factors have been identified that increase risk for candiduria. The first and most important is prior urinary tract instrumentation. Foley catheter insertion or other GU invasive procedures provide opportunity to induce yeast into the urinary tract where it can then colonize. Second, recent antibiotic use also is a risk, when normal flora may be eliminated, allowing overgrowth of *Candida* in the area. The third risk is increased age. It appears that elderly patients have a higher incidence of candiduria than do younger patients.

Candiduria is often seen in the ICUs, where almost every patient has a Foley catheter inserted. Candiduria must be viewed more cautiously in these patients, especially in immunocompromised, neutropenic, and kidney transplant recipients, as *Candida* in the urine may be a marker for hematogenous dissemination.

Diagnosis

Candida generally is not a common contaminant in blood cultures but may contaminate urine from a nonsterile sample due to colonization of the external genitalia. In general, a sterile urine specimen should be sent, ideally from an in-and-out catheter. If a culture becomes positive for *Candida*, a repeat culture should be sent to confirm the presence of yeast in the urine.

Treatment

For all patients, discontinuing the Foley catheter if one is in place is the most appropriate therapy for resolution of candiduria. Just changing the Foley catheter to a new one is not enough; this only results in eradication in <20% of patients. Keeping a foreign body in the urinary tract continues to provide a medium for colonization.

In nonneutropenic patients, there has been no shown value of treatment with antifungal medications. One placebo-controlled trial randomized patients to receive 14 days of 200 mg of fluconazole versus placebo. The patients who received fluconazole (Diflucan) had a negative urine culture earlier, but there was no difference in the percentage of eradication of candiduria between the groups 2 wks after the end of treatment.

Current recommendations are to treat symptomatic patients without a bacterial source, neutropenic patients, low-birth-weight infants, renal transplant recipients, and patients about to undergo a GU procedure. Treatment may also be considered in febrile patients with no other source of infection evident except for candiduria. 7–14 days of treatment with fluconazole, 200 mg PO or IV qd, is recommended. Amphotericin B should only be used if the yeast is resistant to fluconazole; 1–7 days of therapy have been used, but there are no specific guidelines on this regimen. Bladder irrigation or washings with amphotericin are generally not useful. If candiduria persists in immunocompromised patients despite therapy, a CT of the abdomen or renal U/S should be considered to rule out kidney involvement or perinephric abscess.

CATHETER-ASSOCIATED UTIs

Urinary catheter–related infections are a large cause of morbidity and mortality. They are one of the most common reasons for gram-negative sepsis. Indwelling catheters predispose patients to infection for a number of reasons. They provide a conduit of entry for bacteria to travel into the urinary tract. This most often occurs between the interface of the external catheter surface and the urethral meatus and is worse in women. Catheters also provide an environment for a biofilm to form. This biofilm is made up of bacteria, salts, bacterial glycocalyces, and Tamm-Horsfall protein, and it provides protection for the bacteria within it from antibiotic contact. Catheters may also result in inadequate emptying of the bladder contents, allowing residual urine to collect.

Some risk factors have been identified that put patients at an even greater risk of infection in the setting of urinary catheterization. The biggest risk is the duration of catheterization. It is well documented that the risk of bacteriuria increases with each day an indwelling catheter remains in place. Women have a greater risk than men of developing an infection, as well as diabetic patients of both sexes. Poor catheter care overall contributes to bacteriuria development.

Pathophysiology

Most patients are catheterized for only a short time. The majority of bacteriuria in these instances is monomicrobial, and most patients display evidence of pyuria. *E. coli* is again the most common pathogen but is only seen in approximately 25% of cases. Any other nosocomial-related organism may be seen, including *Enterococcus* species, *Pseudomonas*, *Klebsiella*, *Enterobacter*, *Proteus*, and *Staphylococcus* species.

Bacteriuria is a common problem in patients with long-term indwelling urinary catheters. There is a 3–10% chance per day of developing bacteriuria. Up to 95% of these are polymicrobial. The causal pathogens are the same as for short-term catheters, plus more rare organisms may be seen, such as *Morganella morganii*. Bacteriuria in long-term indwelling catheters can lead to symptomatic cystitis, pyelonephritis, and other more serious complications such as urinary stones, chronic renal inflammation, urethral fistulae, prostatitis, or even bladder cancer after many years.

Clinical Manifestations

Patients may range from being asymptomatic to having outright septic features. Many with short-term catheters display the typical UTI symptoms of dysuria, urgency, and suprapubic discomfort. Flank pain is common, especially with concurrent renal stones.

Diagnosis

The workup is the same as for acute uncomplicated cystitis initially, with a UA. A Gram's stain and culture of the urine also should be obtained if the patient really is having symptoms. Additional studies, such as imaging of the GU tract, must be considered, depending on the length of catheterization and the risk of complications associated. If the patient looks very toxic, imaging to rule out an abscess or other problem is indicated.

Differential Diagnosis

Concern over pyelonephritis is high, especially with chronic indwelling catheters. Urinary stones, prostatitis, and other intraabdominal processes such as appendicitis must be considered as well. Chronic renal inflammation, such as interstitial nephritis, may also explain pyuria, along with interstitial cystitis.

Treatment

Asymptomatic Bacteriuria

Antibiotics are not indicated for the presence of bacteriuria without urinary symptoms while the catheter is in place. This may only help to select for resistant bacteria. Therapy is indicated for selected high-risk populations: pregnant or neutropenic patients, transplant recipients, or patients undergoing GU surgery.

Symptomatic UTI

For patients with chronic urinary catheters, when systemic signs of infection such as fever present, a thorough look for other infectious sources should be made first. The catheter should be checked for obstruction, and an evaluation for urethral infections and urinary stones should be done. Urine and blood Gram's stain and cultures should be obtained. 7–10 days of therapy with an agent appropriate for complicated UTI should be chosen (see Complicated UTIs: Treatment). The Foley catheter should also be changed due to the potential biofilm that may be present.

Prevention of Catheter-Related Bacteriuria

The main intervention that can be done to prevent bacteriuria is to remove the urinary catheter as soon as possible. It is known that the chance of bacteriuria increases each day the catheter is in place. Using sterile technique and care on insertion of the catheter also helps in prevention. A closed catheter system, which has become the standard of care, greatly diminishes the colonization of the catheter. It is important to keep the system closed, only drawing samples from the ports available for needle collection of urine. Topical antibiotics on the catheter or when applied to the periurethral tissues have not shown to be effective in decreasing bacteriuria. Prophylactic systemic antibiotics are also not indicated for prevention of bacteriuria, in both short-and long-term catheterized patients. Only in patients who are undergoing GU surgery have prophylactic antibiotics been shown to decrease development of UTI.

Other options to indwelling urinary catheters have been considered. Condom catheters for men are available; although there are no randomized, controlled trials, parallel studies have indicated that the incidence of bacteriuria is decreased compared to Foley catheters. On the contrary, these may also lead to high colonization of the periurethral area if not changed at least daily. Intermittent straight catheterization is also an option and has become the standard of care for some types of patients. These also lead to a very high rate of bacteriuria. Some studies have suggested that they are associated with lower rates of symptomatic UTI development, but there are still no good data. Overall, it is recognized that intermittent catheterization 6–8 times/day is a better option than chronic indwelling catheters, and some evidence suggests PO prophylactic antibiotics, such as nitrofurantoin or TMP-SMX, may also be helpful in reducing bacteriuria in these patients.

KEY POINTS TO REMEMBER

- Resist the temptation to treat asymptomatic bacteriuria, unless the patient is pregnant, undergoing a urologic procedure, or immunocompromised in some way.
- Most lower UTIs in women can be treated with a short 3-day antibiotic course.
- Diabetic patients are more susceptible to UTIs and require longer courses of treatment.
- Treatment of *Candida* in the urine has no benefit unless the patient has symptoms with no bacterial source or the patient is immunocompromised. Foley catheter needs to be removed if present.
- The biggest risk factor for UTI associated with Foley catheters is the length of time the catheter is in place; remove all unnecessary catheters as quickly as possible!

REFERENCES AND SUGGESTED READINGS

Armitage KB, Bologna RA, Horbach NS, Whitmore KE. Best approaches to recurrent UTI. *Patient Care* 1999;Jun:38–69.

Collins MM, MacDonald R, Wilt TJ. Diagnosis and treatment of chronic abacterial prostatitis: a systematic review. *Ann Intern Med* 2000;133:367–381.

Lipsky BA. Prostatitis and urinary tract infection in men: what's new; what's true. *Am J Med* 1999;106:327–334.

Lipsky BA, Schaberg DR. Managing urinary tract infections in men. *Hosp Prac* 2000;35:53–60.

Macfarlane MT. *Urology*, 2nd ed. Baltimore: Williams & Wilkins, 1995:119–123.

McCue JD. Urinary tract infections: treatment guidelines for older women. *Consultant* 1997;Aug:2135–2142.

Nickel JC. The pre and post massage test (PPMT): a simple screen for prostatitis. *Tech Urol* 1997;3:38–43.

Nicolle LE. Asymptomatic bacteriuria in the elderly. *Infect Dis Clin North Am* 1997;11:647–662.

Patterson JE, Andriole VT. Bacterial urinary tract infections in diabetes. *Infect Dis Clin North Am* 1997;11:735–750.

Pewitt EB, Schaeffer AJ. Urinary tract infection in urology, including acute and chronic prostatitis. *Infect Dis Clin North Am* 1997;11:623–645.

Rex JH, Walsh TJ, Sobel JD, et al. Practice guidelines for the treatment of candidiasis. *Clin Infect Dis* 2000;30:662–678.

Ronald AR, Harding GKM. Complicated urinary tract infections. *Infect Dis Clin North Am* 1997;11:583–592.

Sobel JD, Kauffman CA, McKinsey D, et al. Candiduria: a randomized, double-blind study of treatment with fluconazole and placebo. *Clin Infect Dis* 2000;30:19–24.

Spach DH, Stapleton AE, Stamm WE. Lack of circumcision increases the risk of urinary tract infection in young men. *JAMA* 1992;267:679–681.

Stamm WE, Hooton TM. Management of urinary tract infections in adults. *N Engl J Med* 1993;329:1328–1334.

Warren JW, Abrutyn E, Hebel JR, et al. Guidelines from the Infectious Diseases Society of America: guidelines for antimicrobial treatment of uncomplicated acute bacterial cystitis and acute pyelonephritis in women. *Clin Infect Dis* 1999;29:745–758.

Sexually Transmitted Infections

Catherine A. Hermann

APPROACH TO SEXUALLY TRANSMITTED INFECTIONS

The standard clinic approach to sexually transmitted diseases (STDs) is a *syndromic* approach based on the clinical syndrome of presenting symptoms and signs. The common syndromes include genital ulceration, cervicitis, urethritis, vaginitis, and vaginosis. The differential diagnosis, workup, and treatment are based on recognition of the clinical syndrome.

The **history and physical exam** are essential elements of any evaluation for sexually transmitted infections. The reason for the visit and symptoms present should be elicited. Beyond carefully identifying symptoms, it is important to gather a complete sexual exposure history, including number and gender of partners, frequency, types of activity, and contraceptive practices. It is vital to ask these questions even though they may be uncomfortable to the interviewer and the patient. Any history of STDs and treatments is useful information as well. For women, a detailed gynecologic history is necessary. Physical exam should focus on a detailed survey of the skin, oropharynx, external genitalia, lymph nodes, and anus, and for women, a speculum and bimanual exam should be included.

GENITAL ULCER DISEASES

Syphilis, genital herpes, chancroid, lymphogranuloma venereum, and granuloma inguinale (donovanosis) represent the spectrum of diseases that present with some form of genital ulcer. In general, painless ulcers are due to syphilis or the more uncommon granuloma inguinale; however, the lesions associated with granuloma inguinale are typically a beefy-red appearance and are less likely to have regional adenopathy. The remaining ulcerative diseases are associated with a tender ulcer.

GENITAL HERPES

Genital HSV infections can be caused by type 1 or type 2, although genital herpes is typically associated with type 2. Serologic studies indicate that nearly 45 million persons in the United States have been infected with HSV-2.

Pathophysiology

HSV infections are spread by direct contact. Intact skin is fairly resistant to infection, but abraded skin or mucous membranes are more susceptible. The virus attaches to the cell surface and then enters the cell. Viral replication occurs in the cell nucleus and results in cell lysis. Infection may spread by direct cell-to-cell invasion or by sensory nerve pathways. As replication involves nerve endings, the retrograde transport of virions occurs, which allows for infection to occur at other sites (e.g., thighs or buttocks). CNS disease may occur as a result. Latency of virus occurs in sensory and autonomic ganglia. Periodic recurrences due to reactivation of latent virus may occur. Reactivations are site and viral specific. Viral latency and reactivation are not well understood.

Clinical Manifestations

Infection is characterized by small, painful, grouped vesicles in the anogenital region that rapidly ulcerate and form shallow, tender lesions. ***However, virtually any genital lesion may be herpetic regardless of clinical characteristics.*** The initial episode is usually the most clinically severe and may present with fever, myalgias, inguinal adenopathy, headache, and aseptic meningitis. HSV is the second leading cause of erythema multiforme. Beyond mucocutaneous infections, HSV infections may involve ocular disease (blepharitis, keratitis, keratoconjunctivitis), meningitis, encephalitis, Bell's palsy, esophagitis (especially in HIV), and disseminated disease. Recurrent episodes tend to be less severe and may be preceded by a prodromal period associated with pain. Virologic typing is useful in predicting recurrence, as HSV-1 appears less likely to cause recurrent genital ulcerations than HSV-2.

Diagnosis

Diagnosis is suggested by recognizing the clinical syndrome on history and physical exam. ***All genital ulcers not typical for genital herpes (i.e., solitary, painless ulcer) should be evaluated with immediate rapid plasmin reagent and darkfield exam, if available.*** Viral culture and typing are the preferred methods for making a diagnosis of genital HSV infection. Direct fluorescent antibodies of scraped lesions or viral cultures of unroofed vesicles can be used, but these tests are not as sensitive as culture. Type-specific HSV antibodies have recently become available and are useful in determining seroprevalence for epidemiologic studies as well as counseling couples. HSV PCR is most useful in the diagnosis of CNS infections that are otherwise very difficult to diagnose.

Treatment

There are several CDC-recommended treatment regimens for the **initial episode.** Acyclovir (Zovirax), 400 mg PO tid for 7–10 days; famciclovir (Famvir), 250 mg PO tid for 7–10 days; or valacyclovir (Valtrex), 1 g PO bid for 7–10 days, can be used. Treatment can be extended if healing is incomplete. Initiation of therapy during the prodrome or within 1 day of **recurrence** of vesicles has been shown to reduce the severity and duration of the episode. Treatment includes acyclovir, 400 mg PO tid for 5 days (or 200 mg PO qid for 5 days or 800 mg PO bid for 5 days); famciclovir, 125 mg PO bid for 5 days; or valacyclovir, 500 mg PO bid for 5 days. Recurrence can be reduced in frequency by 75% with **chronic suppressive therapy** but does not clear the latent virus; however, chronic suppressive therapy should be restricted to those patients with frequent (>6/yr) or severe recurrences. Treatment options include acyclovir, 400 mg PO bid; famciclovir, 250 mg PO bid; or valacyclovir, 250 mg PO bid (or 500 mg PO qd or 1 g PO qd). To date, studies examining acyclovir have not documented significant resistance with 1 yr or more of suppressive treatment. Asymptomatic viral shedding can occur despite suppressive therapy and appears to be responsible for most transmissions; therefore, it is important to encourage patients to engage in safe sexual practices with barrier methods and to inform partners. The risk of vertical neonatal transmission should also be explained to both men and women.

CHANCROID

Chancroid is caused by *Haemophilus ducreyi*, a fastidious gram-negative bacillus. It is characterized by a painful, nonindurated genital ulcer with undermined edges.

Diagnosis

Diagnosis is made by inguinal lymph node biopsy that demonstrates small, pleomorphic gram-negative bacilli.

Treatment

Treatment options include ceftriaxone, 250 mg IM single dose; erythromycin, 500 mg PO qid for 7 days; azithromycin (Zithromax Z-Pak), 1 g PO single dose; or ciprofloxacin (Cipro), 500 mg PO bid for 3 days.

LYMPHOGRANULOMA VENEREUM

Lymphogranuloma venereum is caused by *Chlamydia trachomatis* serovars L_1, L_2, or L_3. It is characterized by unilateral, tender inguinal lymphadenopathy. The patient may or may not have associated nongonococcal urethritis.

Diagnosis

Diagnosis is made by either type-specific chlamydial serology, but the gold standard is to test acute and convalescent serologies.

Treatment

Treatment can be with doxycycline (Vibramycin), 100 mg PO bid for 3 wks, or erythromycin base, 500 mg PO qid for 3 wks. There are some reports of effective treatment with multiple courses of azithromycin.

GRANULOMA INGUINALE (DONOVANOSIS)

Granuloma inguinale (donovanosis) is an unusual infection caused by the intracellular gram-negative *Calymmatobacterium granulomatis*. It is endemic to many parts of the developing world, including India, Papua New Guinea, southern Africa, and central Australia. The lesions are characterized by a painless, beefy-red vascular ulcerative lesion that tends to bleed when mechanically irritated. There is typically no associated lymphadenopathy.

Diagnosis

Diagnosis is established by tissue crush preparation or biopsy showing bipolar-staining Donovan bodies. The organism cannot be directly cultured.

Treatment

Treatment can be with trimethoprim-sulfamethoxazole (TMP-SMX) (Bactrim, Septra), double-strength tablet PO bid for 3 wks; doxycycline, 100 mg PO bid for 3 wks; ciprofloxacin, 750 mg PO bid for 3 wks; or erythromycin base, 500 mg PO qid for 3 wks. Longer treatment courses may be necessary, and introducing an aminoglycoside may speed resolution.

VULVOVAGINITIS AND VAGINOSIS
Trichomoniasis

Trichomoniasis is caused by *Trichomonas vaginalis*, a protozoal flagellate. It is characterized by an intense pruritus and a malodorous, frothy, yellow discharge. Pelvic exam demonstrates a diffuse erythema of the vaginal walls and cervical inflammation. In men, it is typically asymptomatic in the lower genitourinary tract.

Diagnosis

Diagnosis is established by observing motile trichomonads with flagella on wet-mount light microscopy. Vaginal fluid pH is typically ≥ 4.5.

Treatment

Treatment can be with metronidazole (Flagyl), 2 g PO in a single dose or 500 mg PO bid for 7 days. In the event of treatment failure, another course of 500 mg PO bid for 7 days should be used. Intravaginal metronidazole gel is not effective treatment. There is no safe treatment for pregnant women, although clotrimazole (Mycelex, Gyne-Lotrimin), 100 mg vaginal suppository or cream qd for 7 days, may relieve symptoms. Treatment of both partners is crucial for successful eradication.

Vulvovaginal Candidiasis

Vulvovaginal candidiasis is caused by *Candida* species and is associated with oral contraceptive use, antibiotic therapy, pregnancy, diabetes, and corticosteroid use. Recurrent, especially severe, episodes may be a presentation of HIV infection. The clinical presentation demonstrates thick, cottage-cheese-like vaginal discharge with intense vulvar inflammation, pruritus, and dysuria. The discharge is usually not malodorous.

Diagnosis

Diagnosis is established with the use of 10% potassium hydroxide solution, which dissolves cellular debris except for fungal elements.

Treatment

Treatment can be with over-the-counter intravaginal imidazole creams and suppositories (usually 1-, 3-, or 7-day regimens) or fluconazole (Diflucan), 150 mg PO (single dose).

Bacterial Vaginosis

Bacterial vaginosis is typified by overgrowth of *Gardnerella* species, *Mycoplasma* species, anaerobes, or more likely a polymicrobial infection. Malodorous vaginal discharge may be accompanied by vaginal pruritus; however, there may be no external vaginal irritation or dysuria in many cases. Alterations and overgrowth in the normal vaginal flora and reduction in lactobacilli may be responsible for a homogenous, nonviscous, milky-white fluid that covers the vagina and cervix.

Diagnosis

Diagnosis requires the following criteria: homogenous white vaginal discharge, "clue" cells (vaginal epithelial cells with a stippled appearance due to adherent coccobacilli) on wet smear or Gram's stain, and vaginal fluid pH ≥ 4.5. A positive Whiff test, which is a fishy odor released with the addition of 10% KOH (potassium hydroxide) solution, can aid in the diagnosis.

Treatment

Metronidazole is the standard treatment, and a variety of regimens can be prescribed. Metronidazole (500 mg PO bid for 7 days), metronidazole ER (750 mg PO qd for 7 days), metronidazole (2 g PO and repeat in 48 hrs), and MetroGel (one application intravaginally every night for 5 nights) are all acceptable treatment regimens. Cure rate is >90%. Alcohol should be avoided during treatment because a disulfiram-type relationship can occur. Alternatives include clindamycin (300 mg PO bid for 7 days) or clindamycin 2% cream (apply intravaginally for 7 nights). The treatment of sexual partners is controversial, and there are no standard guidelines at this time. Physicians may opt to treat partner(s) if there is no response to treatment or if recurrences are frequent.

CERVICITIS AND URETHRITIS (INCLUDING GONORRHEA, CHLAMYDIA, AND NONGONOCOCCAL URETHRITIS)

Cervicitis is a clinical diagnosis established by mucopurulent vaginal discharge, dyspareunia, and dysuria. Etiologies may include chlamydia, HSV, *Trichomonas vaginalis*, human papilloma virus (HPV), and gonorrhea. Unsafe sex practices along with having multiple sexual partners can increase the risk of STDs and cervicitis. Cervicitis may also result from a uterine or vaginal infection and is often asymptomatic, although a copious amount of discharge may be present. Other symptoms and signs include postcoital bleeding, cervical erythema and mucopurulent discharge on visual exam, tenderness on bimanual palpation, or easy bleeding with minor instrumentation. Treatment should be directed at the underlying etiology, and barrier methods should be encouraged until the regimen is completed. Sexual partners should also be treated as appropriate.

Urethritis is distinguished by dysuria and a purulent penile discharge. For nongonococcal urethritis, urethral itching can also be present, as can symptoms such as urgency, nocturia, and frequency if there is prostatic involvement. The causative organisms are most frequently *Neisseria gonorrhoeae* and *C. trachomatis* but may also involve *Mycoplasma hominis* or *Ureaplasma urealyticum* (see Trichomoniasis). There is often coinfection with *N. gonorrhoeae* and *C. trachomatis*. In these cases, yellowish-brown discharge, meatal edema, urethral tenderness to palpation, and signs of disseminated gonococcal infection may be present. It should be noted, however, that if urethritis is not treated, patients can become asymptomatic. As with all sexually transmitted diseases, safe sex practices should be encouraged and contacts treated when appropriate. Intercourse should be avoided if possible during the time of treatment to prevent reinfection and recurrences.

As in all STDs, abstinence is the only absolute way to prevent infection. For sexually active patients, condoms are the most effective preventive method. Testing and treatment of all sex partners of an infected patient are also important to prevent reinfection.

Diagnosis

Gonorrhea can be diagnosed with a Gram's stain of the discharge showing polymorphonuclear leukocytes (PMNs) with intracellular gram-negative diplococci. Alternatively, a culture, DNA probe, or PCR test may be used to confirm the diagnosis.

Chlamydia is diagnosed with DNA probe, PCR, direct fluorescent antibody, or by culture. All patients who test positive for gonorrhea or chlamydia should also be tested for syphilis and HIV.

Nongonococcal urethritis is typically caused by *C. trachomatis*, although the aforementioned organisms can play a role. The discharge is less purulent than gonococcal infections and may be mucoid. The diagnosis is established with ≥2 of 3 criteria being met: (a) symptoms of urethral discharge/dysuria, (b) purulent/mucopurulent urethral discharge, or (c) urethral Gram's stain showing ≥5 PMNs per high-powered field. A urine specimen may show leukocyte esterase and ≥10 WBCs per high-powered field. It is important to obtain both gonococcal and chlamydial cultures or probes at that time.

Treatment

Treatment of both gonorrhea and chlamydia is recommended due to the high coinfection rate, especially in patients without adequate follow-up. Single-dose antigonococcal therapies include ofloxacin (Floxin), 400 mg PO; ciprofloxacin, 500 mg PO; ceftriaxone, 125 mg IM; cefixime (Suprax), 400 mg PO; or spectinomycin, 2 g IM. Antichlamydial therapy includes azithromycin, 1 g PO in a single dose; doxycycline, 100 mg PO bid for 7 days; or erythromycin stearate, 500 mg PO qid (or enteric-coated erythromycin base, 666 mg PO tid) for 7 days. Azithromycin or doxycycline are suitable regimens for nongonococcal urethritis.

MUCOPURULENT CERVICITIS

Mucopurulent cervicitis is also caused by *N. gonorrhoeae* or *C. trachomatis*. There is a mucopurulent cervical discharge and associated inflammation showing cervical friability, edema, ectopy, and PMNs. Vaginal discharge, dyspareunia, and postcoital or intermenstrual bleeding are more nonspecific patient concerns.

Diagnosis

Diagnosis must include an endocervical Gram's stain demonstrating ≥15 PMNs per high-powered field and at least one of the following: purulent endocervical discharge, cervical ectopy, or endocervical bleeding with gentle swabbing. There must be no evidence of other infection, such as HSV, trichomoniasis, candidiasis, and especially gonorrhea.

Treatment

Treatment should be based on lab results. Empiric therapy may be necessary in patients with unlikely or poor follow-up and should include the following regimens: azithromycin, 1 g PO single dose; doxycycline, 100 mg PO bid for 7 days; or erythromycin base or stearate, 500 mg PO qid for 7 days. Alternatively, enteric-coated erythromycin base, 666 mg PO tid for 7 days, can be used. Single-dose gonococcal treatment should be considered as well.

PELVIC INFLAMMATORY DISEASE

Pelvic inflammatory disease (PID) refers to an upper genital tract infection, such as endometritis, salpingitis, ovarian abscess, tuboovarian abscess, pelvic peritonitis, and perihepatitis. It most frequently affects sexually active women 15–24 yrs of age. The vast majority are community acquired; however, recent instrumentation, such as dilation and curettage or induced abortion, is associated with an increased risk. Untreated PID can result in infertility, ectopic pregnancies, and chronic pain.

Diagnosis

Patients present with pelvic pain, dyspareunia, vaginal discharge, abnormal menses, and fever. On exam, lower abdominal tenderness, adnexal tenderness, and cervical motion tenderness are hallmark findings that occur in only 20% of patients. Fever is reported in approximately one-third of patients. As with cervicitis, cultures or probes for gonorrhea and chlamydia should be obtained. A pelvic U/S can be used to confirm the diagnosis of an abscess; however, the absence of any findings does not preclude PID. Criteria for hospitalization include an uncertain diagnosis, suspected pelvic abscess, PID in pregnancy, adolescence, PID with HIV infection, severe nausea or vomiting, intolerance of PO medication, lack of follow-up, and failure to respond to outpatient therapy.

Treatment

Many options exist for treatment. Inpatient therapy should include either cefoxitin, 2 g IV q6h, or cefotetan, 2 g IV q12h, plus doxycycline, 100 mg IV or PO q12h; or clindamycin, 900 mg IV q8h, plus gentamicin, 2-mg/kg loading dose followed by 1.5-mg/kg maintenance dose q8h (extended-interval dosing of gentamicin may also be used). Both IV regimens should be continued for >48 hrs after the patient shows signs of improvement; subsequent treatment should include doxycycline, 100 mg PO bid for 14 days. For outpatient therapy, several regimens are effective: (a) cefoxitin, 2 g IM, with probenecid, 1 g PO, plus doxycycline, 100 mg PO bid for 14 days; (b) ceftriaxone, 250 mg IM, plus doxycycline, 100 mg PO bid for 14 days, plus metronidazole, 500 mg PO bid for 7 days; or (c) ofloxacin, 400 mg PO bid for 14 days, plus metronidazole, 500 mg PO bid for 14 days. IUDs should be removed. Patients should abstain from sexual intercourse during therapy. All patients must receive follow-up within 72 hrs to ensure adequate response to therapy. Partner screening is recommended.

MISCELLANEOUS SEXUALLY TRANSMITTED INFECTIONS

Pediculosis Pubis

Pediculosis pubis is often referred to as **crabs** and is caused by lice, *Phthirus pubis*. Typically intense pruritus of the pubic region and inflammation are noted. Lice should be visible on the skin, and eggs should be visible on hair shafts. Treatment options include lindane 1% shampoo for 4 mins, permethrin 1% creme rinse for 10 mins, or pyrethrins with piperonyl butoxide for 10 mins to all skin between the chest and thighs, including the axillae. Environmental cleanup is essential to prevent reinfection; patients should be advised to launder in hot water and dry with high heat all clothes, sheets, and other linens.

HBV and HCV

See Acute Hepatitis: HBV and Acute Hepatitis: HCV in Chap. 7, Infections of the Hepatobiliary System.

Molluscum Contagiosum

Molluscum contagiosum is a poxvirus. Infection consists of flesh-colored, dome-shaped papules with central umbilication. These papules are typically a few millimeters in diameter but may attain a sizable appearance in patients with AIDS. Diagnosis is typically by inspection of the characteristic skin lesion. The infection is typically self-limited in immunocompetent individuals; however, any mechanical approach, such as curettage, cryotherapy, or laser, can be used in instances in which cosmesis is a factor. Cantharidin, a blistering agent, can be used as well. Effective control of HIV is necessary for resolution of molluscum in patients with AIDS.

Genital Warts

Genital warts (condylomata acuminata) are associated with HPV. The appearance can vary considerably; usually, they are verrucous papules approximately 1 cm in diameter. They may have a spontaneous remission and recurrence. Treatment is designed to induce as long of a wart-free interval as possible. Anogenital warts are usually treated with either 25% podophyllum resin tincture or the purified resin, podofilox.

KEY POINTS TO REMEMBER

- Remember to use the syndrome classification of STDs in your differential diagnosis, as it greatly simplifies the approach to treatment.
- Nearly all genital ulcer disease in the United States is caused by HSV and syphilis, even if atypical symptoms and signs are present.
- Patients treated empirically for cervicitis/urethritis should receive therapy for **both** gonorrhea and chlamydia.
- All patients with a new diagnosis of HSV, gonorrhea, chlamydia, or other genital ulcer diseases should also be tested for HIV and syphilis.
- Remember to test and treat all partners!

REFERENCES AND SUGGESTED READINGS

Aliotta PJ. Urethritis and nongonococcal urethritis. In: Ferri FF, ed. *Ferri's clinical advisor: instant diagnosis and treatment*. St. Louis: Mosby, 2002:734, 735.

Centers for Disease Control and Prevention. 2002 Guidelines for treatment of sexually transmitted diseases. *MMWR Recomm Rep* 2002;51(RR-6):1–78.

Danakas GT. Cervicitis. In: Ferri FF, ed. *Ferri's clinical advisor: instant diagnosis and treatment*. St. Louis: Mosby, 2002:158.

Winters K, Diemer K. Women's health. In: Lin TL, Rypkema SW, eds. *The Washington manual of ambulatory therapeutics*. Philadelphia: Lippincott Williams & Wilkins, 2003:528–550.

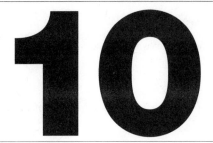

Skin and Soft Tissue Infections

Behzad Razavi

CELLULITIS

Skin is the major barrier between human hosts and the environment. Therefore, skin and soft tissue infections are common problems. Although skin infections may be caused by viruses, fungi, rickettsia, and parasites, **bacterial infection** is the most common form. The skin is composed of the epidermis, the dermis, and SC fat. Infection of specific layer(s) results in different clinical syndromes. Therefore, knowledge of the anatomy of the skin and thorough history and physical exam are the key to accurate diagnosis and therapy. Cellulitis is an acute spreading infection of the skin and SC tissue without involvement of the fascia or muscle.

Pathophysiology

The infection usually results from microscopic or evident breakdown in the skin barrier. The most common pathogens are group A *Streptococcus* (GAS) and *Staphylococcus aureus*. Patients with diabetes mellitus, chronic venous insufficiency, and lymphedema are more prone to (recurrent) cellulitis. The initial local infection can spread rapidly and involve deeper layers and the regional lymphatic system ("red streaks"). Cellulitis can be complicated by bullae, abscess, and ulcer formation.

Clinical Manifestations

The involved area is usually painful, warm, and erythematous. In contrast to erysipelas, the borders are not raised or sharply demarcated. Fever, chills, and malaise may be present. Tender regional lymphadenopathy is a frequent finding. Erysipelas, a clinical variant of cellulitis, is caused by group A beta hemolytic *Streptococcus* (GABHS) that involves the dermis and lymphatics. It is characterized by sudden onset of painful, shiny, erythematous, and indurated swelling of the face or extremities. On the face, it commonly involves the cheeks and the nasal bridge, resulting in a butterfly rash. Erysipelas can be complicated by bullae formation. In contrast to cellulitis, erysipelas typically has sharply demarcated and raised borders. Risk factors for erysipelas are venous stasis, diabetes mellitus, and alcohol use. Isolation of GABHS from involved skin is uncommon.

Diagnosis

A thorough history and physical exam are crucial. Leukocytosis with a left shift is almost always present. Plain films of the involved areas should be done to rule out osteomyelitis and gas within soft tissue (suggestive of necrotizing process). Any fluid collection or abscess should be aspirated and evaluated for Gram's stain and cultures. Blood cultures should be obtained because bacteremia can occur. If the lower extremity is involved, Doppler U/S should be done to rule out deep venous thrombosis. Demarcation of the involved area should be outlined, and serial clinical assessments should be performed for rapidly advancing lesions and deeper tissue involvement that may need immediate surgical intervention. *Remember, get a surgical consult sooner rather than later!*

Differential Diagnosis

The differential diagnosis includes impetigo (initially, vesicular; later, crusted superficial skin infection), erysipelas, osteomyelitis, acute gout, pseudogout, erythema nodosum, vasculitis, thrombophlebitis, and drug reactions.

Treatment

Mild infections (localized, superficial, no constitutional symptoms) can be treated with PO antibiotics. Dicloxacillin, 500 mg PO q6h; cephalexin (Keflex), 500 mg PO q6h; or clindamycin (Cleocin), 450–600 mg PO q8h, are all reasonable choices. Serious or rapidly progressing infections require hospitalization and IV antibiotics. Cefazolin (Ancef), 1 g IV q8h; nafcillin/oxacillin, 1–2 g IV q4–6h; or clindamycin, 600 mg IV q8h, are appropriate initial therapies. The usual duration of therapy is 10–14 days but should be based on clinical response to treatment. Good attention to foot and nail care (i.e., treat tinea or onychomycosis if present), tight blood glucose control in diabetics, and control of lymphedema or venous stasis (i.e., with compression wraps) can all be helpful in prevention. Traumatic breaks in the skin should be thoroughly cleansed.

NECROTIZING FASCIITIS

Necrotizing fasciitis (NF) is a serious, invasive, and rapidly progressing infection with necrosis of the skin, SC fat, and fascia. It is uncommon but often potentially life-threatening, with a mortality rate of 20–47%.

Pathophysiology

NF often results from breakdown in the normal mucocutaneous or cutaneous barriers through trauma, perforation (i.e., diverticulitis), or infected ulcers. The initial local infection results in an inflammatory and necrotizing process, which can rapidly spread at a rate of 3 cm/hr. Individuals with impaired host defense, such as those with advanced age, diabetes, malignancy, and receipt of immunosuppressive therapies, are at higher risk for development of NF. The exotoxin-producing GABHS can cause a severe septic picture via release of cytokines, such as tumor necrosis factor, interleukin (IL)-1, IL-2, and IL-6.

Clinical Manifestations

On physical exam, the involved areas usually resemble cellulitis. However, patients with NF have exquisite tenderness. The skin may appear normal or have an erythematous or dusky hue. Bullae and crepitus (SC air due to gas producing anaerobes) may be appreciated. The patients often appear more toxic than one would expect from the superficial appearance of the skin and may exhibit hypotension and high fevers. Leukocytosis is commonly present.

Diagnosis

A high index of suspicion is required for early diagnosis, especially in patients with "mild"-appearing cellulitis. The affected area should be demarcated, and frequent clinical assessments should be done to evaluate for rate of progression. Plain films may show gas within tissue. However, *the absence of gas does not exclude the diagnosis.* CT or MRI may play a major role for diagnosis. Anaerobic and aerobic blood cultures should be collected. Bacteriologic evaluation of wound exudate and bullae fluid is essential. A wound exudate with gram-positive rods and few polymorphonuclear leukocytes (PMLs) is characteristic of clostridial infection.

Differential Diagnosis

The differential diagnosis includes impetigo, erysipelas, osteomyelitis, thrombophlebitis, and drug reactions. Most cases are polymicrobial in origin with both anaerobes (i.e., *Bacteroides* and *Peptostreptococcus* species) and gram-variable aerobes, such as GABHS, *Escherichia coli*, and *Klebsiella* species. NF can affect any body part but most commonly affects the extremities, abdominal wall, perianal area, and groin (Fournier's gangrene). The key to successful treatment is early diagnosis and rapid medical and surgical interventions.

Treatment

If NF is suspected, an immediate surgical consultation should be obtained. IV fluids and broad-spectrum antibiotics should be initiated. Aggressive débridement of the necrotic area is essential for a favorable outcome. Generally, antibiotic combinations are used that are active against anaerobes and gram-positive and -negative aerobes. Clindamycin or metronidazole (Flagyl) can be used in combination with a third-generation cephalosporin, such as ceftriaxone (Rocephin). Clindamycin is believed to have antitoxin effects and should be included in cases of suspected or proved GABHS NF ("the Eagle effect"). Other antibiotic choices include imipenem (Primaxin), piperacillin-tazobactam (Zosyn), or ampicillin-sulbactam (Unasyn), preferably in combination with clindamycin or metronidazole. High-dose PCN G is the drug of choice for clostridial infections. The use of adjunctive hyperbaric oxygen therapy is controversial, although some studies have shown benefit in selected patients.

DECUBITUS ULCER

Decubitus ulcers are caused by prolonged pressure at weight-bearing sites that results in ischemic necrosis of the skin and underlying soft tissue. They occur among individuals with prolonged immobility, such as those with stroke, quadriplegia, paraplegia, or sensory deficits as in diabetes.

Pathophysiology

Decubitus ulcers are most common at the sacrum and heels due to high weight-bearing pressure and short skin-to-bone distance. They may become secondarily infected with skin or GI flora, with anaerobes and gram-negative rods being the most common isolates. Low serum albumin, urinary or fecal incontinence, perspiration, and poor wound care are all risk factors for infection.

Clinical Manifestations

Infected ulcers are a common source of fever and leukocytosis. The affected area may have a surrounding cellulitis. The infected ulcer frequently has a foul-smelling, yellowish drainage. In severe cases, the underlying bone can be exposed, which is equivocal to osteomyelitis.

Diagnosis

Each ulcer should be examined carefully and thoroughly. The extent of the ulcer should be probed with a sterile glove, cotton swab, or wooden probe. The WBC count and ESR are elevated in most cases. Plain bone films, CT, or MRI of the involved areas should be done to identify the extent of the disease and to rule out osteomyelitis. In most cases, culture of the ulcer reveals mixed microbial flora. However, the culture will not distinguish between colonization and true infection. (That's our job!)

Differential Diagnosis

The differential diagnosis is pyoderma gangrenosum (biopsy required for diagnosis) and osteomyelitis.

Treatment

Treatment of decubitus ulcers needs a multidisciplinary approach, including surgeons (preferably plastic surgeons), infectious disease specialists, wound care specialists, and excellence in nursing care. All necrotic tissue must be débrided to allow proper healing. Skin grafting or muscle flaps are sometimes required to repair extensive ulcerations. Systemic antibiotics are required when fever, bacteremia, osteomyelitis, severe cellulitis, or increasing drainage is present. Antibiotics should have broad-spectrum coverage, including skin flora and aerobic and anaerobic GI flora. A 2- to 3-wk course of ampicillin-sulbactam, piperacillin-tazobactam, imipenem, and ciprofloxacin with clindamycin or metronidazole is reasonable for empiric therapy of infected decubitus ulcers. If osteomyelitis is present, a longer period (often 6–8 wks) of parenteral antibiotics is required based on results of bone cultures. Frequent turning and the use of special beds (air mattress) play a key role in preventing future pressure sores.

DIABETIC FOOT

Foot problems are the leading cause of hospitalization among individuals with diabetes mellitus. It is estimated that 15% of all diabetics develop a serious foot condition at some time in their lives. Common problems include infection, ulceration, or gangrene that may lead, in severe cases, to amputation. Diabetes is the most common cause of amputation in the United States. Many of these problems are preventable through proper care and adequate diabetes management.

Pathophysiology

Foot infections in persons with diabetes are usually the result of three primary factors: neuropathy, poor circulation, and decreased resistance to infection. Charcot foot deformity occurs as a result of decreased sensation and maldistribution of pressure leading to tissue ischemia, necrosis with formation of calluses, and ulcers. Unnoticed microfractures in the bones result in disfigurement, chronic swelling, and additional bony prominences. Neuropathy predisposes patients to trauma, which is the triggering event in most cases. Poor circulation is the result of hyperglycemia and other comorbidities, such as smoking, HTN, and hyperlipidemia, which lead to accelerated atherosclerosis. Poor glycemic control (blood glucose levels >200 mg/dL) is associated with decreased neutrophil function.

Clinical Manifestations

Local signs and symptoms predominate the clinical picture of the diabetic foot ulcer. There may be a surrounding cellulitis, and the wound may have a purulent exudate. Tenderness is minimal or absent due to symmetric distal neuropathy. Patients may have diminished distal pulses and often report claudication symptoms. Fever is uncommon, and patients rarely appear toxic. In a study of patients with life-threatening limb infections, only 36% had a fever >100.4°F (38°C). Blood cultures are positive in 10–15% of patients. The WBC count may be minimally elevated or normal, but the ESR is usually elevated.

Diagnosis

A careful physical exam, including testing for distal pulses and neuropathy by monofilament, is mandatory. Lack of lower extremity hair often reflects vascular insufficiency. Routine labs and blood cultures should be obtained in all patients. Plain films of the involved foot should be performed to rule out GABHS within soft tissue and osteomyelitis. Measurement of arm-ankle indices should be done to identify poor circulation. Diabetic wounds are often chronic and frequently colonized with organisms that are not the causative pathogen (i.e., staphylococci or enterococci). Deeper tissue cultures are preferred. CT and MRI are frequently used to identify abscesses and bony involvement. Bone and labeled leukocyte scans can sometime detect occult osteomyelitis. However, bone biopsy remains the gold standard for the diagnosis of osteomyelitis in these patients.

Differential Diagnosis

The differential diagnosis includes arterial ulceration, venous stasis ulceration, and osteomyelitis.

Treatment

Successful treatment of diabetic foot problems is **multifactorial. Proper control** of hyperglycemia and concomitant HTN or hyperlipidemia can help to reduce the ongoing risks of peripheral vascular disease and altered host defenses. **Careful daily inspection of the feet** by the patient is one of the easiest, least expensive, and most effective measures for preventing foot complications—at least among those without visual deficits. **Gentle cleansing** with soap and water, followed by the application of topical moisturizers, helps to maintain healthy skin. **Early recognition of the ulceration,** avoidance of weight-bearing activities, and avoidance of "closed-in" shoes play a major role for favorable outcome. Custom-made shoes help to take pressure off the wound area. Optimal ulcer healing requires **adequate tissue perfusion.** Thus, arterial insufficiency should be suspected if an ulcer does not heal, and vascular surgery consultation and possible revascularization should be considered when present. **Smoking cessation** is essential for preventing the progression of occlusive disease. Once an ulcer has occurred, early surgical, infectious disease, and wound care specialist **consultations** are recommended for optimal management. Empiric broad-spectrum antibiotics commonly are used and should cover staphylococci, enteric gram-negatives, and anaerobes. Options include ampicillin-sulbactam (3 g IV q6h), piperacillin-tazobactam (3.375 g IV q6h), ceftriaxone (1 g IV qd) in combination with clindamycin (600 mg IV q8h) or metronidazole (1 g IV q12h), and imipenem (0.5 g IV q6h). (This dosing information is provided as a sample; many diabetics need variable renal dosing of these medications.) The final regimen may be modified based on deep tissue or bone culture results. The optimal duration of therapy is unknown and depends on the severity and extent of infection. Bony involvement usually requires 6 wks of IV antibiotics. Surgical removal of all necrotic tissue, including bone, is essential for proper healing. In severe cases, amputation may be necessary to salvage the limb.

PYOMYOSITIS

Pyomyositis is an acute bacterial infection of the skeletal muscle caused by *S. aureus.* Most cases occur in tropical areas, although there has been an increasing frequency of pyomyositis among HIV-positive individuals in the United States. Local trauma is a predisposing factor. The infection usually involves a single muscle group, and toxic symptoms are rare.

Pathophysiology

Pyomyositis results from primary infection of the muscle, presumably due to transient bacteremia, and is not secondary to involvement of adjacent skin, soft tissue, or bone. Predisposing factors include trauma, diabetes, alcoholism, and immunosuppressed states (e.g., HIV, steroids, malignancy). The primary infection is followed by a local inflammatory response with pus formation.

Clinical Manifestations

A single muscle group is most commonly affected, so the symptoms are localized pain and swelling. Signs of inflammation may not be evident initially due to the deep location of the infection. Frequently, the area is indurated and has a woody or brawny appearance. Fever and chills are common. In 20–50% of cases, patients report recent blunt trauma or vigorous exercise. The most commonly involved sites are the large muscles of the lower extremities (quadriceps and gluteal muscles). Lab studies usually show a leukocytosis with evidence of rhabdomyolysis with myoglobinuria and acute renal failure. However, serum muscle enzyme levels may be normal, even despite gross muscle destruction. Approximately 5–30% of patients have positive blood cultures.

Diagnosis

MRI or CT with contrast usually reveals the location and extent of the infection. Diagnosis is usually made by needle aspiration under U/S or CT guidance. In the United States, *S. aureus* is responsible for 66% of all cases, whereas GABHS accounts for up to 5% of cases.

Differential Diagnosis

Differential diagnosis includes muscle hematoma, osteomyelitis, severe cellulitis, vasculitis, and Kaposi's sarcoma.

Treatment

Surgical drainage of any fluid collection is essential. Antibiotic therapy should be guided by the interpretation of the Gram's stain of the aspirated fluid. The initial empiric antibiotic therapy should cover *S. aureus*. Because of the increasing number of PCN-resistant isolates, administration of a beta-lactamase–resistant PCN, such as nafcillin, is recommended. Pyomyositis may be complicated by compartment syndrome and may require additional surgical drainage or even fasciotomy.

GAS GANGRENE

Gas gangrene is usually a rapidly progressive and life-threatening infection characterized by muscle necrosis and systemic toxicity. It is caused by *Clostridium perfringens* in 80% of cases and usually occurs after muscle injury.

Pathophysiology

The infection occurs after penetrating (knife or gunshot wounds) or crushing muscle injury that creates an anaerobic environment with contamination of soil or other material containing spores of *C. perfringens*. Despite the high frequency of clostridial contamination in major traumatic wounds, the incidence of gas gangrene is only 1–2%, reflecting the insult from hypoperfused devitalized tissue. Other clinical scenarios associated with posttraumatic gas gangrene are abdominal surgery, retained placenta, iatrogenic abortion, and intrauterine fetal demise. It appears that the toxins produced by *C. perfringens* are major virulent factors associated with myonecrosis and impaired local host defenses. Spontaneous or nontraumatic gas gangrene is associated with the more aerotolerant *Clostridium septicum*.

Clinical Manifestations

The mean incubation period is usually <24 hrs. The first and most important symptom is pain, which can be excruciating. Systemic toxicity is frequent, and patients may quickly develop shock and multiorgan failure with fatal outcome if not properly treated. The skin may initially appear pale but quickly changes to bronze. Local swelling and tenderness are prominent. If the wound is open, swollen muscle may be visible. The wound typically has a foul odor and a serosanguineous discharge that may be culture-positive for the inciting pathogen. Crepitance can be noted on physical exam, and the overlying skin frequently shows fluid-filled bullae.

Diagnosis

Anemia results from brisk intravascular hemolysis. Leukocytosis is common, and bacteremia occurs in approximately 15% of patients with gas gangrene. Gram's stain of the wound discharge usually shows gram-positive rods with typically few or no PMLs. Usually, NF and skin necrosis are also present. Liquid anaerobic cultures should be obtained and observed for gas production. Plain films of the involved area typically show extensive gaseous dissection of muscle and fascial planes.

Differential Diagnosis

The differential diagnosis includes other gas-forming, nonclostridial infections of the soft tissue, which are more gradual in onset and progression.

Treatment

Prompt and extensive surgical exploration, with fasciotomy and débridement of all necrotic tissue, is the cornerstone of therapy. Systemic antibiotics are an important adjunct to surgery. Although many antibiotics, including PCN, clindamycin, tetracycline, metronidazole, chloramphenicol, and many cephalosporins, have good *in vitro* activity against *C. perfringens*, the combination of PCN G (1–2 million units IV q2–4h) and clindamycin (600 mg IV q6–8h) is the preferred regimen. PCN should not be used in combination with metronidazole, because it antagonizes the effect of the latter. A fluoroquinolone or higher-generation cephalosporin should be added to the regimen if the initial Gram's stain also shows gram-negative organisms. Clindamycin with chloramphenicol (Chloromycetin) is an alternative regimen for PCN-allergic patients. Although some studies showed benefit with the use of hyperbaric oxygen in patients with gas gangrene, its use is still controversial and should never delay immediate surgical exploration and débridement.

PROSTHETIC JOINT INFECTIONS

Joint replacements, particularly of the hip and knee, are frequent orthopedic procedures, with approximately 450,000 arthroplasties performed each year in the United States. Major indications for joint replacement are severely damaged and incapacitating joints from infection (septic arthritis), degenerative joint disease changes, or systemic illnesses such as rheumatoid arthritis. Infection is a rare but serious complication of these procedures and occurs in 1–2% of all cases.

Pathophysiology

The pathogenesis of prosthetic joint infections involves local or systemic introduction of organisms and impaired local host defense. Prosthetic joint infections can be classified as *early* (within the first 3 mos), *delayed* (within the first 2 yrs), and *late* (after 2 yrs). Early infections usually develop from an infected wound or hematoma. Delayed infections result from contamination of the prosthetic device or wound at the time of surgery or other events, such as unrecognized (line-related) bacteremias. Late infections generally occur through hematogenous spread from another focus, such as UTI, cellulitis, pneumonia, or colitis. The organisms adhere to the prosthetic device and cause a local inflammatory reaction. Major risk factors for development of prosthetic joint infections are advanced age, prior joint surgery, postop wound infection, and compromised immune status (e.g., rheumatoid arthritis and diabetes mellitus). *S. aureus* and coagulase-negative staphylococci are the most important organisms, accounting for approximately 50% of all prosthetic joint infections. Gram-negative rods are isolated in 25% of all cases.

Clinical Manifestations

The most common presenting symptoms of prosthetic joint infection are joint pain and fever followed by periarticular swelling and wound drainage. Pain is the prominent symptom and is generally constant, progressive, and exacerbated by weight bearing. A wide spectrum of the severity of the inflammatory response can be seen. Early infections are usually associated with fever and marked joint inflammation. Some may have an obvious infected wound or hematoma with draining sinus tracts. Delayed or late infections frequently present with a long and indolent course, with pain as the sole complaint without any local or systemic signs of inflammation. Sometimes patients report a history of recurrent wound infection treated with several courses of antibiotics. Routine lab tests may be nonspecific. However, the ESR is elevated in >90% of patients.

Diagnosis

A complete history, including the nature and duration of pain, and a thorough physical exam are essential. The key is to distinguish prosthesis infection from mechanical problems. However, an infection should always be considered until proved otherwise. Patients may require surgical exploration to obtain diagnostic tissue and to rule out prosthesis infection. Plain radiographs may show prosthesis loosening or osteomyelitis. MRI or CT is of little value due to metal artifact. Bone scans are limited due to their inability to distinguish infection from prosthesis loosening, and abnormal results are routinely seen for ≥6 mos after arthroplasty. Definite diagnosis requires isolation of the organism from aspirated joint fluid or surgically obtained tissue. The presence of polymorphonuclear cells on Gram's stain usually suggests infection. Arthrocentesis reveals the organisms in 85–98% of cases.

Differential Diagnosis

Noninfectious causes of joint pain and inflammation, such as gout, pseudogout, prosthesis loosening, or hemarthrosis, should be included in the differential diagnosis.

Treatment

Treatment of prosthetic joint infection generally consists of drainage of any fluid collection, removal of the prosthesis, and a long course of antibiotics, followed by implantation of a new device with continued antibiotics. Single surgical débridement with retention of the prosthesis along with a 6-wk course of antibiotics has been successful in approximately 70% of selected patients with prosthesis infection within 1 mo of implantation. The empiric antibiotic therapy should cover gram-positive organisms. Penicillinase-resistant PCN (e.g., nafcillin) and first-generation cephalosporins (e.g., cefazolin), vancomycin, or ciprofloxacin in combination with rifampin are all reasonable initial choices pending the results of microbiologic and sensitivity tests. Clindamycin or amoxicillin-clavulanate (Augmentin) is the preferred agent if anaerobes are cultured. Patients who cannot tolerate surgery may require lifelong suppressive antibiotic therapy. Other strategies to prevent infections are antibiotic-impregnated devices or cement, use of filtered laminated airflow ("ultraclean air") in ORs, and short-term postsurgical antibiotic prophylaxis to prevent superficial and deep wound infections.

OSTEOMYELITIS

Osteomyelitis is an infection of the bone that is characterized by progressive inflammatory destruction of bone resulting in ischemia, necrosis, and new bone apposition. It can be clinically divided into two groups: hematogenous osteomyelitis from bacteremia or contiguous-focus osteomyelitis through spread from an infected adjacent tissue. Osteomyelitis is most often caused by pyogenic bacteria but may be also due to other pathogens, such as mycobacteria and fungi. Acute osteomyelitis usually represents the first presentation, whereas the chronic form usually evolves from acute osteomyelitis or represents relapse of a previously identified or treated infection.

Pathophysiology

Infection of the bone usually occurs as a result of very large inocula, trauma, or the presence of foreign body. Certain bacteria, such as *S. aureus,* express receptors for components of bone matrix, allowing them to adhere to bone. The local inflammatory response, mediated by the offending organism, leads to release of various cytokines (IL-1, IL-6, tumor necrosis factor), toxic oxygen radicals, and proteolytic enzymes that lyse surrounding tissue. This leads to pus formation and increased intraosseous pressure. The result is impaired blood flow leading to ischemic bone necrosis, with separation of devascularized fragments ("sequestra"). Primary hematogenous osteomyelitis occurs primarily in infants and children and involves metaphysis of long bones (tibia and femur). In adults, secondary hematogenous osteomyelitis from a quiescent focus of infection during childhood, after injury or fracture, or infected prosthesis is more common.

Clinical Manifestations

Acute osteomyelitis presents with fever, chills, malaise, and bone pain. Erythema, swelling, and limited motion may be present over the involved joint/bone. **Chronic** osteomyelitis has an indolent course, with vague constitutional symptoms of 1–3 mos' duration. Patients do not appear toxic, and increasing pain may be the only symptom. Sinus tract formation with purulent drainage may develop over time. Patients with **vertebral** osteomyelitis typically present with neck/back pain and fever. Referred pain due to nerve root irritation may mislead the examiner from the actual site of infection. Neurologic deficits, such as lower extremity weakness, have been reported in approximately 50% of patients. Therefore, patients with vertebral osteomyelitis should have frequent neurologic exams.

Diagnosis

Physical exam may show evidence of cellulitis or sinus tract formation with purulent discharge. Leukocyte counts and ESR are frequently elevated. Blood cultures are positive in approximately 50% of patients with acute hematogenous osteomyelitis. Although plain films of the involved bone may show soft tissue edema and periosteal elevation, they may be normal in some cases. Both CT and MRI have excellent resolution and help to identify the extent and severity of disease involvement, including soft tissue abscesses. MRI is particularly helpful in the diagnosis of vertebral disease. Bone scan (technetium 99) is a sensitive test for detection of early osteomyelitis. Definite diagnosis is made by isolation of the pathogen from bone biopsy, particularly in vertebral osteomyelitis in which blood cultures are usually sterile. The microbiology of osteomyelitis is age dependent. Although *S. aureus* and streptococci are typically isolated from infants, *S. aureus* is also isolated among older patients. There is increasing incidence of osteomyelitis due to gram-negative rods among the elderly population. Osteomyelitis due to *S. aureus, Staphylococcus epidermidis,* and *Pseudomonas aeruginosa* (vertebral) is common among IV drug users. Fungal osteomyelitis is rare and often the result of prolonged neutropenia or catheter-related fungemia. Patients with sickle cell disease are prone to *Salmonella* and *Proteus* species osteomyelitis, whereas diabetics frequently have mixed infections. Sinus tract cultures are often not reliable and misleading. Therefore, cultures should be taken at débridement surgery or from deep bone biopsies.

Differential Diagnosis

The differential diagnosis includes malignancy, histiocytosis X, fractures, and connective tissue diseases such as rheumatoid arthritis.

Treatment

Once the diagnosis of osteomyelitis is made, a combined antimicrobial and surgical approach should be considered. Abscesses should be drained and dead tissue and bone débrided to allow proper healing. Generally, a 6-wk course of parenteral antibiotic is recommended from the last débridement or positive blood culture. PCN G (4 million units IV q4h) or first-generation cephalosporin (cefazolin, 2 g IV q6h) is the drug of choice for sensitive staphylococci and streptococci. Nafcillin or oxacillin (2 g IV q4–6h) is used for PCN-resistant strains. Vancomycin is reserved for documented methicillin-resistant or PCN-allergic patients. Because of its excellent bone penetration, rifampin can be used in osteomyelitis due to oxacillin-susceptible *S. aureus*, oxacillin-resistant *S. aureus*, or coagulase-negative staphylococci, particularly if the first course of antibiotics has failed. However, rifampin should be used only in combination with these antibiotics because of rapid development of resistance to this drug when used as monotherapy. Clindamycin (600 mg PO/IV q6h) is the preferred drug if anaerobes are involved. Fluoroquinolones (ciprofloxacin, 750 mg PO q12h or 400 mg IV q12h) or third-generation cephalosporins (ceftriaxone, 2 g IV q24h) are used for gram-negative osteomyelitis. The ESR is usually measured serially to monitor response. IV antibiotic therapy is generally preferred for the entire duration of therapy of osteomyelitis. However, in compliant patients with susceptible organisms, or in those with difficult IV access, the antibiotics can be switched to PO after 2 wks of IV course. Fluoroquinolones alone or in combination with rifampin (Rifadin, Rimactane) have been successful in a few studies as PO alternatives. Adjunctive hyperbaric oxygen therapy may be useful in the treatment of chronic osteomyelitis.

BACTERIAL ARTHRITIS

Infectious arthritis is an inflammation of a joint space caused by one or more of many different infectious agents. The incidence of these infections in adults is relatively low; however, they can cause significant morbidity as a result of pain, immobility, and loss of joint function. There are an estimated 20,000 cases/yr in the United States; 56% of cases occur in men, and 45% of patients are >65 yrs. Disseminated gonococcal infection (DGI) is the leading cause of hospitalization for infectious arthritis in the United States. Risk factors include rheumatoid arthritis, diabetes mellitus, malignancy, old age, HIV infection, and situations that increase the risk of bacteremia, such as IV drug abuse and indwelling catheters. Risk is also increased with prior surgery or trauma, as well as with intraarticular injections and arthroscopy. DGI occurs most frequently among sexually active, menstruating women. The male to female ratio is 1:4.

NONGONOCOCCAL ARTHRITIS

Pathophysiology

Nongonococcal arthritis most frequently results from hematogenous seeding of the joint space. Bacteremia may be either primary or secondary, with an identifiable focus found in approximately 50% of cases. Direct inoculation is another mechanism of infection. The risk of bacterial arthritis after arthrocentesis is reported to be 0.002–0.007% and 0.04–0.40% after arthroscopy. After bacteria have entered the joint space, PMLs enter, and destruction of articular cartilage occurs due to the inflammatory process. *S. aureus* is the most common etiologic agent. In patients with rheumatoid arthritis, nearly 80% of cases are due to *S. aureus*. Group B streptococcal infection is more likely in patients with diabetes, and gram-negative bacilli are more common in the elderly and debilitated. Coagulase-negative staphylococci infection occurs after medical procedures. Anaerobic infection is rare except for that occurring after human or animal bites. *Mycoplasma* species may cause infections in hypogammaglobulinemic patients.

Clinical Manifestations

Typically, nongonococcal arthritis is monoarticular and has an acute presentation. However, a polyarticular infection with *S. aureus* occurs approximately 15% of the time. Nearly all patients describe pain and limitation of joint motion. Fever is common but not usually high grade. Physical exam usually reveals a warm, tender joint with an effusion. Active and passive ranges of motion are typically decreased. However, these findings may be absent in patients with rheumatoid arthritis or ongoing immunosuppression. Clinical findings can be difficult to ascertain in infections of the shoulder and hip as well.

Diagnosis

The history and exam may lead to high index of suspicion for infection, but a positive synovial fluid culture is the only definitive method for diagnosing bacterial arthritis. Blood cultures are positive in up to 70% of patients and should be obtained. The majority of patients have elevated ESR and c-reactive protein levels; however, these tests are nonspecific. The diagnostic procedure of choice is arthrocentesis. This should be done immediately once the diagnosis is suspected and ideally before antimicrobial therapy is initiated. If fluid cannot be obtained by blind aspiration (i.e., possible hip infection), a radiologist can obtain a sample under fluoroscopy.

Synovial fluid is often cloudy or purulent in appearance. The fluid should routinely be examined for cell count, differential, and uric acid and calcium pyrophosphate crystals. A Gram's stain and aerobic culture should be performed. Anaerobic cultures should be sent when clinically indicated. The leukocyte count is often >100,000 cells/mm^3, with >75% PMNs. The Gram's stain is positive approximately 50% of the time, and synovial fluid cultures are positive in approximately 90% of cases of nongonococcal arthritis.

Differential Diagnosis

In adults with possible infectious arthritis, the main differential is with gout and pseudogout. Other potential diagnoses include nonbacterial infectious arthritis, rheumatic fever, reactive arthritis, infectious bursitis, Lyme disease, and connective tissue disease. Nongonococcal arthritis should be suspected in patients at risk for the disease.

Treatment

Initial antimicrobial therapy should be based on the results of the Gram's stain and the clinical setting. If no microorganisms are seen on Gram's stain, empiric therapy for *S. aureus* and streptococci should be initiated. Therapy with oxacillin or nafcillin, 2 g IV q4h, or cefazolin, 1 g IV q8h, is appropriate initial therapy. If rates of methicillin-resistant *S. aureus* are high, empiric therapy with vancomycin, 1 g IV q12h, is indicated. Vancomycin levels should be followed to ensure proper dosing. Most experts would treat with IV therapy for 2–4 wks; in most cases, this can occur as an outpatient.

GONOCOCCAL ARTHRITIS

Pathophysiology

Gonococcal arthritis occurs in sexually active, usually young persons (<30 yrs) as a result of DGI caused by *Neisseria gonorrhoeae*. It is most common in menstruating women but also occurs during pregnancy and the peripartum period.

Clinical Manifestations

DGI typically presents with fever, migratory polyarthralgias, tenosynovitis (typically involving the hands and fingers), and skin lesions. The skin lesions may be maculopapular, vesicular, or necrotic. This has been described as the *arthritis-dermatitis syndrome*. Asymmetric joint involvement is common. The knee, elbow, wrist, and metacarpophalangeal joints are most commonly involved. If untreated, the patient will present later with a monoarticular arthritis.

Diagnosis

The history and exam lead to high index of suspicion for infection. Again, the diagnostic procedure of choice is arthrocentesis. This should be done immediately once the diagnosis is suspected and ideally before antimicrobial therapy is initiated. However, synovial fluid cultures are positive in only approximately 25–30% of patients with DGI. Nearly 80% of patients have a positive test for DNA of *N. gonorrhoeae* from the cervix, urethra, rectum, pharynx, or urine, and swabs from these sites should be obtained as clinically indicated. Blood cultures are positive only 5% of the time.

Differential Diagnosis

DGI must be differentiated from meningococcemia, other bacterial arthritis, reactive arthritis, secondary syphilis, and connective tissue diseases.

Treatment

In the appropriate clinical setting, empiric therapy for DGI should be initiated, as the Gram's stain will likely be negative. Therapy with ceftriaxone, 1 g IV q24h, for 24–48 hrs after clinical improvement followed by cefixime (Suprax), 400 mg PO q12h; ciprofloxacin, 500 mg PO q12h; or ofloxacin (Floxin), 400 mg PO q12h, to complete 1 wk of treatment.

VIRAL ARTHRITIS

Arthritis is a common complication of infections with HBV, parvovirus B19, rubella virus, and the alpha viruses. Arthritis can also occur with HSV, mumps, enteroviruses, and adenoviruses. Most commonly, there is joint invasion during a period of viremia; however, immune complex deposition has been postulated to play a role. There is no specific pattern that is unique to a given viral etiology. Diagnosis is based on clinical clues and viral serologies. The disease is typically self-limited but may rarely progress to chronic arthropathy. Prevention is dependent on vaccination.

KEY POINTS TO REMEMBER

- Necrotizing fasciitis is a rapidly progressing and potentially fatal disease. Check your patient frequently. Get the surgeons involved as soon as you suspect NF.
- Always do a thorough foot exam in your diabetic patients. A foot ulcer should always be evaluated for the possibility of osteomyelitis. Toenail clipping and callus removal by a podiatrist are important preventive measures as is daily foot exam by the patient.
- Gas gangrene is associated with a high rate of mortality. Look for crepitance on exam and air in x-rays. Immediate surgical consult and antibiotics are crucial for favorable clinical and microbiologic outcomes.
- Osteomyelitis is a difficult-to-treat infection. Prolonged course(s) of antibiotic therapy is needed for optimal treatment. IV therapy is the preferred route. Check periodic ESR to monitor the patient's response to therapy. Generally, parenteral antibiotic therapy is continued for 6 wks, possibly followed by switch to a PO regimen.

REFERENCES AND SUGGESTED READINGS

Caputo GM, Cavanagh PR, Ulbrecht JS, et al. Assessment and management of foot disease in patients with diabetes. *N Engl J Med* 1994;331:854–860.

Gillespie WJ. Prevention and management of infection after total joint replacement. *Clin Infect Dis* 1997;25:1310–1317.

Lew DP, Waldvogel FA. Osteomyelitis. *N Engl J Med* 1997;336:999–1007.

Lipsky BA. Osteomyelitis of the foot in diabetic patients. *Clin Infect Dis* 1997;25:1318–1326.

Nichols RL, Florman S. Clinical presentations of soft-tissue infections and surgical site infections. *Clin Infect Dis* 2001;33[Suppl 2]:S84–S93.

Swartz MN. Skin and soft tissue infections. In: Mandell GL, Bennett JE, Dolin R, eds. *Mandell, Douglas, and Bennett's principles and practice of infectious diseases,* 5th ed. Philadelphia: Churchill Livingstone, 2000.

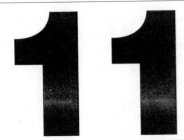

Eye Infections

Kristin Mondy

INTRODUCTION

Infections of the eye have typically been categorized at the tissue level and include conjunctivitis, keratitis, infections of periorbital structures, and infections of deeper intraocular structures (endophthalmitis, uveitis, and retinitis). There are also numerous noninfectious causes of eye inflammation; thus, the initial patient history and physical exam should include recent noninfectious exposures (chemical irritants, trauma, allergens, foreign bodies, and medications), other systemic diseases, and specific ocular diseases such as glaucoma. Suspected infections that are immediately sight-threatening or involve deeper ocular structures should be referred emergently to an ophthalmologist for more detailed slit-lamp exam and initiation of intraocular therapy if needed. Before referral, nonophthalmologists should perform a detailed exam of the eye that includes visual acuity, cranial nerve function, funduscopic exam, and careful inspection of the pupil, conjunctiva, cornea, and periorbital structures.

EYELID INFECTIONS

Eyelid infections are some of the most common infections and include hordeola (sty) and blepharitis (usually a chronic inflammation of the eyelid margins). Both are usually due to staphylococci. Patients often present with redness and swelling at the eyelid margin, as well as pain or itching.

Treatment

Blepharitis can be a risk in persons with chronic skin or eye conditions and should be treated with hygienic measures (warm compresses and scrubbing with diluted baby shampoo) as well as prolonged therapy with a topical antibiotic ointment, such as bacitracin. If symptoms are still present after 2–3 wks, then further measures such as surgical incision and drainage or intralesional steroids may also be appropriate. Relapses can be frequent. Hordeola are usually treated with hot soaks unless located internally in a meibomian gland, in which pain and swelling may be more pronounced, and the addition of an oral antistaphylococcal antibiotic (e.g., dicloxacillin, 500 mg PO qid) may be required. HSV and VZV may occasionally infect the eyelids. Antiviral therapy is not required unless corneal involvement is suspected.

LACRIMAL SYSTEM INFECTIONS

Clinical Manifestations

The lacrimal system (canaliculi, sac, and ducts) can be predisposed to infection due to stasis of tear flow from an anatomic defect, trauma, or local disease. Canaliculitis often presents with pain and tenderness in the inner canthus. Dacryocystitis, or inflammation of the lacrimal sac, may present either acutely with local pain, erythema, and swelling or chronically as a block in tear drainage.

Diagnosis

A variety of viruses, fungi, and bacteria can cause this infection, but it is most frequently due to *Actinomyces israelii*. Pressure over the punctum and expression of exudate containing characteristic microscopic granules on Gram's stain confirm the diagnosis.

Treatment

Therapy consists of drainage and irrigation with fluid containing PCN. For dacryocystitis, treatment usually requires drainage as well as systemic antibiotic therapy (directed against common colonizing nasal and skin flora) in acute cases.

PERIORBITAL CELLULITIS

Clinical Manifestations

Patients may present with upper or lower lid edema; with orbital involvement, there may be proptosis, reduced eye mobility, and even vision loss.

Diagnosis

Blood cultures should be obtained before initiation of broad-spectrum parenteral antibiotics and CT or MRI performed to determine the extent of orbital involvement and need for possible débridement. A rare but extremely serious cause of orbital cellulitis is mucormycosis. Patients are usually diabetic with ketoacidosis or otherwise immunosuppressed.

Differential Diagnosis

Common pathogens include streptococci, staphylococci, and *Haemophilus influenzae* (in children) and are acquired via contiguous spread, usually from the sinuses.

Treatment

Treatment with ceftriaxone (Rocephin, 2 g IV q24h) empirically should be initiated. Emergent ENT consultation for diagnostic biopsy and surgical débridement is usually required, along with high doses of amphotericin B in cases of suspected mucormycosis.

CONJUNCTIVITIS

Conjunctivitis is most likely due to a viral, bacterial, or allergic etiology. Viral conjunctivitis is most commonly seen and is usually due to adenovirus.

Clinical Manifestations

Patients typically present with itching, watery discharge; follicular reaction at the lids; redness; tearing; and preauricular lymphadenopathy over a period of 2 days to 2 wks. Bacterial conjunctivitis usually presents as an acute process with marked hyperemia, lid edema, and a purulent exudate.

Differential Diagnosis

HSV (usually type 1) can be a common viral cause in children but is rare in adults (in whom it usually presents as keratitis). Lid or oral vesicles/ulcers are sometimes present, and patients should be seen by an ophthalmologist to rule out corneal involvement if HSV is suspected. The classic lesion in HSV is a corneal dendritic lesion. Routine Gram's stain and culture can be taken of any purulent discharge; otherwise, therapy is generally empiric.

Treatment

Treatment is supportive and consists of cold compresses and lubricants. Most cases of bacterial conjunctivitis are due to streptococcal and staphylococcal species and are treated empirically with eyedrops, such as bacitracin–polymyxin B (Polysporin), trimethoprim, or ciprofloxacin (Cipro), until symptoms resolve.

Prevention

The virus is extremely contagious via hand/eye/fomites, and a work or school excuse for up to 2 wks from the day of onset should be considered. Health care workers should be removed from direct patient contact until symptoms resolve. Cultures and immunofluorescent testing should be taken for neonatal, chronic, unusual, or severe cases in which *Neisseria gonorrhoeae* or *Chlamydia trachomatis* may be etiologies. Adult chlamydial conjunctivitis, termed *inclusion conjunctivitis*, can present insidiously with minimal inflammation and the presence of large, lush follicles. All oculogenital cases are supported by the patient's history and require additional systemic therapy [7 days ceftriaxone (Rocephin) for gonorrheal infection; up to 3 wks doxycycline for inclusion disease], frequent ophthalmologic referral, and treatment of mother or sexual partner. A rare type of bacterial conjunctivitis is oculoglandular (Parinaud's) syndrome, a granulomatous inflammation (usually unilateral) associated with preauricular lymphadenopathy and most commonly seen in cat-scratch disease or tularemia. Resolution usually occurs with systemic treatment of the underlying disease.

KERATITIS

Infections that cause keratitis, or inflammation of the cornea, are usually sight-threatening and require urgent ophthalmologic referral. HSV-1 is the most common adult cause of keratitis in the developed world. Cases are most likely due to recurrence of latent infection triggered by factors such as fever, sunlight, or trauma, and there may be accompanying vesicles or ulcers elsewhere. Bacterial keratitis may present with corneal clouding and ciliary hyperemia in addition to the clinical symptoms noted above. Risk factors include contact lens wear with poor lens hygiene, trauma or surgery, dry eye, and immunosuppression (including diabetes or corticosteroid use).

Clinical Manifestations

Patients frequently present acutely with unilateral eye pain, photophobia, tearing, and blurred vision. Discharge is usually absent. Acanthamebic keratitis usually progresses insidiously over several weeks.

Diagnosis

HSV and other viral causes are diagnosed by visualization of characteristic dendritic branching seen on the cornea after staining with fluorescein. Common causes of bacterial keratitis in non–contact lens wearers include staphylococci, streptococci, and Enterobacteriaceae, whereas *Pseudomonas* is most frequently associated with the use of soft contacts. Diagnosis of bacterial keratitis is made by Gram's stain and culture of corneal scrapings. For fungal keratitis, diagnosis requires microscopic visualization of characteristic cysts from scrapings stained with calcofluor white. Fungal keratitis may require corneal biopsy as well as scraping for definitive diagnosis.

Differential Diagnosis

Infectious causes of keratitis include viral, bacterial, fungal, or parasitic (*Acanthamoeba*) pathogens. Corneal trauma (usually of plant origin) or immunosuppression predisposes to fungal keratitis, most commonly caused by *Aspergillus*, *Fusarium*, or *Candida* species. *Acanthamoeba* are ubiquitous in soil and water and are usually acquired via contamination of contact lens solutions or trauma.

Treatment

Treatment of viral keratitis includes the use of a topical suppressive HSV agent, such as trifluridine (Viroptic), for up to 3 wks. Occasionally, epithelial débridement is also required. Recurrences are common and may be reduced with the use of suppressive oral acyclovir (Zovirax) therapy. VZV keratitis may occur in ≥50% of patients with herpes zoster who have trigeminal ganglion involvement; thus, treatment should be focused on prevention of this complication with the use of oral acyclovir as soon as possible after the appearance of facial lesions. For presumptive treatment of bacterial keratitis, topical broad-spectrum therapy with more than one antibiotic [i.e., piperacillin plus tobramycin or vancomycin plus ceftazidime (Fortaz)] is usually begun before microbial confirmation. Antibiotics are initially given q15–60 mins around the clock for 1–3 days, with subsequent taper over several weeks. Débridement may also be necessary. For fungal keratitis, therapy often consists of combined topical and system therapy. Therapy is usually empiric, with natamycin (Natacyn) drops and débridement if necessary. Response is poor compared with bacterial keratitis.

ENDOPHTHALMITIS

Although it is uncommon, endophthalmitis is a serious threat to vision that involves the vitreous humor and other deep intraocular structures. It is categorized into several subgroups based on clinical setting and route of acquisition, including acute postop (within 2 wks); delayed-onset (after 2 wks); trauma-related; conjunctival filtering bleb-associated; and endogenous (by hematologic spread) sources.

Clinical Manifestations

Clinical symptoms may vary greatly depending on the timing and mode of infection; thus, a high index of suspicion and urgent ophthalmologic referral are very important. In all cases, the vitreous humor is involved and usually appears abnormal with increasing haziness.

Diagnosis

Definitive diagnosis usually requires that both the aqueous and vitreous humor be aspirated before therapy for appropriate stains and culture. Many organisms that cause infection can otherwise be normal colonizing flora of the ocular, nasal, and facial areas.

Differential Diagnosis

Acute infections are most commonly due to coagulase-negative staphylococci, followed by *Staphylococcus aureus,* streptococci, and, more rarely, gram-negatives. Delayed-onset infections are more likely due to indolent organisms, such as *Propionibacterium acnes, Staphylococcus epidermidis,* and *Corynebacterium* species, whereas bleb-associated infections are commonly due to streptococcal species and *H. influenzae.* Posttraumatic infections are often polymicrobial and can include *Clostridium* species, *S. aureus,* and *Bacillus cereus.* Endogenous infection is usually associated with another distant site of infection and is often seen with streptococci, *S. aureus,* Enterobacteriaceae, and *Neisseria meningitidis. Candida* species and other fungi are common in injecting drug users and immunosuppressed conditions.

Treatment

Therapy consists of early use of both intravitreal and systemic therapies against suspected and confirmed pathogens. Duration of therapy is variable. Up to 50% of patients may have substantial vision loss within 24–48 hrs of onset of infection. Adjunctive vitrectomy and topical steroids may also help; thus, close collaboration with ophthalmology is needed.

RETINITIS AND UVEITIS

Although the retina and uveal tract (choroid, iris, and ciliary body) often overlap with other intraocular structures discussed above, they are highly vascularized tissues and are thus prone to hematogenous spread from a variety of systemic infections.

Clinical Manifestations

Common symptoms include "floaters," changes in vision, photophobia, and pain. Any patient describing these symptoms should be referred to an ophthalmologist for a slit-lamp exam.

Diagnosis

A slit-lamp exam can usually isolate the lesion and provide assistance in narrowing the differential diagnosis and obtaining appropriate material for culture and pathology. Additional tests, including chest x-ray, CBC, ESR, serologic tests (e.g., VDRL, fungal battery, Lyme), and HLA-B27 antigen can be helpful. Syphilitic ocular infection may be suspected when uveitis worsens with steroid treatment. If serum serologic tests are subsequently positive, then a lumbar puncture and HIV test should also be performed.

Differential Diagnosis

Potential causes include (a) congenital infections (including toxoplasmosis, which may remain asymptomatic until later in life); (b) CMV retinitis or progressive outer retinal necrosis due to VZV (typically in patients with AIDS); (c) HSV; (d) secondary syphilis; (e) late Lyme disease; (f) *Toxocara canis*; (g) *Bartonella henselae*; (h) *Mycobacterium tuberculosis*; and (i) fungi, including *Candida* species and *Histoplasma capsulatum*. Uveitis is also a complication of many autoimmune and rheumatologic systemic diseases. Patients with advanced HIV may be particularly prone to infectious causes of retinitis and uveitis. CMV retinitis is most common, but other diseases, such as VZV, HSV, *Pneumocystis*, mycobacteria, and fungi, may infect these eye structures. Uveitis may also be a complication of rifabutin therapy in HIV-infected patients receiving other medications that elevate rifabutin levels. Patients receiving ethambutol are at risk for a retrobulbar neuritis and should receive visual acuity and red-green color perception testing at baseline and every 4 wks while taking this drug.

Treatment

Treatment varies for these conditions and should be guided with infectious disease input and ophthalmologic consultation.

KEY POINTS TO REMEMBER

- Ocular infections require close consultation between the infectious disease specialist and the ophthalmologist to ensure proper diagnosis, treatment, and response to therapy. Emergent referral is advised.
- Orbital/periorbital cellulitis should be further evaluated with periorbital CT or MRI to look for postseptal involvement.

REFERENCES AND SUGGESTED READINGS

Barza M, Baum J. Ocular infections. *Infect Dis Clin North Am* 1992;6:769–1003.

Baum J. Infections of the eye. *Clin Infect Dis* 1995;21:479–488.

Duker JS, Barza M. Infectious retinitis and uveitis. In: Armstrong D, Cohen J, eds. *Infectious diseases*. London: Harcourt, 1999.

Herbert L. Conjunctivitis, keratitis, and infections of periorbital structures. In: Armstrong D, Cohen J, eds. *Infectious diseases*. London: Harcourt, 1999.

O'Brien TP. Eye infections. In: Mandell GL, Bennett JE, Dolin R, eds. *Mandell, Douglas, and Bennett's principles and practice of infectious diseases*, 5th ed. Philadelphia: Churchill Livingstone, 2000.

Tsai L, Kamenetzky S. Ophthalmology. In: Lin TL, Rypkema SW, eds. *The Washington manual of ambulatory therapeutics*. Philadelphia: Lippincott Williams & Wilkins, 2003:584–597.

Whitby M, Hirst L. Endophthalmitis. In: Armstrong D, Cohen J, eds. *Infectious diseases*. London: Harcourt, 1999.

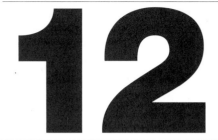

Central Nervous System Infections

Erin K. Quirk

ACUTE MENINGITIS

The spectrum of disease in acute meningitis is quite variable in terms of the etiologic agents, severity of symptoms, and prognosis for recovery. In general, this entity is defined as an inflammatory condition of the meninges that is usually manifested over the course of hours to days and is accompanied by the presence of a CSF pleocytosis. **Acute bacterial meningitis** with encapsulated organisms is an **infectious disease emergency** requiring prompt antimicrobial therapy, whereas viral or aseptic meningitis is typically a self-limiting illness that requires only supportive treatment.

Pathophysiology

The infectious etiologic agents of acute meningitis can be divided among bacterial, viral, fungal, and protozoan organisms. The **encapsulated upper respiratory pathogens** have historically been the most important and common bacterial agents of acute bacterial meningitis, accounting for approximately 80% of cases. Whereas pneumococcus and meningococcus remain the most common causes, *Haemophilus influenzae* B has become a much less common agent of meningitis since the introduction of vaccines against this organism in 1987. The discussion of bacteria causing community-acquired meningitis is best approached by categorizing patients according to age group (Table 12-1).

Risk factors for gram-negative bacterial meningitis include head trauma, neurosurgical procedures, immunosuppression, gram-negative sepsis, and extremes of age (neonates and the elderly).

Other bacteria have been well defined as agents of meningitis. Nocardial meningitis usually occurs in patients with malignancy, sarcoidosis, and other chronic granulomatous disease; patients with history of head trauma or CNS procedures; and in those taking immunosuppressant medications. Diphtheroids and *Staphylococcus epidermidis* are frequently associated with meningitis resulting from CNS shunt and ventriculostomy infections. Syphilitic meningitis is the earliest stage of neurosyphilis, and invasion into the CNS by *Treponema pallidum* is believed to occur in ≥10% of cases of primary syphilis. Approximately 15% of Lyme disease cases have CNS involvement with *Borrelia burgdorferi*. *Leptospira* is another spirochete that has been associated with outbreaks of meningitis resulting from contact with infected water, most notably in triathletes swimming in contaminated lake water. *Mycobacterium tuberculosis* is the most common agent of mycobacterial meningitis, although CNS infections with *Mycobacterium avium* complex, *Mycobacterium kansasii*, *Mycobacterium gordonae*, and *Mycobacterium genavense* are well described, particularly among immunocompromised hosts. A number of rickettsial pathogens can cause meningitis as a part of the systemic syndromes of Rocky Mountain spotted fever and epidemic (louse-borne), endemic (murine), and scrub typhus. *Ehrlichia chaffeensis*, *Ehrlichia ewingii*, and the agent of human granulocytic ehrlichiosis also cause meningitis and encephalitis, although usually in the context of the systemic syndrome of ehrlichiosis.

The virulence factors of meningococcus and pneumococcus leading to meningitis have been well studied. **Nasopharyngeal colonization** via fimbriae is the primary event. The

TABLE 12-1. BACTERIA CAUSING COMMUNITY-ACQUIRED MENINGITIS

Age group	Common bacterial agents
0–4 wks	Group B streptococci, *Escherichia coli*, *Listeria monocytogenes*, *Klebsiella pneumoniae*, *Enterococcus*, *Salmonella*
4–12 wks	Group B streptococci, *E. coli*, *L. monocytogenes*, *Haemophilus influenzae*, *Streptococcus pneumoniae*, *Neisseria meningitidis*
3 mos–18 yrs	*H. influenzae*, *N. meningitidis*, *S. pneumoniae*
18–50 yrs	*S. pneumoniae*, *N. meningitidis*
≥50 yrs	*S. pneumoniae*, *N. meningitidis*, *L. monocytogenes*, enteric gram-negative bacilli

bacterial capsule also aids in attachment and evasion of host immunity, particularly in patients with complement deficiencies and in asplenic hosts in whom phagocytic immune cell response is attenuated. The mechanisms for meningeal invasion by encapsulated bacteria are poorly understood, although it is clear that once organisms are present in the subarachnoid space, the local host defense mechanisms and resultant neutrophilic inflammatory response are unable to control these highly lethal infections. Group B streptococci colonize the nasopharyngeal mucosa of neonates born to vaginally colonized mothers during delivery, although mechanisms of CNS infection are poorly understood with this pathogen as well. Screening for group G streptococci at 35–37 wks' gestation and use of perinatal prophylaxis with ampicillin among positive carriers have proved effective in preventing *Streptococcus agalactiae* sepsis and meningitis in neonates [1].

The higher predominance of **gram-negative** meningeal infections among neonates and the elderly is poorly understood. Direct invasion or inoculation is the mechanism of gram-negative infection occurring as a result of head trauma or neurosurgical procedures.

Viruses are the most common agents of aseptic meningitis. Enteroviruses account for ≥85% of these infections. Other notable agents of viral meningitis include the herpesviruses (HSV-1 and -2, HHV-6, EBV, VZV, and CMV), lymphocytic choriomeningitis virus, and acute HIV infection. After initial infection, these viruses invade the CNS via a variety of mechanisms, such as direct invasion of the cells constituting the blood–brain barrier and the choroid plexus. Herpesviruses are believed to gain access to the CNS via afferent nerves. Other viral meningitides are believed to follow viremic periods. Once viral particles enter the subarachnoid space, recruitment of inflammatory cells and activation of cytokine cascades occur, resulting in the typical signs and symptoms of meningitis.

Acute meningitis can occur with *Cryptococcus*, *Aspergillus*, and *Candida* species, typically in **immunosuppressed hosts.** These fungal organisms gain access to the CNS, usually after respiratory infection in cases of *Cryptococcus* and *Aspergillus* and after fungemic episodes usually from primary bloodstream infections or other focal sites of infection in cases of *Candida*.

Parasitic meningitis is rare in the United States. The ameba *Naegleria fowleri* is the protozoan most commonly associated with primary amebic meningitis. Infection occurs typically in children via exposure to fecally contaminated water, although asymptomatic carriers have been described. *Angiostrongylus cantonensis* is the classic agent of eosinophilic meningitis that occurs after dissemination of adult worms from GI infection, which is fairly prevalent in Southeast Asia and perpetuated by exposure to the fecal material of rats. *Strongyloides stercoralis* can also cause meningitis typically in the setting of the hyperinfection syndrome and subsequent overwhelming parasitemia in HIV patients.

Clinical Manifestations

The hallmark symptoms of acute meningeal irritation are **headache** and **neck stiffness.** Most patients also report **fever.** Acute bacterial meningitis typically progresses to altered levels of consciousness, whereas aseptic meningitis typically does not progress beyond mild confusion. A history consistent with pneumonia or URI may be elicited in cases of *S. pneumoniae* or *H. influenzae* meningitis.

Fever is usually present in all forms of acute meningitis. Bacterial meningitis may present with hypotension and tachycardia. The bilateral adrenal hemorrhage characteristic of the Waterhouse-Friderichsen syndrome that can accompany meningococcal meningitis must also be considered in patients who present with hypotension. Some degree of nuchal rigidity is usually present in all forms of acute meningitis. A diffuse petechial rash with predilection for the extremities is the classic physical exam finding of meningococcal meningitis. The neurologic exam can be quite variable, ranging from normal to nonspecific alterations in level of cognitive function to focal weakness.

Diagnosis

Performance of the **lumbar puncture and analysis of CSF** are crucial. Meningitis, by definition, is an inflammation of the meninges; therefore, the demonstration of inflammatory cells within the CSF is the hallmark of diagnosis. CT of head or MRI of brain and spinal cord with IV contrast typically reveals meningeal enhancement.

Treatment

When acute bacterial meningitis is suspected, **IV antibiotics should be administered immediately** and should not be delayed by diagnostic testing, including head CT and lumbar puncture. High-dose cephalosporins that cross the blood–brain barrier, such as ceftriaxone, 2 g IV q12h, are typically the empiric treatment of choice in cases of acute bacterial meningitis. Vancomycin, 15 mg/kg IV q12h, is typically added to cover for beta-lactam–resistant *S. pneumoniae* infections until susceptibilities are available. Patients with acute bacterial meningitis, particularly pneumococcal, may benefit from adjunctive dexamethasone (10 mg IV q6h for 4 days, begun early *before* antibiotics) [2]. Ampicillin may be administered in cases of *L. monocytogenes* meningitis. Aseptic meningitis is usually treated with acyclovir, 10 mg/kg IV, until HSV infection can be ruled out. A delay in administration of acyclovir of >72 hrs after onset of symptoms of HSV-1 meningitis is associated with poor outcome. Supportive care is the typical treatment of nonherpetic aseptic meningitis, which usually resolves spontaneously. Amphotericin B is the usually recommended treatment of fungal meningitis, although some cases of cryptococcal meningitis can be treated with 5-fluorouracil or high-dose fluconazole.

CHRONIC MENINGITIS

The syndrome of chronic meningitis is typically defined as symptoms and signs of meningoencephalitis with evidence of meningeal inflammation that persists or progresses over the course of **4 wks.** Routine bacterial pathogens are less common etiologic agents than are mycobacterial or fungal organisms. Infectious chronic meningitis is fairly rare, and noninfectious entities are important to consider. Most cases of chronic meningitis in areas where TB is not endemic are noninfectious.

Pathophysiology

The most common organism causing chronic meningitis in endemic areas is *M. tuberculosis*. Atypical mycobacteria can also cause chronic CNS infection, usually in the setting of systemic disease in the immunocompromised host. Fungi are also important agents of chronic meningitis, particularly *Candida* species, cryptococcosis, histoplasmosis, coccidioidomycosis, and blastomycosis. *Sporothrix schenckii* has clearly been reported to cause chronic meningitis but is quite uncommon. The bacteria most commonly associated with chronic meningitis are *T. pallidum* (secondary and tertiary syphilis), *B. burgdorferi* (Lyme disease), and *Brucella*. The specific means by which these pathogens invade the CNS has not been definitively elucidated; however, it is assumed that systemic infection is present in most cases.

Clinical Manifestations

Patients typically present with the subacute or insidious onset of headache, neck stiffness, fever, confusion, and often cognitive changes. Overt sepsis is uncommon as an initial presentation. Nausea and vomiting are frequently present as signs of increased ICP. Per the definition of chronic meningitis, these symptoms are present for several weeks and may wax and wane but should not entirely resolve.

History of potential exposure to certain etiologic agents is often key to making the diagnosis of infectious chronic meningitis. A family history of or exposure to TB must be actively sought. Travel to the San Joaquin Valley of the southwestern United States may invoke the possibility of coccidioidomycosis, whereas exposure to tick bites in New England may suggest late Lyme disease.

There are no true pathognomonic physical findings in chronic meningitis. Fever should be documented. Nuchal rigidity is often present. Neurologic exam can vary from normal to evident cranial nerve palsies, gait disruption, ataxia, lethargy, and alterations in speech and memory. It is important to evaluate the fundi for papilledema, as this is evidence of increased ICP and reason to defer lumbar puncture. The skin exam is particularly important, and any acute or subacute finding, such as nodules, abscesses, and rashes, should be noted, as biopsy of these lesions may prove to be diagnostic.

Diagnosis

It is often difficult to arrive at the definitive diagnosis of chronic meningitis. According to some case series, 30–85% of cases go undiagnosed. Nevertheless, every effort should be made to obtain CSF and often brain or meningeal biopsy for culture when possible.

The CSF profile may vary, but a lymphocytic pleocytosis and elevated protein are almost always present. **Lumbar puncture** should be performed on multiple occasions to demonstrate persistent meningeal inflammation over time and to increase the diagnostic microbiologic yield. Fluid should be sent for routine, fungal, and mycobacterial cultures, which should be held for up to 6 wks. Testing for histoplasma antigen and cryptococcal antigen from CSF is indicated. Serum cryptococcal antigen is also indicated, although a negative test does not rule out meningeal disease. Concomitant routine, fungal, and mycobacterial cultures of blood, sputum, and urine should also be performed. PPD skin testing is indicated in all cases and should be repeated in 2–4 wks if negative. There is no clear role for fungal antigen skin testing.

All patients with evidence of chronic meningitis should undergo **HIV testing** as the presence of HIV/AIDS broadens the differential diagnosis significantly. **Neuroimaging** in the form of head CT with IV contrast or brain MRI with gadolinium contrast should also be performed to define focal mass lesions or particular areas of meningeal enhancement to guide invasive neurosurgical biopsy for culture and further diagnostic testing in the case of a negative workup as above. Any focal finding, such as skin lesions, hepatomegaly, or hematopoietic disturbance, should be investigated by biopsy of the organ system of interest. Specimens should be sent for routine, fungal, and mycobacterial cultures as well as pathologic exam and other indicated diagnostic testing, as these may be the key to diagnosis.

Treatment

Empiric therapy of chronic meningitis is indicated when the clinical course decompensates in the midst of workup or when comprehensive evaluation has been negative. A four-drug antituberculous regimen is typically the first choice for empiric therapy. If there is definitive proof of tuberculous meningitis, glucocorticoid therapy at 0.5–1.0 mg/kg PO should be considered. A full course of therapy as for pulmonary TB should be completed if cultures become positive for *M. tuberculosis*, CSF polymerase chain reaction (PCR) confirms the presence of TB, or if patients respond clinically.

Treatment is otherwise guided by identification of the causative organism. Cryptococcal meningitis can be treated with fluconazole at a minimum dose of 400 mg/day for ≥6 mos. Other forms of fungal meningitis are typically treated with long courses of amphotericin B. Lumbar puncture should be repeated periodically to document resolution of pleocytosis, normalization of CSF protein, and failure of the organism to grow in culture over time. High-dose PCN IV is indicated for tertiary syphilis, and resolution of CSF VDRL positivity must be documented.

BRAIN ABSCESS

A brain abscess is a suppurative fluid collection that initially begins as a cerebritis. Approximately 1500–2500 cases occur in the United States each year. Before the availability of antimicrobial medicines and sophisticated neuroimaging and neurosurgical techniques, this diagnosis was almost uniformly fatal. Currently, mortality rates range from 0% to 42%.

The greatest risk factor for brain abscess is **immunosuppression.** Advanced HIV, bone marrow transplant (BMT), and solid organ transplant patients are those most frequently affected. A second group at risk for developing brain abscess includes patients with severe or chronic cardiopulmonary disease, particularly those with chronic pyogenic lung disease, congenital cyanotic heart disease (e.g., tetralogy of Fallot and transposition of the great vessels), and hereditary hemorrhagic telangiectasia with pulmonary arteriovenous malformations. Patients with penetrating head trauma, particularly gunshot wounds, compose another cohort at risk for brain abscess. Postcraniotomy patients have an appreciable but much smaller risk. Brain abscess is a relatively uncommon complication of bacterial endocarditis.

Pathophysiology

Microbial pathogens infect the CNS by three major routes. **Contiguous spread** from infected structures (e.g., sinusitis, otitis, and dental abscesses) comprises an estimated 50% in nonimmunocompromised hosts. Approximately 25% of all cases result from **hematogenous spread** of organisms, which is the major mechanism of disease in immunosuppressed individuals. **Reactivation of latent infection** is the major cause of CNS toxoplasmosis, which typically occurs in immunocompromised patients, particularly those with AIDS. 20–30% of cases are "cryptic" brain abscesses in which no clear sources of infection can be identified.

The microbiology of brain abscesses is best discussed in terms of the immunologic state of the host. Brain abscess in **immunocompetent** patients typically results from bacterial infection, which is a polymicrobial process in 60% of cases. Streptococci, the most common organisms found in brain abscess, are demonstrated in 70% of bacterial cases. The most frequently isolated of these are the *Streptococcus milleri* group, which includes *Streptococcus anginosus*, *Streptococcus intermedius*, and *Streptococcus constellatus*. The next most commonly identified bacteria are anaerobes, particularly *Bacteroides* and *Prevotella* species, which are present in 40–100% of cases, depending on the reported case series. Enteric gram-negative organisms are isolated in 20–33% of cases and are more common in immunocompromised patients. *Staphylococcus aureus* is found in approximately 10–15% of pyogenic brain abscesses and often is introduced by penetrating trauma, neurosurgical procedures, and bacterial endocarditis. In developing countries, an important, nonbacterial, etiologic agent of brain abscess in immunocompetent patients is the larval form of the pork tapeworm *Taenia solium*, which causes neurocysticercosis.

The spectrum of microbial agents causing brain abscess in **immunocompromised** hosts is quite different. BMT patients are at particular risk for fungal brain abscess, especially with *Aspergillus* and *Candida* species. *Toxoplasma gondii* CNS infections are very common in patients with AIDS who are also at risk for brain abscess caused by *Cryptococcus neoformans*, *Nocardia* species, *Candida* species, mycobacteria, and *L.*

monocytogenes. Solid organ transplant patients tend to be affected by the same spectrum of organisms as HIV patients. Brain abscess in neutropenic patients can be caused by enteric gram-negative bacteria or other bacteria previously discussed. These patients also are at particular risk of fungal involvement with *Aspergillus* species, *Candida* species, or the molds included in the Mucoraceae family (*Rhizopus*, *Absidia*, and *Mucor*). The Mucoraceae are also notorious for causing orbital cellulitis in diabetics that can rapidly invade the CNS and cause brain and cavernous sinus abscess in these patients.

Clinical Manifestations

Headache, fever, and **focal neurologic deficit** comprise the classic symptomologic triad of brain abscess. In clinical practice, however, <50% of patients present with this complete triad. Most patients with brain abscess report headache (present in 70% of cases). Other prominent symptoms include mental status changes, seizures, nausea, vomiting, and nuchal rigidity. Although this profile of symptoms seems similar to that seen in acute meningitis, the onset of these complaints in brain abscess tends to be less acute, and focal neurologic signs are usually more pronounced, which may help to distinguish between the diagnoses. Sudden worsening of a prior subacute headache with the onset of meningismus is an important clue to the possibility of abscess rupture into a ventricular space, a complication that carries a poor prognosis.

Fever is frequently absent in patients with brain abscess; therefore, a normal temperature does not exclude the diagnosis. It is important to note the level of alertness of the patient, as those with increased ICP (also evidenced by gait disturbance on neurologic exam) typically require more prompt neurosurgical attention. A careful HEENT exam revealing evidence of a sinus, middle ear, or dental process may be a clue to the diagnosis of brain abscess. The funduscopic exam is particularly important, as up to 25% of cases present with papilledema, which again indicates increased ICP and necessitates prompt neurosurgical evaluation. The patient should be evaluated for nuchal rigidity. A complete neurologic exam is crucial to determine whether focal neurologic signs are present. Common findings include hemiparesis, hemisensory deficits, aphasia, and ataxia, although any deficit is possible depending on the location of the abscess within the brain.

Diagnosis

Standard lab exam should include a CBC in which the WBC count is often normal. ESR can be elevated or within the normal range. Lumbar puncture can be dangerous due to risk of brain herniation from space-occupying lesions often associated with increased ICP, and it is rarely helpful in maintaining the diagnosis of brain abscess. The exception to this is in cases of CNS toxoplasmosis in which PCR of CSF can amplify *T. gondii* DNA, a very sensitive and specific diagnostic procedure.

The development of sophisticated neuroimaging techniques in the late 20th century has revolutionized the diagnosis and treatment of brain abscess. The CT appearance of these lesions typically shows a hypodense center in the peripheral ring enhancement with IV contrast. MRI of the brain is more sensitive for early cerebritis and associated satellite lesions and therefore has become the imaging procedure of choice for brain abscess. Of note, the lack of contrast enhancement of brain abscesses on either CT or MRI is a poor prognostic sign, as it indicates an inability of the host to mount the appropriate inflammatory mechanisms to encapsulate and isolate the offending organism.

Treatment

Resection or **aspiration** of suspected brain abscess with culture of tissue for routine bacterial as well as fungal and mycobacterial organisms is the preferred management. At times, this may not be possible due to the anatomic locations of the lesions and risks to the patient. In such cases, empiric antimicrobial therapy is guided by the organisms most likely to be the causative agent of disease according to the patient population as discussed above. In those cases resulting from direct spread of sinusitis or otitis, a regimen of a third-generation cephalosporin [cefotaxime (Claforan) or ceftriaxone is usually recommended given the ample data for CNS penetration with these agents] in conjunction with metronidazole is typically used. PCN can be added in cases resulting from dental or lung abscess. Vancomycin is often recommended as an additional agent in cases believed to originate from penetrating trauma, bacterial endocarditis, or congenital heart disease to cover for methicillin-resistant *S. aureus*. Cefepime (Maxipime) is frequently substituted for cefotaxime or ceftriaxone when nosocomially acquired gram-negative bacilli are suspected, although the CNS penetration of this drug has yet to be formally established. Antibiotic therapy can be tailored when the culture and susceptibility data are finalized. Appropriate neurosurgical excision or stereotactic aspiration is recommended for lesions >2.5 cm in any one dimension, when possible.

In patients with advanced HIV who present with multiple ring-enhancing lesions on magnetic resonance and with positive anti-*Toxoplasma* IgG serology or CSF PCR, there is rarely need for neurosurgical intervention for diagnostic purposes. **CNS toxoplasmosis** is typically treated with pyrimethamine (Daraprim) and sulfadiazine (Microsulfon) or clindamycin (Cleocin) in sulfa-allergic patients. Folinic acid supplementation (i.e., leucovorin, 10 mg PO qd) is required during pyrimethamine therapy. Lesions exerting significant symptomatic mass effect or with evidence of impending herniation require prompt neurosurgical intervention.

Optimal therapy of **fungal brain abscess** usually includes a combined medical and surgical approach. Amphotericin B preparations are the agents of choice for all fungal CNS infections, with 5-flucytosine adjunctive therapy for *Candida* and *Cryptococcus* infections. Aggressive surgical débridement is important for cerebral mucormycosis and in *Pseudallescheria boydii* brain abscess. Successful treatment with high-dose itraconazole (Sporanox) as well as caspofungin (Cancidas) for *Aspergillus* CNS infection has been reported, but these agents are not generally recommended as first-line therapy. Corticosteroids are important adjunctive agents in all patients with increased ICP from brain abscess.

ENCEPHALITIS

Most infectious encephalitides are **viral** in nature. The most serious of these is HSV encephalitis, which is the most life-threatening and the most likely to cause long-term neurologic sequelae. Before the availability of antiviral therapy, HSV encephalitis carried a 70% mortality rate, and <10% of infected patients regained full neurologic function.

A host of arboviruses, including Japanese encephalitis virus, eastern equine encephalitis virus, western equine encephalitis virus, St. Louis encephalitis virus, California encephalitis virus, and West Nile encephalitis virus (see West Nile Virus), can cause human encephalitis. These infections are all transmitted by mosquitoes and are typically rare with the exception of Japanese encephalitis virus, of which there are 50,000 annual case reports in Asia. The HIV virus can replicate in the CNS and cause encephalitis in both acute HIV infection and advanced HIV disease. Rabies, which is rare in the United States, is an important and fatal viral cause of encephalitis.

Nonviral causes of infectious encephalitis include tick-borne illnesses, such as Lyme disease, Colorado tick fever, ehrlichia, relapsing fever, and typhus, and often include an encephalitic picture. Tertiary syphilis is becoming less common but has historically been an important cause of encephalitis.

Pathophysiology

HSV encephalitis is usually caused by HSV-2. (Note that HSV-2 CNS infection is usually characterized by a self-limited aseptic meningitis rather than a true encephalitis.) One-third of cases arise during primary HSV-1 infection, one-third of cases occur during reactivation of mucocutaneous HSV-1, and one-third of cases arise in previously infected individuals with no cutaneous manifestation of HSV reactivation.

Arboviral encephalitis usually occurs during the summer months when people are exposed to biting mosquitoes. Regional epidemics of these viral infections have been well described in many cases. Most cases of rabies in the United States occur after the bite of a skunk, raccoon, or bat. In fact, if a person has been in close proximity to a bat (e.g., awakened with the animal in the room), even without clear evidence of a bite, rabies prophylaxis is warranted.

Although it has long been known that HSV has a particular predilection for the temporal lobes, the mechanisms by which HSV and arboviruses infect parenchymal cells of the brain and how they gain access to the CSF are poorly understood. The major pathophysiologic mechanism in these infections is the host's immune response to virally infected cells resulting in cell death and local inflammation.

Clinical Manifestations

Fever, headache with or without meningeal signs or symptoms, and **cognitive dysfunction** displayed as speech, memory, or behavior disturbances are the common presenting signs of viral encephalitides. Potential exposure to mosquitoes is an important factor in arboviral encephalitis.

Temporal lobe seizures are a particular manifestation of HSV encephalitis. Untreated HSV encephalitis can progress to change in level of consciousness, which is a poor prognostic sign. Presence of preceding herpetic mucocutaneous lesions is present in only one-third of cases.

Elevated temperature is a common but not exclusive finding. Nuchal rigidity can be present. Mental status exam usually reveals cognitive dysfunction and, at times, altered levels of alertness. Focal neurologic signs can be present. Poor short-term memory and aphasia are particularly characteristic of HSV encephalitis. The typical skin rashes of Rocky Mountain spotted fever, Lyme disease, and ehrlichiosis can be clues to these diagnoses.

Diagnosis

The most important diagnostic test is the **lumbar puncture** and **CSF analysis.** A pleocytosis is usually present but is variable, with a range of zero to thousands of WBCs. CSF profile typically shows an elevated protein and normal glucose. Elevated RBC count is particularly common in later-stage HSV disease. A normal CSF profile does not rule out early viral encephalitis. The peripheral blood can show an elevated WBC count, but this is not a sensitive or specific indicator of disease.

The current gold standard for the diagnosis of HSV encephalitis is PCR of viral DNA performed on CSF samples. This test is readily available at multiple centers and carries a high sensitivity and specificity, compared to the <15% sensitivity of viral culture of CSF. Noncontrast head CT is not usually helpful. CT of the head with contrast and MRI of the brain typically show inflammation, usually in the temporal lobe(s), which extends across both white and gray matter. Concomitant meningitis is often demonstrated as well with enhancement of the meninges. The CSF profile typically shows a normal protein and glucose, a normal or slightly elevated WBC count, and an elevated RBC count, particularly in later-stage disease. EEG demonstrating temporal lobe seizure activity adds further credibility toward the diagnosis of HSV meningitis and can be useful in directing anticonvulsant therapy.

Arboviral encephalitis is usually diagnosed by serology, and convalescent studies are sometimes required to definitively diagnose these disorders as well as many of the tick-borne illnesses. Human rabies remains a clinical and postmortem diagnosis. Patients presenting with headache and symptoms of encephalitis with recent potential exposures to HIV and negative HIV ELISA tests should undergo p24 antigen assay or HIV DNA PCR to rule out acute HIV.

Treatment

For HSV encephalitis, the treatment of choice is acyclovir, 10 mg/kg IV for 10 days to 3 wks, depending on the severity of the illness. Studies have shown that acyclovir can decrease morbidity and mortality from HSV encephalitis if administered early (i.e., before the onset of mental status changes). Therefore, if HSV encephalitis is suspected, acyclovir should be started before performing or awaiting diagnostic testing.

Even with acyclovir therapy, HSV encephalitis has significant mortality and morbidity, with only 25–40% regaining full neurologic function.

There is little available therapy for other viral encephalitides other than supportive care. HIV encephalitis should be treated with antiretroviral agents that have good CNS penetration, particularly zidovudine (Retrovir) and nevirapine (Viramune).

WEST NILE VIRUS

West Nile virus (WNV) was first isolated and identified in 1937 in a febrile person in the West Nile district of Uganda. Before 1999, the virus was found only in the eastern hemisphere, with wide distribution in Africa, Asia, the Middle East, and Europe. There were infrequent reports of human outbreaks, mainly associated with mild febrile illnesses, in Israel and Africa. One notable outbreak in Israeli nursing homes in 1957 was associated with severe neurologic disease and death. Since the mid-1990s, the frequency and apparent clinical severity of WNV outbreaks have increased. Outbreaks in Romania (1996), Russia (1999), and Israel (2000) involved hundreds of persons with severe neurologic disease. West Nile virus was first described in the United States in New York City in 1999 and has since spread across the country.

Pathophysiology

WNV is a single-stranded RNA virus of the family Flaviviridae, genus *Flavivirus*. WNV is a member of the Japanese encephalitis virus antigenic complex, which includes several medically important viruses associated with human encephalitis: Japanese encephalitis; St. Louis encephalitis; Murray Valley encephalitis; and Kunjin, an Australian subtype of WNV. The close antigenic relationship of the flaviviruses, particularly those belonging to the Japanese encephalitis complex, accounts for the serologic cross-reactions observed in the diagnostic laboratory. WNV is maintained in nature in a **transmission cycle that primarily involves birds and mosquitoes.** Humans and other mammals are incidental hosts. Age is by far the most important risk factor for developing neuroinvasive WNV infection.

Clinical Manifestations

The majority of persons infected with WNV experience no symptoms or clinical illness. Those who experience symptoms frequently develop West Nile fever, a syndrome consisting mostly of headache, fever, fatigue, and, on occasion, truncal rash and adenopathy. Severe neuroinvasive disease develops in a small minority of patients and is most commonly a meningoencephalitis, but patients may exhibit only meningeal signs without symptoms of encephalitis (i.e., confusion or focal neurologic signs). Features of severe disease include fever, diarrhea, ataxia and extrapyramidal signs, focal neurologic signs, seizures, and mental status changes. A minority of patients with severe disease develop a maculopapular or morbilliform rash involving the neck, trunk, arms, or legs. Flaccid paralysis has been described and can be very debilitating.

Total leukocyte counts in peripheral blood are mostly normal or elevated, with lymphopenia and anemia also occurring. Hyponatremia is sometimes present, particularly among patients with encephalitis. Exam of the CSF shows pleocytosis, usually with a predominance of lymphocytes. Protein is universally elevated. Glucose is normal. CT is not useful in the diagnosis of WNV infection but is useful in excluding other etiologies of acute meningoencephalitis. Brain MRI is often normal but sometimes displays leptomeningeal enhancement or parenchymal signal changes.

Diagnosis

WNV infection can be suspected based on clinical symptoms and patient history. Lab testing is required for a confirmed diagnosis. The most efficient diagnostic method is detection of IgM antibody to WNV in serum collected within 8–14 days of illness onset or CSF collected within 8 days of illness onset using the IgM antibody-capture, enzyme-linked immunosorbent assay (MAC-ELISA). Because IgM antibody does not cross the blood–brain barrier, presence of IgM in CSF strongly suggests CNS infection. The serologic tests for WNV cross react with other closely related flaviviruses (Japanese encephalitis, St. Louis encephalitis, yellow fever, dengue), and this should be kept in mind in recently immunized patients (yellow fever) or if other arboviruses are active in the community. Neutralization assays (plaque reduction neutralization tests) are more specific and should be considered if any of these other infections are suspected. The diagnosis of WNV infection relies on a high index of clinical suspicion and on results of specific laboratory tests. WNV or other arboviral diseases, such as St. Louis encephalitis, should be seriously considered in adults ≥50 yrs of age who have onset of unexplained encephalitis or meningitis in late summer or early fall.

Treatment

No specific treatment is available. Severe cases require supportive care that often involves hospitalization, IV fluids, respiratory support, and prevention of secondary infections. Several clinical trials are ongoing, including treatment with IV immunoglobulin and interferon. The risk of severe illness and death is highest for people >50 yrs old. Lasting sequelae in those with severe disease have been described.

SUPPURATIVE INTRACRANIAL PHLEBITIS

Occurring after infection of the cranial sinus, middle ear, mastoid sinus or bone, or oropharynx, suppurative intracranial phlebitis results from venous spread of bacterial infection or from concomitant epidural abscess, subdural empyema, or meningitis. *S. aureus* is the most frequent causative organism, although any number of other bacteria can cause suppurative intracranial phlebitis. **Clinical presentation** varies according to the vein or venous sinus involved:

- Cortical vein: progressive loss of consciousness, seizures, increased ICP if collateral blood flow is compromised. Otherwise, disease may have no neurologic signs or symptoms.
- Cavernous sinus: unilateral periorbital edema; papilledema; decreased pupillary reactivity; decreased corneal reflex; decreased sensation in the regions of cranial nerves VI and VII; and palsies of cranial nerves II, IV, V, and VI.
- Lateral sinus: fifth and sixth cranial nerve palsies, facial pain, facial sensory deficits, and papilledema (if bilateral disease is present).
- Superior sagittal sinus: bilateral leg weakness and increased ICP.
- Superior petrosal sinus: temporal lobe seizures and ipsilateral pain or sensory deficit.
- Inferior petrosal sinus: ipsilateral pain and sensory deficit, sixth cranial nerve palsy.
- Gradenigo's syndrome (otorrhea, headache, diplopia, and retroorbital pain).

Risk factors for septic intracranial venous thrombosis include hypercoagulable states, sickle cell disease, trauma, mucormycosis, HIV, and CMV infection. **Diagnosis** is typically made by MRI or CT of brain demonstrating intracranial venous thrombosis in a patient with fever and leukocytosis and a predisposing sinus or HEENT infection. Plain films of the skull are not helpful. Magnetic resonance angiography is the diagnostic procedure of choice.

Antimicrobial agents directed at staphylococci and streptococci are the best choices for **empiric therapy.** Culture of the blood and primarily infected craniofacial structure can provide directed antibiotic therapy. Neurosurgical consultation is recommended, as surgical removal of the infected thrombus may be necessary as well as relief of intracranial HTN in the form of a CSF shunt, lumbar puncture, or diuretics. Anticoagulant therapy is often recommended, although no data exist regarding its use. The prognosis for any intracranial venous thrombosis is poor, with an overall mortality of 34% [3].

KEY POINTS TO REMEMBER

- Empiric initial therapy for bacterial meningitis should include ceftriaxone and vancomycin if pneumococcal resistance rates are higher than 4–5% in your community.
- Coverage for *Listeria* should be added (ampicillin, 2 g IV q4h) for patients at the extremes of age or for immunocompromised patients until Gram's stain and culture results are available.
- Close contacts (i.e., housemates, people with exposure to nasopharyngeal secretions) of patients with *Neisseria* meningitis should receive antibiotic prophylaxis (i.e., ciprofloxacin, 500 mg PO in one dose).
- Patients with aseptic meningitis may warrant empiric therapy with acyclovir until HSV can be ruled out.

REFERENCES

1. Tunkel AR, Scheld WM. Acute meningitis. In: Mandell GL, Bennett JE, Dolin R, eds. *Mandell, Douglas, and Bennett's principles and practice of infectious disease,* 5th ed. Philadelphia: Churchill Livingstone, 2000.
2. de Gans J, van de Beek D; European Dexamethasone in Adulthood Bacterial Meningitis Study Investigators. Dexamethasone in adults with bacterial meningitis. *N Engl J Med* 2002;347:1549–1556.
3. Bleck TP, Greenlee JE. Suppurative intracranial phlebitis. In: Mandell GL, Bennett JE, Dolin R, eds. *Principles and practice of infectious diseases,* 5th ed. Philadelphia: Churchill Livingstone, 2000:1034–1036.

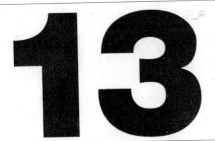

Oncologic Infections

Erik Dubberke

PREDISPOSITION TO INFECTION

Many cancer patients are predisposed to infections, and infections are among the leading causes of death in cancer patients. The increased risk of infection may be due to an alteration of immune function secondary to the malignancy, treatment of the malignancy, or disruption of the body's integument.

DIMINISHED T-CELL AND MONONUCLEAR PHAGOCYTE FUNCTION

Patients with Hodgkin's disease and non-Hodgkin's lymphoma have impaired T-cell function (the former more so than the latter). This impairment often persists after a complete remission has been achieved. Certain types of antineoplastic chemotherapy also impair T-cell function. Corticosteroids have profound effects on the distribution and function of neutrophils, monocytes, and lymphocytes. T-cell activation is inhibited, and T cells are redistributed out of the circulation leading to a peripheral lymphopenia as well as a peripheral monocytopenia. In addition to causing immunosuppression, corticosteroids directly stimulate the growth of *Aspergillus fumigatus in vitro*.

Fludarabine and other purine analogues, such as cladribine, are lymphotoxic, particularly to CD4⁺ T cells, and can induce a clinical situation similar to AIDS. The combination of fludarabine and corticosteroids is more immunosuppressive than either alone, and the immunosuppression may persist for months after completion of therapy. Methotrexate (Folex, Rheumatrex, Trexall), an inhibitor of dihydrofolate reductase, is highly immunosuppressive to T cells as well.

Diminished T-lymphocyte function leads to a predisposition to a wide variety of infections. Bacterial infections that are more common in this population include *Mycobacteria tuberculosis* and nontuberculous mycobacteria, *Listeria*, *Nocardia*, *Legionella*, and *Salmonella* infections. Herpesvirus infections are common (HSV, CMV, EBV, VZV), and viruses that are common respiratory pathogens, such as RSV and adenovirus, can cause life-threatening pneumonitis. Fungal pathogens include *Candida* species; *Cryptococcus neoformans*; and geographic dimorphic fungi, such as *Histoplasma*, *Coccidioides*, and *Blastomycosis*. Parasitic infections can occur at increased frequency as well, and these include *Pneumocystis jiroveci*, *Toxoplasma gondii*, *Giardia*, *Entamoeba*, *Cryptosporidium*, and *Strongyloides*.

DIMINISHED B-CELL FUNCTION AND OPSONIZATION

Impaired Ig production occurs whenever lymphocyte function is abnormal. This is more pronounced when mainly B cells are affected. Cancers associated with significant B-cell impairment include multiple myeloma and chronic lymphocytic leukemia. At high doses, corticosteroids also inhibit Ig generation by B cells.

Sinopulmonary infections are more common and more severe in patients with abnormal B-cell function. Encapsulated bacteria predominate, such as *Streptococcus pneumoniae, Haemophilus influenzae, Escherichia coli, Pseudomonas aeruginosa*, and *Salmonella* species. In addition, these patients are predisposed to infections caused by *C. neoformans*.

144

SPLENECTOMY

Splenectomized patients are at increased risk of overwhelming sepsis by encapsulated organisms, particularly *S. pneumoniae*, *H. influenzae*, and *Neisseria meningitidis*.

Splenectomized patients with Hodgkin's disease or non-Hodgkin's lymphoma are becoming less common with the use of CT for staging instead of splenectomy. Other less common pathogens associated with a more fulminant course in asplenic individuals include *Capnocytophaga* species, babesiosis, malaria, and *Salmonella* species. Patients without a spleen should be vaccinated against pneumococcus, *H. influenzae*, and *Neisseria*, preferably before the spleen is removed.

NEUTROPENIA

See Neutropenic Fever in Chap. 2, Febrile Syndromes.

OTHER ORGAN DYSFUNCTION

Tumors themselves may lead to infection by local organ dysfunction. Solid tumors often cause obstruction of natural passages, which leads to inadequate drainage of excretory or secretory fluids from nasal sinuses, bronchi, bile ducts, and so forth. Tissue invasion by solid tumors can also lead to connections between normally sterile areas and the outside world. CNS involvement is associated with an increased risk of infection due to (a) a diminished cough reflex or inability to swallow, or (b) being unable to completely void the bladder of urine. Necrotic tissue within the tumor, as a result of overgrowth of its blood supply or in response to chemotherapy, can create a protected nidus for infection.

Diagnosis

Patients with neutropenia should be managed according to Neutropenic Fever in Chap. 2, Febrile Syndromes. Patients with infection suspected to be secondary to worsening tumor invasion should receive CT or MRI scanning of the area to rule out occult abscess, fistula, or infection secondary to obstruction. Patients with lung cancer may warrant a chest x-ray to rule out postobstructive pneumonia.

Treatment

Patients with neutropenia should be managed according to Neutropenic Fever in Chap. 2, Febrile Syndromes. Nonneutropenic patients should receive antibiotic therapy based on the suspected site of infection (i.e., lung, biliary system; see corresponding chapters).

Prevention

Patients with neutropenia may benefit from cessation of chemotherapy and the use of granulocyte colony-stimulating factor until neutropenia has resolved. Patients with certain leukemias or lymphomas and recurrent infections should have a CD4 count and quantitative immunoglobulins checked. If the CD4 count is ≤200, then *Pneumocystis* pneumonia prophylaxis is a good idea. If immunoglobulin levels are low, the patient may benefit from IV immunoglobulin; collaboration with the patient's oncologist is advised if such therapy is considered.

KEY POINTS TO REMEMBER

- Patients with suspected infection and neutropenic fever should be started on broad antibiotics, and immunosuppression should be reversed if possible.
- It is important to be familiar with a patient's chemotherapy regimen (consult with an oncologist if needed), as the patient may be at risk for certain infections based on the type of chemotherapy used.

- Infections suspected secondary to tumor invasion should be assessed with additional imaging (e.g., CT, MRI, U/S, and so forth).

REFERENCES AND SUGGESTED READINGS

Segal BH, Walsh TJ, Holland SM. Infections in the cancer patient. In: DeVita VT, Jr., Hellman S, Rosenberg SA, eds. *Cancer: principles and practice of oncology,* 6th ed. Philadelphia: Lippincott Williams & Wilkins, 2001:2851–2868.

DePauw BE, Donnelly JP. Infections in the immunocompromised host: general principles. In: Mandell GL, Bennett JE, Dolin R, eds. *Mandell, Douglas, and Bennett's principles and practice of infectious disease,* 5th ed. Philadelphia: Churchill Livingstone, 2000:3079–3089.

DePauw BE, Meunier F. Infections in patients with acute leukemia and lymphoma. In: Mandell GL, Bennett JE, Dolin R, eds. *Mandell, Douglas, and Bennett's principles and practice of infectious disease,* 5th ed. Philadelphia: Churchill Livingstone, 2000.

Fauci AS, Dale DC, Balow JE. Glucocorticosteroid therapy: mechanism of action and clinical considerations. *Ann Intern Med* 1976;84:304–315.

Thomas CR Jr, Wood LV, Douglas JG, et al. Common emergencies in cancer medicine: infectious and treatment-related syndromes, part I. *J Natl Med Assoc* 1994;86:765–774.

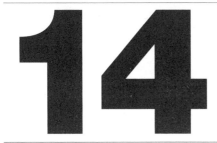

Bone Marrow Transplant Infections

Erik Dubberke

INTRODUCTION

Bone marrow transplant (BMT) patients go through four phases of predictable, sequential suppression of host defenses. Infection and graft-vs-host disease (GVHD) remain major causes of morbidity and mortality in BMT patients. The severity and type of infection depend on the type of transplant (allogeneic or autologous), presence and degree of histocompatibility mismatch, T-lymphocyte manipulation (depletion), type of GVHD prophylaxis used, severity of GVHD, and viral and fungal infections occurring before transplant.

PHASE I: PRETRANSPLANTATION

The pretransplantation phase consists of the time from conditioning to transplant.

Risk of Infection

The risk of infection during the pretransplantation period is highly variable. It depends on the underlying disease, prior chemotherapy exposures, degree of immuno-suppression, and infection history. The crucial determinants of infection during this period are the degree of neutropenia and the existence of compromised anatomic barriers. Approximately 12% of infections occur during the pretransplantation phase.

Types of Infection

The majority of infections are caused by gram-negative bacilli (GNB). 60% are local infections of the skin and soft tissue, oral cavity, or urinary tract. Sepsis and pneumonia (24% and 10%, respectively) occur less commonly. Fatal infections are unusual. Development of infection before transplant does not alter the success of transplant or delay the time to engraftment.

PHASE II: PREENGRAFTMENT

The preengraftment phase consists of days 0–30.

Risk of Infection

The major host defect during this phase is profound, prolonged neutropenia as a side effect of the conditioning chemotherapy. Another major side effect of the conditioning that predisposes to infection is disruption of the barrier protection provided by the skin and mucous membranes. Certain conditioning regimens may predispose to certain infectious complications as well (e.g., total body irradiation, increased incidence of diarrhea and bacteremia, and increase in late-occurring herpes zoster). Neutropenia and mucositis both start on approximately days 7–10 and resolve on approximately days 20–30 after the conditioning is started. The main causes of infection during this phase include bacteria, fungi, and HSV.

Bacterial Infections

Bacteremia

Bacteremia occurs in 15–50% of patients during this phase. Over the last few decades, there has been a shift in causative organisms from GNB to gram-positive cocci (GPC). Staphylococcal infections, particularly *Staphylococcus epidermidis*, may be related to increased use of indwelling catheters as well as respiratory and GI tract colonization at some centers. Streptococcal infections have become more common with the presence of severe mucositis and the use of certain prophylactic antibiotics (e.g., TMP-SMX and fluoroquinolones). Although typically GPC bacteremia tends not to have as fulminant a course as GNB, *Streptococcus mitis* bacteremia is associated with high rates of sepsis, ARDS, and death. In addition to primary bacteremia, other common bacterial infections during the preengraftment period are catheter-associated bacteremia and pneumonia. Catheter-associated bacteremias are most commonly caused by GPC, and the majority (60–90%) can be cured with antibiotics alone. See Chap. 2, Febrile Syndromes, for therapy and Chap. 16, Bacteremia and Sepsis, for details.

Pneumonia

Although most bacterial pneumonias occur late in the course of transplantation, up to 35% occur during the preengraftment phase. Infection is documented in only 20% of those with a pulmonary infiltrate, but GNB are the predominant causes of bacterial pneumonia during this phase. Fungal pneumonia, HSV pneumonia, pulmonary edema, toxic effects from chemotherapy or radiation, extension of the patient's underlying disease, and diffuse alveolar hemorrhage may also present with pulmonary infiltrates in the preengraftment phase.

Neutropenic Enterocolitis (Typhlitis)

A less common bacterial infection in the preengraftment period is neutropenic enterocolitis. The symptoms are nonspecific: nausea, vomiting, abdominal pain, and diarrhea. U/S and CT may show thickening of the bowel wall, a cecal mass, or pneumatosis coli. Surgery should be considered in rapidly progressive cases. Typical organisms include *Clostridium* species, *Pseudomonas* species, *Escherichia coli*, *Klebsiella* species, *Streptococcus bovis*, *Citrobacter* species, *Bacillus fragilis*, *Enterobacter* species, *Acinetobacter* species, and *Candida* species. Mortality rates are reported at 50–100%. The differential diagnosis includes *Clostridium difficile* colitis, mucositis, antibiotic-associated diarrhea, and viral enterocolitis.

Fungal Infections

Patients in the preengraftment period may have a number of risk factors for fungal infections: prolonged neutropenia, exposure to corticosteroids and broad-spectrum antibiotics, presence of indwelling catheters, GVHD, advanced age, poor histocompatibility match, and transplantation of T-lymphocyte–depleted bone marrow. The median onset to fungal infection during this phase is 2 wks, typically caused by *Candida* species or *Aspergillus* species.

Candida

Candida infection occurs in approximately 11% of BMT patients. *Candida albicans* is the most common pathogen, although *Candida tropicalis* is the causative agent in up to 25% of cases. *Candida krusei* remains uncommon, but the incidence is rising with the use of fluconazole fungal prophylaxis. Candidal infections can be localized to the GI tract (esophagitis) or genital area, or they can be disseminated, as demonstrated by positive blood cultures or histologic evidence of tissue invasion. Disseminated candidal infections may present with diffuse, erythematous, tender nodules. The mortality of candidemia alone is 39%, and it is 90% when tissue invasion is involved.

Filamentous Fungi

Filamentous fungi can present with pulmonary, sinus, or CNS disease or skin lesions such as ecthyma gangrenosum. *Aspergillus* is the most common filamentous fungi to cause infection in BMT patients, although other pathogens reported in the preengraftment period include *Scopulariopsis* species; *Fusarium* species (presents with fevers, sinusitis, and occasionally endophthalmitis and pyomyositis; blood cultures are positive >60%); *Trichosporon* species (presents in a fashion similar to disseminated candidiasis); *Pseudallescheria boydii* (resistant to amphotericin B); *Alternaria* species; and *Pityrosporum* species (presents with a disseminated skin rash and on biopsy; the fungi are localized to the skin follicle without tissue invasion, and treatment is topical). *Aspergillus* infections occur in 4–20% of BMT recipients, and they tend to occur in a bimodal time distribution, with peaks at 20 days and 80 days after transplant. Risk factors for early *Aspergillus* infection include prolonged neutropenia, donor type (allogeneic vs. autologous), male gender, transplantation during the summer months, and lack of laminar airflow rooms. In the preengraftment period, the risk increases from 1%/day for the first few weeks to >4%/day after 3 wks of neutropenia.

PULMONARY DISEASE. The main clinical manifestation of invasive *Aspergillus* is pulmonary disease, although it is not uncommon for patients to present with sinus or CNS disease. Diagnosis can be difficult because radiographic abnormalities are often nonspecific (although nodular and cavitary lesions on chest x-ray and the halo sign are suggestive) and blood cultures are positive <5% of the time. A definitive diagnosis is made by biopsy and culture.

SINUS DISEASE. Early signs of fungal sinusitis include pale or graying nasal mucosa and turbinates, hypesthesia to light touch, and absence of bleeding with abrasion. Sinus CT can confirm the diagnosis as well as provide evidence of bony invasion. Sinus puncture and aspiration for culture should be performed.

HSV

80% of patients seropositive for HSV-1 not on prophylaxis develop clinical disease during the preengraftment period. 85% of patients with HSV disease present with gingivostomatitis (and HSV causes 50% of all oral lesions during this period as well). Oral HSV lesions are a risk factor for bacterial infection as well as HSV of the esophagus and lungs. The most severe form of HSV is pneumonitis. This usually occurs in the setting of mucocutaneous disease, with onset of fevers, cough, dyspnea, hypoxemia, and infiltrates on chest x-ray. Contiguous spread from the oropharynx produces multifocal infiltrates, whereas diffuse infiltrates are the result of seeding after viremia.

Prophylaxis

Use of antifungal and antibacterial prophylaxis remains controversial. Antifungal and antibacterial prophylaxis has reduced the incidence of infections in BMT patients, but survival has been improved only in patients with aplastic anemia. High-efficiency particulate air filters have been shown to reduce the incidence of *Aspergillus* infections, particularly if there is construction at the medical center. Prophylactic amphotericin B during episodes of neutropenia in patients who have had prior fungal pulmonary infections significantly reduces the rate of reactivation. In contrast to the questionable efficacy of antibacterial and antifungal prophylaxis, HSV prophylaxis is very effective for patients who are seropositive for HSV. Growth factors have been shown to decrease the length of neutropenia and the rate of bacterial infections in BMT patients.

PHASE III: POSTENGRAFTMENT

The postengraftment phase consists of days 30–100.

Risk of Infection

The postengraftment phase starts when neutropenia and mucositis resolve. The rate and extent of recovery of the host's new immune system, presence of GVHD, and immunosuppression to treat GVHD are the major determinants of infection during this phase. Infections related to cell-mediated immunity are most common during this phase.

CMV

CMV is the greatest infectious cause of morbidity and mortality in BMT patients. 15–20% of those who develop CMV infection (defined as viral shedding or seroconversion) die. The major determinant of CMV infection is the serologic status of the donor and recipient. Before blood products were screened for CMV or leukocyte poor, 20% of seronegative recipients of seronegative transplants, 57% of seronegative recipients of seropositive transplants, and 70% of seropositive recipients developed CMV infection. Risk factors for developing CMV infection include the use of blood products not screened for CMV, advanced age, HLA mismatch, acute GVHD, total body irradiation, and multiagent conditioning regimens. Use of seronegative or leukocyte-reduced blood products has decreased the rate of CMV infection in seronegative recipients of seronegative transplants to <3%, and preemptive antiviral therapy has reduced the rate of CMV disease in seropositive recipients to <20% of patients who develop CMV viremia. CMV disease occurs when there is documented tissue involvement. CMV disease can manifest as pneumonitis (63%), enterocolitis (26%), retinitis (5%), or less commonly with hepatitis, cystitis, or esophagitis. The most severe manifestation of CMV disease is pneumonitis. It occurs in 50% of patients not on prophylaxis and has a mortality of 30–50%. CMV disease is treated with ganciclovir (Cytovene), 5 mg/kg bid for 14–21 days and then 5 mg/kg qd until day 100 posttransplant. In addition, pneumonitis is treated with IV immunoglobulin, 500 mg/kg qd for 14–21 days.

Adenovirus

Adenoviral shedding occurs in 3–21% of BMT patients, and 1.0–6.5% of these patients develop disease. Adenovirus has been reported to cause pneumonia, hepatitis, cystitis, GI disease, and disseminated disease. Adenovirus infection is associated with a 60% mortality in BMT patients. Treatment is supportive.

Viral Gastroenteritis

Viral gastroenteritis is typically caused by rotavirus and coxsackievirus (as well as adenovirus) in BMT patients. Cases parallel community outbreaks but are associated with a mortality of 55%. There are no good therapies, and treatment is symptomatic.

Respiratory Viruses

Common respiratory viruses in BMT patients include RSV, parainfluenza virus, and, less commonly, influenza virus, rhinovirus, and corona virus. RSV typically occurs in the winter, and pneumonia occurs in as many as 50% of patients, with a subsequent mortality of 80%. Use of aerosolized ribavirin appears to improve survival in patients with a positive nasopharyngeal swab if started before hypoxemia develops. Parainfluenza virus occurs year-long and is associated with a mortality of 30–35% if pneumonia develops.

Fungal Infections

Candida

The main form of candidal disease in the postengraftment period is hepatosplenic candidiasis; *Candida* seeds the patient's liver and spleen during the neutropenic period. Patients present with fever, abdominal complaints, and an elevated alkaline phosphatase after neutrophil recovery. MRI is the most sensitive radiographic procedure, and a definitive diagnosis requires a liver biopsy. IV amphotericin B is the drug of choice, and often >2 g is necessary for cure.

Aspergillus

As mentioned above, *Aspergillus* occurs in a bimodal fashion, with a second peak at approximately day 80 after transplant. Risk factors for late *Aspergillus* include construction in the vicinity of the hospital, acute GVHD, and corticosteroid use. The 1-yr survival rate for BMT patients with invasive aspergillosis is <10%.

Bacterial Infections

Bacterial infections are less common during the postengraftment period. Most bacterial infections are GPC bacteremias associated with indwelling catheters. Patients with gut GVHD may also develop infections with GNB, such as intraabdominal abscesses and bacteremia.

Pneumocystis jiroveci

In the past, *P. jiroveci* was associated with 5–32% of cases of intersitial pneumonia during days 40–80. This has been greatly reduced with the use of prophylaxis. PCP presents with cough, dyspnea, and bilateral infiltrates on chest x-ray.

Toxoplasmosis

Toxoplasmosis has been reported to reactivate in BMT patients. In France, where the seroprevalence is 70%, the incidence of toxoplasmosis is 2–3% in BMT patients. Risk factors for toxoplasmosis are seropositivity for *Toxoplasma gondii* before transplantation, allogeneic transplant, and GVHD.

Prophylaxis

There are two well-studied methods for CMV prophylaxis. Preemptive therapy involves following weekly blood CMV shell vial cultures or CMV polymerase chain reaction (PCR) and, if positive, initiating ganciclovir at 5 mg/kg IV bid for 7–14 days, then continuing that dose qd until day 100. The prophylactic method involves starting GCV at engraftment at the induction dose for 5 days, then continuing that dose qd until day 100. Development of a CMV-specific T-lymphocyte response is necessary for protection against late CMV disease. The use of prophylactic GCV may delay that response and is associated with a 10% incidence of CMV occurring after day 100.

PCP prophylaxis typically involves TMP-SMX, 1 DS tablet PO three times per week, with a subsequent decrease in PCP to an incidence of 0.15%. This also provides prophylaxis for toxoplasmosis.

PHASE IV: LATE POSTTRANSPLANT PERIOD

The late posttransplant period consists of the time beyond day 100.

Risk of Infection

The late posttransplant period is the phase in which chronic GVHD becomes apparent. The effects of GVHD on target organs and the associated delay in immune system recovery are the major determinants of infection during this period. Chronic GVHD occurs in 30–50% of HLA-identical sibling transplants. Chronic GVHD typically involves multiple organ systems, most commonly the skin, mouth, and liver, with subsequent disruption of anatomic barriers. Patients with chronic GVHD also demonstrate abnormal humoral and cell-mediated immune function as well as functional asplenia. Infection in the absence of chronic GVHD is uncommon.

VZV

VZV is the most common cause of infections during this period, accounting for >40% of infections. VZV infection occurs in 20–50% of both allogeneic and autologous transplant recipients. Most infections represent reactivation, and 85% occur >1 yr after transplant. Zoster accounts for 86% of cases and varicella the remaining 15%. Patients with varicella are more likely to have dissemination and deep organ involvement; however, up to 36% of cases of zoster develop disseminated cutaneous disease.

The mortality rate of varicella/disseminated zoster before effective therapy is 10%. Risk factors for VZV disease include acute and chronic GVHD, allogeneic transplant, and lymphoma as the underlying disease. Risk factors for dissemination include the presence of acute GVHD and occurrence within the first year of transplant. Both IV acyclovir (Zovirax) and vidarabine (Vira-A) are effective for VZV infection.

Bacterial Infections

Patients with chronic GVHD have decreased reticuloendothelial function with subsequent functional asplenia, as well as a decreased IgG response to polysaccharide antigens. This leads to a predisposition to infections caused by encapsulated bacteria (*Streptococcus pneumoniae, Haemophilus influenzae,* and *Neisseria meningitidis*). The majority of bacterial infections are caused by GPC and involve the upper and lower respiratory tracts.

Fungal Infections

Oropharyngeal candidiasis is the most frequent fungal infection, and systemic fungal infections are rare.

Prophylaxis

Acyclovir is effective at decreasing the incidence of VZV infection, although the effect of acyclovir lasts for as long as it is used. Because of the high incidence of pneumococcal infection in patients with chronic GVHD, TMP-SMX twice weekly has been used as prophylaxis. Pneumococcal vaccine appears to be of little benefit.

CLINICAL INFECTION SYNDROMES IN BONE MARROW TRANSPLANT PATIENTS

The likelihood of the different pathogens mentioned depends on which phase of transplant the patient is in.

Hemorrhagic Cystitis

Hemorrhagic cystitis can have an infectious or noninfectious etiology. Most infectious causes are viral. BK virus and JC virus are most common, followed by adenovirus. HSV and CMV can cause hemorrhagic cystitis as well. There is no specific therapy for BK virus or JC virus infections. Noninfectious etiologies include GVHD and toxic effects of chemotherapy.

Hepatitis

Infectious hepatitis must be distinguished from hepatitis of noninfectious origin, including hepatic dysfunction secondary to the conditioning regimen, GVHD, chemical hepatitis, and venoocclusive disease of the liver. Important viral causes of hepatitis after BMT include acquisition or reactivation of HBV or HCV, adenovirus, CMV, or disseminated VZV.

Pneumonia

Noninfectious pulmonary complications of BMT that can be confused with pneumonia include pulmonary edema, diffuse alveolar hemorrhage, drug pulmonary toxicity, ARDS, idiopathic interstitial pneumonia, bronchiolitis obliterans, and chronic GVHD. Infectious causes include bacteria, TB, atypical mycobacteria, *Nocardia, Actinomyces,* PCP, CMV, HSV, VZV, and respiratory viruses.

Diarrhea

Diarrhea is associated with infection <15% of the time in BMT patients. The common infectious etiologies include *C. difficile,* adenovirus, rotavirus, coxsackievirus, and CMV.

Rash

Vesicular lesions should be unroofed and cultured for VZV and HSV. Catheter-related exit site or tunnel infections should be cultured for bacteria, atypical mycobacteria, and *Nocardia*. Focal nodular lesions should be biopsied and cultured for bacterial and fungal infections.

KEY POINTS TO REMEMBER

- Infections in BMT patients vary according to the phase of engraftment. In general, bacterial infections are most common in the preengraftment phase, and infections related to diminished T-cell–mediated immunity are more common postengraftment.
- An aggressive, rapid workup (i.e., blood/urine cultures, chest x-ray, CT scans) is very important, as these patients deteriorate very quickly. Close consultation with a BMT and ID specialist is advised.
- Carefully review a patient's prophylactic regimen, as inadequate prophylaxis may predispose to a certain infection.

REFERENCES AND SUGGESTED READINGS

Sable CA, Donowitz GR. Infections in bone marrow transplant recipients. *Clin Infect Dis* 1994;18:273–284.

Van Burik JH, Weisdorf DJ. Infection in recipients of blood and marrow transplantation. *Hematol Oncol Clin North Am* 1999;13:1065–1089.

Walter EA, Bowden RA. Infection in the bone marrow transplant recipient. *Infect Dis Clin North Am* 1995;9:823–847.

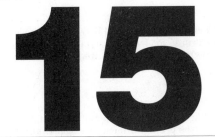

Solid Organ Transplant Infections

Erik Dubberke

INTRODUCTION

The major factor in improved clinical outcomes in solid organ transplant (SOT) patients is a decline in deaths due to infection. Factors involved include improved operative techniques, organ preservation, and postop care; pretransplant evaluation by infectious disease experts; immunizations; primary antibiotic prophylaxis; improved diagnostics; preemptive antibiotics in high-risk patients; more selective immunosuppressive agents; and more attention to CMV disease. Despite these advances, infection remains a major cause of morbidity and mortality in SOT recipients. The risk of infection is related to the interplay between the net state of immunosuppression and epidemiologic exposures. The net state of immunosuppression is related to the nature of the immunosuppressive therapy, the presence of defects in the mucocutaneous surfaces of the body (e.g., intravascular catheters, Foley catheters, surgical wounds), the presence of neutropenia, metabolic abnormalities (malnutrition, uremia, hyperglycemia), and the presence of immunomodulatory viruses (herpesviruses, hepatitis viruses, HIV). Periods of infectious risks in SOT patients can be divided into three categories. The *early period* (<1 mo posttransplant) is characterized by infections related to the transplant procedure and postop course (e.g., wound infection, allograft infection, IV catheter infection, ventilator-associated pneumonia). The only significant viral cause of infection is HSV. The *middle period* (mos 1–6 posttransplant) is characterized by maximal T-cell suppression. Intracellular pathogen, viral, and fungal infections typically occur during this period. Reactivation of *Mycobacterium tuberculosis* (MTB) and endemic mycosis typically occurs during this period as well. Infections that occur during the *late period* (>6 mos posttransplant) are dependent on the net state of immunosuppression. Patients experiencing recurrent or chronic rejection of the allograft requiring excessive doses of immunosuppression remain at risk for intracellular, fungal, and viral infections. Patients on minimal immunosuppression are at risk for community-acquired infections, such as influenza or pneumococcal disease. In addition, cryptococcal disease and CMV retinitis may occur despite minimum immunosuppression.

BACTERIAL INFECTIONS

Most bacterial infections occur during the early posttransplant period. Common infections include surgical site and allograft infections, ventilator-associated pneumonia, central venous catheter (CVC) infections, UTIs, and *Clostridium difficile* colitis. *Listeria monocytogenes* and *Nocardia* may occur during the middle period, and the late period is characterized by an increased risk of pneumococcal disease.

RENAL TRANSPLANT

There has been a dramatic decrease in the incidence of early posttransplant infections with the use of prophylactic antibiotics (TMP-SMX, quinolones).* Before prophylaxis, UTIs occurred in 60% of patients, with a 40% incidence of bacteremia. The incidence of UTI has decreased to 5–10%. Most centers continue antibiotic prophylaxis for 4

---

*Dosing guidelines and duration of prophylaxis are not standard.

mos. However, despite prophylaxis, UTI remains a significant cause of bacterial infection, and 50% of bacteremic episodes originate in the urine. Symptoms may be absent early in the course of UTI, so routine surveillance cultures are often indicated.

LIVER TRANSPLANT

The incidence of bacterial infection after liver transplantation is >50%, with a mortality of approximately 10%. >80% of bacterial infections occur within 8 wks. Intraabdominal infection (14–30%), wound infection (14–22%), pneumonia (10–13%), and UTI (12%) all occur regularly and are associated with bacteremia. Prolonged surgical time, retransplantation, prolonged hospitalization, rejection, reoperation, CMV infection, renal failure, and hyperbilirubinemia are all associated with an increased risk of bacterial infection in liver transplant patients. Choledochojejunostomy increases the risk of sepsis. Bile duct leaks are associated with secondary bacterial peritonitis, and bile duct strictures are associated with bacteremia and liver abscess formation. Bacteremia occurs in 20% of liver transplant patients and is associated with a 36% mortality. >50% of bacteremias are related to CVC infections. The majority of CVC infections are caused by gram-positive cocci, including coagulase-negative *Staphylococcus*, *Staphylococcus aureus*, and *Enterococcus*. *Enterococcus* isolates are becoming more frequent, including vancomycin-resistant *Enterococcus*. Vancomycin-resistant *Enterococcus* bacteremia is associated with an increase in mortality, tends to be monomicrobial, occurs later in the posttransplant course, and is more likely to come from an endovascular source when compared to vancomycin-sensitive *Enterococcus* bacteremia. Gram-negative bacilli bacteremia typically occurs in the setting of intraabdominal or biliary tract infections. *Enterobacter* and *Pseudomonas aeruginosa* are the major pathogens. Gram-negative bacilli bacteremia occurring several weeks after liver transplantation is usually associated with a liver abscess secondary to a biliary stricture or a hepatic artery thrombosis. Strategies to prevent bacterial infections in liver transplant patients include selective bowel decontamination, periop antibiotics, and administration of antibiotics before cholangiography or ERCP.

LUNG TRANSPLANT

The acute onset of hypoxemia and pulmonary infiltrates in the early posttransplant period in a lung transplant patient may be caused by a nosocomial pneumonia, aspiration, or acute rejection. Fever and nonproductive cough may also be present. *Klebsiella*, *Escherichia coli*, *Pseudomonas*, and *Enterobacter* are the causative organisms for the majority of bacterial pneumonias. HSV, *Aspergillus*, and toxoplasmosis can also cause early necrotizing pneumonia. Chronic rejection leads to bronchiolitis obliterans, which is associated with increased colonization with *Pseudomonas* and *Acinetobacter* and subsequent pneumonia. Bacteremia occurs in 25% of lung transplant patients and is an independent predictor of mortality. The majority of bacteremias originate in the lungs.

HEART TRANSPLANT

Risk factors for severe bacterial infections in heart transplant patients include age >50 yrs, ventilator support at the time of transplant, prolonged extracorporeal bypass, and the presence of a ventricular assist device. The most common bacterial infection is nosocomial pneumonia. *Pseudomonas* and *S. aureus* are the major pathogens. Bacteremia occurs in 10–20% of patients, with the lungs, CVC, and wound infections being the most common sources. Bacterial wound infections are relatively common in heart transplant patients, with an incidence of 8%. Common organisms include *S. aureus*, coagulase-negative *Staphylococcus*, and *Enterobacter*. Culture-negative sternal wound infections should raise the index of suspicion for fungal, atypical mycobacterial, and *Legionella* infections. Community-acquired pneumonia secondary to pneumococcus in heart transplant patients occurs at 10 times that found in the general population.

PANCREATIC AND SMALL BOWEL TRANSPLANTATION

One-third of pancreas transplantations are complicated by intraabdominal or wound infections. Bacterial infections occur in >90% of small bowel transplant patients. Many of these are the result of surgical complications, such as bowel wall perforation and anastomotic leaks. Episodes of rejection are commonly associated with bacteremia. See Intraabdominal Abscess in Chap. 6, Infections of the Gastrointestinal Tract, for more information on pathogens and treatment.

SPECIFIC AND SELECT OPPORTUNISTIC BACTERIA

Legionella Species

Legionella infection in SOT patients typically causes severe pneumonitis. Heart-lung and lung transplant recipients are at greatest risk. Community- or nosocomially acquired infection can occur after exposure to environmental or potable water sources in which *Legionella* is found. Chest x-ray findings are variable and nonspecific. Diagnosis is made by isolating the organism from respiratory secretions. Urine *Legionella* antigen may be of use as well. The preferred macrolide for therapy is azithromycin (Zithromax, Zithromax Z-Pak) because it has the least effect on cyclosporine levels.

Nocardia Species

Nocardia infection is characterized typically by pulmonary infection. Chest x-ray may reveal reticulonodular infiltrates, cavitary lesions, abscesses, or lobar infiltrates. Empyema is present 25% of the time. Dissemination is common, and the brain is the most commonly involved metastatic site (45%). Classically, CNS involvement is characterized by brain abscesses, although meningitis has been reported. Other sites of dissemination include the skin, retina, bones, joints, and heart. The diagnosis is suggested by histologic exam of infected material revealing partially acid-fast, gram-positive, beaded, branching rods. Definitive diagnosis is made by culture. Risk factors for *Nocardia* infection include multiple episodes of rejection, high-dose corticosteroids, and uremia. The treatment of choice is high-dose sulfonamides. Cefotaxime (Claforan), imipenem (Primaxin), amikacin (Amikin), and aminoglycosides may also be effective.

Listeria Species

The most common bacterial cause of CNS infection in SOT patients is *L. monocytogenes*. Two-thirds of patients have meningitis; the others can have meningoencephalitis, rhomboencephalitis, or brain abscesses. CSF reveals a neutrophilic pleocytosis in two-thirds of cases with meningitis. Hypoglycorrhachia is found 40% of the time. Gram-positive bacilli resembling diphtheroids occur 40% of the time. Blood cultures are positive the majority of the time. Ampicillin (Principen, Totacillin) is the drug of choice; TMP-SMX and vancomycin (Vancocin) are alternatives. PCP prophylaxis with TMP-SMX may prevent *Listeria* infection in SOT patients.

Rhodococcus Species

Rhodococcus equi, a gram-positive bacillus, can cause infection in SOT patients. Infection can occur in the early period, but most commonly it occurs during the middle or late periods. Pulmonary infection is the most common cause of pulmonary nodules or cavities. Purulent pericarditis and vertebral osteomyelitis have been reported. Blood cultures are positive 25% of the time. Treatment is based on susceptibility testing, although beta-lactams, vancomycin, and quinolones have been used with success.

FUNGAL INFECTIONS

The type, incidence, and severity of fungal infections vary among specific SOT recipients. *Candida* and *Aspergillus* species account for 80% of fungal infections. Other pathogens include endemic dimorphic fungi, *Cryptococcus,* and Zygomycetes. Risk factors of fungal infections include the level of immunosuppression, use of broad-spectrum antibiotics, high-dose corticosteroids, community and hospital exposures, and technical aspects of the surgical procedure. Although fungal infections are less common than bacterial and viral infections, they cause the highest infection-related mortality in SOT patients. This is likely multifactorial because early diagnosis of fungal infections is difficult and often requires invasive procedures, antifungal therapy has multiple toxicities and drug-drug interactions, and decreasing immunosuppression may be required, thus putting the allograft at risk for rejection.

Candida Species

Candida species account for the majority of fungal infections in liver, pancreas, and small bowel allograft recipients and 30–60% of fungal infections in renal, lung, and heart-lung recipients. *Candida albicans* is the most common cause of invasive disease, although multiple other *Candida* species have been described as well. Most infections occur within 2 mos of transplantation, and the majority develop from endogenous sources. Risk factors for *Candida* infection include depressed cell-mediated immunity, neutrophil dysfunction, diabetes mellitus, prior antibiotic use, CVC, Foley catheters, GI surgery, early *Candida* colonization, renal failure, prolonged operation time, and retransplantation. Mucocutaneous disease is the most common form of *Candida* infection, although sepsis and dissemination may occur. Intraabdominal infection, abscess, and wound infection are common after liver, pancreas, and small bowel transplantation. Cystitis, pyelonephritis, and ureteral obstruction from fungus ball formation can complicate renal transplantation. Infection of vascular anastomotic sites can occur, as well as mediastinitis, endocarditis, CVC infection, septic arthritis, and brain abscess.

Aspergillus Species

Mortality is >75% for invasive pulmonary disease and approaches 100% for disseminated and CNS disease. A pseudomembranous tracheobronchitis can occur in lung transplant recipients and is associated with a 30% mortality. Invasive disease varies from 0.7% in renal transplant recipients to 10% in lung transplant recipients to 18% in heart-lung transplant recipients. Risk factors among liver transplant patients include neutropenia, retransplantation, renal failure, augmented immunosuppression, poor allograft function, and concurrent CMV infection. Additional risk factors in lung transplant patients include single-lung transplantation and increased colonization associated with recurrent episodes of rejection. *Aspergillus* infection is seen starting 2 wks posttransplantation. The peak incidence in heart transplant patients is at 1 mo; >75% of cases in liver transplant recipients occur within 3 mos, but it is not uncommon to see disease >3 mos after lung transplantation. The portal of entry typically is the respiratory tract, and patients present with nonproductive cough, shortness of breath, and pleuritic chest pain. Radiography is nonspecific, but CT scan may identify lesions 5 days earlier than a standard chest x-ray. Dissemination is common, and potential metastatic sites include the CNS, liver, spleen, blood vessels, heart, eye, GI tract, bones, and joints. Although brain abscesses in SOT recipients are relatively uncommon (0.6%), 78% are caused by *Aspergillus*. Diagnosis is difficult. Blood cultures are rarely positive, even in cases of endocarditis. Colonization of the respiratory tract and surgical wounds is common, and as many as 40% of patients with invasive pulmonary aspergillosis have negative British antilewisite cultures.

Cryptococcus Species

Infection due to *Cryptococcus neoformans* is rare <6 mos posttransplant, and early infection suggests allograft transmission. *Cryptococcus* most commonly is inhaled where it causes asymptomatic infection in the lungs with subsequent hematogenous spread. Subacute meningitis is the most common clinical presentation with fever, confusion, headache, seizures, and focal neurologic findings. Lumbar puncture reveals an elevated opening pressure, a lymphocytic pleocytosis, hypoglycorrhachia, and elevated protein.

Other potential areas of dissemination include the genitourinary tract, skin, bones, joints, and retina. Multiple skin lesions have been described, including cellulitis, necrotizing vasculitis, nodules, plaques, and papules. Suspicious skin lesions should be biopsied and cultured. Serum and CSF cryptococcal antigen are useful in making a rapid diagnosis.

Endemic Dimorphic Fungi

Histoplasmosis and coccidioidomycosis reactivation or primary infection is the most common endemic dimorphic fungi to cause infection in SOT patients. The incidence of histoplasmosis in renal transplant patients in endemic regions is 0.4–2.1%, and the incidence of coccidioidomycosis in Arizona ranges from 4.5% in heart transplant recipients to 7.0% in renal transplant recipients. Blastomycosis is rare in SOT patients, with only five reported cases (four in renal transplant patients and one in a heart transplant patient). Histoplasmosis typically presents subacutely to chronically with fevers, night sweats, and cough, but progressive disease with dissemination may occur. Although inoculation occurs through the lungs, chest x-ray shows infiltrates in only 50% of cases. Mucocutaneous lesions are common. Hepatosplenomegaly and cytopenias may occur as well. The diagnosis is made by culture and histopathologic exam of involved sites. Urine histoplasma antigen may be of diagnostic value in the appropriate clinical setting. Coccidioidomycosis commonly presents with disseminated disease from a respiratory portal of entry. Areas commonly affected include the CNS, genitourinary tract, liver, skin, spleen, and musculoskeletal system. Mortality is >50% in disseminated disease. Diagnosis is made by culture and histopathologic exam of involved sites.

Zygomycosis

Now rarely reported, the incidence of zygomycosis was once as high as 9%. This is due to the use of more selective immunosuppression. Most cases occur 1–6 mos posttransplant, and risk factors include augmented immunosuppression, diabetes mellitus, metabolic acidosis, and neutropenia. Ubiquitous in nature, the portal of entry typically is through the nose and sinuses. Rhinocerebral disease is most common, presenting with either the rhino-orbital-cerebral type or the rhino-maxillary type. Diagnosis should be suspected in patients with black nasal discharge or necrotic palatal lesions. The involved genera, *Rhizopus*, *Mucor*, *Cunninghamella*, and *Absidia*, have a vascular tropism and frequently invade blood vessels and cause thrombosis and infarction. Cavitary pneumonia, invasive cutaneous disease, and GI disease with perforation have been described. Histopathology reveals vascular invasion by broad, nonseptate hyphae.

MYCOBACTERIAL INFECTIONS

Mycobacterium tuberculosis

MTB causes infection in 0.35–15% of SOT recipients. Reactivation is most common, although primary infection and allograft transmission do occur. The median time to onset is 9 mos posttransplant. The diagnosis requires a high index of suspicion because it has atypical presentations in SOT patients. Lung involvement occurs in 70% of infected patients, with dissemination in 20%. The most common radiographic finding is a focal infiltrate, and a pulmonary cavity is present in only 4% of cases. 30% of patients with MTB have extrapulmonary disease. The most common sites of involvement include the GI tract, liver, bones, kidney, and genitourinary tract. MTB-related mortality is 30%. Treatment is difficult because of drug toxicities and drug-drug interactions. Allograft loss occurs in 27% of SOT patients being treated for MTB. In one review, discontinuation of isoniazid due to hepatotoxicity occurred in 2.5% of renal transplant patients, 4.5% of heart transplant patients, and 41% of liver transplant patients (although the incidence in the liver transplant patients is likely overestimated because biopsy to rule out rejection or viral hepatitis was not performed). All potential transplant patients should be screened for MTB and receive prophylaxis if there is ≥5 mm induration, if the patient has received inadequate prophylaxis or treatment in the past, has had close contact with active MTB, or chest x-ray abnormalities are consistent with prior MTB without prior therapy.

Atypical Mycobacteria

Atypical mycobacteria cause infection in the late transplant period, with a mean time to diagnosis of 48 mos. Cutaneous disease is most common, and dissemination is rare. *Mycobacterium kansasii* and *Mycobacterium avium* complex commonly present with pulmonary disease.

HERPESVIRUSES

The herpesviruses cause significant morbidity and mortality in SOT recipients. They can cause direct tissue invasion and facilitate oncogenesis, and their immunomodulatory capacity increases the likelihood of opportunistic infection and allograft injury.

HSV

Reactivation of HSV occurs in 25% of seropositive SOT patients not receiving prophylaxis. Mucocutaneous disease during the early posttransplant period is the most common presentation. Primary infection from a sick contact or the allograft is more likely to result in disseminated disease. Pulmonary involvement is associated with a 75% mortality. Other sites of dissemination include the liver, skin, and GI tract. HSV pneumonitis can develop in intubated patients with active orolabial disease. Likewise, esophageal involvement can occur in patients with active orolabial disease.

VZV

Zoster reactivation occurs in 15% of seropositive SOT recipients, usually within 1 yr of transplant. Patients typically have localized skin lesions confined to one or two dermatomes, although patients on augmented immunosuppression are at greater risk for dissemination. Varicella infection is associated with higher rates of disseminated disease as well. Disseminated VZV can cause hemorrhagic pneumonia, hepatitis, encephalitis, skin lesions, and widespread visceral involvement. Pretransplant vaccination of seronegative patients has not been evaluated. Exposed seronegative SOT patients should receive varicella zoster immune globulin as soon as possible.

Epstein-Barr Virus

The majority of EBV disease in SOT recipients represents reactivation, usually within 4 mos posttransplant. It may present with a mononucleosis-like syndrome, although the most severe complication is EBV-related posttransplant lymphoproliferative disease (PTLD). 1% of renal transplant recipients, 10% of lung transplant recipients, and 18% of small bowel transplant recipients develop EBV-related PTLD. Patients at increased risk for PTLD include patients who received antilymphocyte globulin (ALG) or anti-CD3 monoclonal antibody (OKT3) as induction immunosuppression, patients on tacrolimus-based immunosuppression, and patients with primary CMV infection. Clinical presentation is quite variable, and extranodal involvement is common. PTLD can range from a benign polyclonal process to a highly malignant monoclonal immunoblastic lymphoma with a mortality of 50–80%. Diagnosis is made by histopathology that reveals a clonal B-cell proliferation with the presence of EBV DNA, RNA, or protein. Treatment involves decreasing immunosuppression, and this may be all that is required for benign forms of PTLD. Cytotoxic chemotherapy may be required for more malignant forms. EBV-related PTLD does not respond to antiviral therapy.

CMV

CMV is the most important viral pathogen affecting SOT recipients. Symptomatic infection develops in 50% of SOT patients, usually 2–6 mos posttransplant, although late CMV retinitis can occur in patients on minimal immunosuppression. Primary infection in seronegative patients has the greatest risk of developing severe disease. Use of ALG/OKT3 and coinfection with human herpesvirus (HHV-6) are risk factors for developing symptomatic disease. Although CMV disease is rarely fatal, it is associated with an increase in opportunistic infection (severe bacterial infections, *Aspergillus*), allograft injury (premature atherosclerosis in heart transplants, bronchiolitis obliterans in lung transplants, and vanishing bile duct syndrome in liver transplants), and an increase in 1-yr mortality. Organ involvement is common, and it tends to have a predilection for the allograft. Diagnosis is made by histopathology and viral culture. Prevention of CMV disease involves screening blood products given to seronegative patients for CMV, administering leukocyte-depleted blood products, and preemptive therapy with ganciclovir in patients with evidence of CMV infection by positive CMV PCR of the blood or in patients at high risk for developing CMV disease (use of ALG/OKT3 in seropositive patients).

Human Herpesvirus-6

Reactivation of HHV-6 usually occurs within 2 mos posttransplant, although the pathogenicity in SOT patients has been questioned. HHV-6 has been implicated as the cause of pneumonitis, hepatitis, and encephalitis. The most common manifestations are fever and leukopenia. HHV-6 is an independent risk factor for developing CMV disease in liver and renal transplant patients and allograft rejection and invasive fungal disease in liver transplant patients. Diagnosis is made by isolating the virus from peripheral mononuclear cells, shell vial assay, detection of HHV-6 antigens in the blood, or PCR. Treatment is not defined, but HHV-6 is susceptible to ganciclovir and foscarnet *in vitro*.

Human Herpesvirus-8

HHV-8 infection in SOT recipients places them at risk for developing Kaposi's sarcoma. The median time to onset is 29–31 mos. The incidence of Kaposi's sarcoma in low-seropositive populations is 0.5% and 5.3% in high-seropositive populations. Patients can present with localized skin lesions or disseminated disease with multiorgan involvement. Treatment requires a decrease in immunosuppression and may require cytotoxic chemotherapy. Antiviral therapy is not helpful.

PARASITIC INFECTIONS

Pneumocystosis

There has been a dramatic decline in PCP with the use of TMP-SMX prophylaxis. Most commonly, disease presents during the middle period posttransplant, although 35% of patients presents >1 yr posttransplant. PCP currently occurs only in patients on augmented immunosuppression and not on prophylaxis.

Strongyloidiasis

Strongyloides stercoralis can produce life-threatening disseminated disease in SOT patients. Patients often have subclinical disease before transplant and develop a hyperinfection syndrome characterized by enterocolitis and pulmonary symptoms with the onset of immunosuppression. Dissemination to the lungs, heart, CNS, and skin can occur. 50% of patients with strongyloidiasis have evidence of invasive enteric bacterial infection caused by the passage of organisms through the disrupted intestinal mucosa.

Toxoplasmosis

Unlike disease caused by *Toxoplasma gondii* in AIDS patients, toxoplasmosis in SOT patients usually represents primary infection transmitted from the allograft. *T. gondii*–

seronegative recipients of heart transplants from seropositive donors are at greatest risk. 60% will become seropositive, and 50% of these will develop symptomatic disease. Necrotizing pneumonitis, encephalitis, myocarditis, chorioretinitis, and hepatitis can occur, generally within 3 mos posttransplant. Reactivation is usually asymptomatic, although late-onset retinitis has been described. Diagnosis requires identification of trophozoites and inflammation in tissue specimens.

KEY POINTS TO REMEMBER

- When evaluating fever in solid organ transplant recipients, always evaluate the transplanted organ and surgical site, as infection is most likely to occur at these sites.
- Review patient's prophylaxis regimen and medication compliance, as improper prophylaxis can predispose to certain infections.
- Routine blood/urine/sputum cultures may not detect many infections due to atypical bacteria, fungi, and viruses.
- In patients with suspected infection and negative cultures or scans, consider getting a tissue sample for culture and histologic exam.

REFERENCES AND SUGGESTED READINGS

Knotoyiannis DP, Rubin RH. Infection in the organ transplant recipient. *Infect Dis Clin North Am* 1995;9:811–822.

Pelletier SJ, Crabtree TD, Gleason G, et al. Characteristics of infectious complications associated with mortality after solid organ transplantation. *Clin Transplant* 2000;14:401–408.

Simon DM, Levin S. Infectious complications of solid organ transplantations. *Infect Dis Clin North Am* 2001;15:521–549.

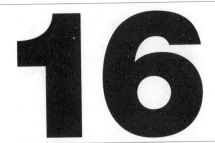

Bacteremia and Sepsis

Erik Dubberke

There are >200,000 cases of bacteremia per year in the United States and the incidence is increasing. This is likely related to multiple factors: increased use of central venous catheters (CVCs) and invasive procedures and increased seriousness of underlying illness in hospitalized patients.

GRAM-NEGATIVE BACILLI

Gram-negative bacilli (GNB) bacteremia is associated with 20–25% mortality. Traditionally the most common etiologic agent of bacteremia, recent data show a change in this trend. GNB remain the most common cause of community-acquired bloodstream infections (BSI). Gram-positive cocci (GPC) are now the most common cause of nosocomial BSI (64%), followed by GNB (27%) and *Candida* species (8%).

Organisms

Of positive blood cultures, Enterobacteriaceae account for nearly all cases of bacteremia originating from the urinary tract. Two-thirds of cases originate from gastroenteritis, and one-third of cases are a component of sepsis. The most common organisms in community-acquired bacteremia are *Escherichia coli, Klebsiella pneumoniae, Proteus mirabilis, Haemophilus influenzae,* and *Bacteroides* species. Organisms commonly associated with nosocomial GNB bacteremia include *E. coli, Klebsiella* species, *Enterobacter* species, *Serratia* species, and *P. aeruginosa.* A concerning trend in nosocomial GNB bacteremia is that the incidence of more sensitive organisms (e.g., *E. coli* and *Klebsiella* species) is decreasing and the incidence of more resistant organisms (e.g., *Serratia* species and *Enterobacter* species) is increasing. Approximately 15% of GNB bacteremias are polymicrobial.

Risk Factors

Increased risk of GNB bacteremia is associated with advanced age, prolonged hospitalization, prior antimicrobial use, and severe underlying disease [e.g., malignancy, end-stage renal disease, cirrhosis, diabetes mellitus, congestive heart failure, and skin lesions (decubitus ulcers, burns)]. GNB bacteremia is also associated with urinary tract manipulation, corticosteroid use, respiratory tract manipulation, and surgical procedures. The greatest risk factor for GNB bacteremia is neutropenia starting with an absolute neutrophil count of <1000 cells/mm^3. Risk of GNB bacteremia increases with magnitude and duration of neutropenia. Some studies indicate that GNB bacteremia is an opportunistic infection and not related to an intrinsic virulence factor.

Clinical Manifestations

GNB bacteremia should be suspected in any patient with fevers, rigors, and a known predisposing condition, such as pyelonephritis or cholecystitis, typically caused by GNB. One should also have a high index of suspicion in the elderly and in neutropenic patients. Certain subpopulations at high risk for GNB bacteremia may have a decreased fever response, such as those with advanced age, uremia, corticosteroid use, and severe debilitation. These patients may manifest with more subtle clinical changes consistent ith sepsis (hypothermia, hypotension, tachycardia, tachypnea, mental status changes, cute respiratory distress syndrome, leukopenia, thrombocytopenia, hyperbilirubin-mia, DIC, hypoglycemia, metabolic acidosis, respiratory alkalosis, oliguria). There is an ncreased incidence of shock at presentation in patients of advanced age, with prior ntineoplastic chemotherapy or corticosteroid use, azotemia, or congestive heart fail-re. At times, patients with GNB bacteremia present with colorful cutaneous manifes-ations. Ecthyma gangrenosum is considered the pathognomonic lesion of *Pseudomonas eruginosa* bacteremia and is present in 5–25% of cases, although it has been associated ith *Aeromonas hydrophilia* bacteremia as well. Skin lesions have also been described ith *E. coli, Klebsiella, Enterobacter,* and *Serratia* bacteremia. Other lesions described nclude colorful vesicular/bullous lesions, cellulitis, diffuse erythematous reactions, and etechiae. Skin lesions are easily aspirated for Gram's stain and culture.

ources

he most common source of GNB bacteremia, both community and nosocomially cquired, is the urinary tract. Other possible sources include the lungs, the hepatobil-ry tract, abdominal cavity, intravascular catheters, pelvic infections, and skin infec-ons. Depending on the definition of source of bacteremia, up to 30% of cases have nknown origins. The site of origin of bacteremia may suggest which organism is nost likely. *E. coli* typically causes >50% of bacteremias originating from the urinary ract. Up to one half of GNB originating from the respiratory tract are either *Kleb-iella* or *Pseudomonas*. Up to 75% of bacteremias originating in the abdomen are *E. oli, Bacteroides* species, or mixed. Also, there is a relationship between bacterial spe-ies and site of origin. 80% of *E. coli* bacteremias originate in the urinary or GI tracts. 0% of *Pseudomonas* bacteremias originate in the urinary or respiratory tracts. *Kleb-iella* is twice as likely to originate in the urine and then in the lung. *Bacteroides* bac-eremias almost exclusively originate in the abdomen. Comorbid conditions may also id in identifying the source of bacteremia. As the severity of the underlying illness ncreases, so does the frequency of bacteremias originating from the abdomen or skin.

valuation

he diagnosis should be confirmed, and the underlying source should be identified. wo to three sets of blood cultures should be obtained from separate venipuncture ites over 15–30 mins. Thorough evaluation of known common sources of GNB bacte-emia is warranted (urinary tract, hepatobiliary tract, and pelvis). All possible sources f infection should be cultured. Identification of the organism on blood culture may elp to identify the source of the infection. Neutropenic patients often have more sub-le presentations because of dampened immune response and inflammation, and the ource may be translocated across the intestinal epithelium.

entral Venous Catheter or Implanted Device–Associated Infection

Nontunneled catheters should be removed, and empiric antibiotics (e.g., cefepime, 1–2 g V q12h, or imipenem, 500 mg IV q6h) covering *Pseudomonas* should be started. If the atient responds to therapy, it should be continued for 10–14 days. If the catheter is emoved but there is prolonged bacteremia, antibiotics should be continued for 4–6 wks. If he catheter is tunneled or is unable to be removed, salvage therapy can be attempted ith 14 days of systemic antibiotics as well as antibiotic lock therapy. The initial addition f vancomycin as an antistaphylococcal agent may also be appropriate in patients with ndwelling CVCs. If there is no response, then the catheter should be removed, and antibi-tics should be continued for 10–14 days. If the CVC infection is complicated (e.g., endo-arditis, metastatic infection, and septic thrombophlebitis), the catheter must be emoved, and antibiotics should be continued for 4–6 wks. Due to poor response to salvage herapy, all CVC or implanted device–associated infections associated with *Pseudomonas* pecies other than *P. aeruginosa, Burkholderia* species, *Stenotrophomonas* species, *Agro-acterium* species, and *Acinetobacter baumanii* (as well as *Bacillus* species or *Corynebacte-ium* species) should prompt removal of the device.

Treatment

Community hepatobiliary tract infections with bacteremia can empirically be treated with ampicillin-sulbactam (Unasyn); piperacillin-tazobactam (Zosyn), clindamycin (Cleocin), and gentamicin; or aztreonam, ciprofloxacin (Cipro), or a third-generation cephalosporin plus metronidazole (Flagyl). Community-acquired UTI can be empirically treated with ampicillin and gentamicin, ciprofloxacin, aztreonam, or a third-generation cephalosporin. Nosocomial GNB bacteremias can be empirically treated with antipseudomonal PCN/cephalosporin, aztreonam, or imipenem with or without an aminoglycoside. Any obstruction should be relieved. Supportive measures should be implemented (see Sepsis).

GRAM-POSITIVE COCCI

GPC have become the most common overall cause of bacteremia. This is mainly related to increased use of intravascular devices. In one study involving 49 hospitals over a 3-yr period, coagulase-negative *Staphylococcus* (CoNS) accounted for 32% of nosocomial BSI; *Staphylococcus aureus* accounted for 16%; and *Enterococcus* accounted for 11%.

Organism: *Staphylococcus aureus*

S. aureus is a GPC that grows in clusters and is catalase as well as coagulase positive. It can survive for several months on dry surfaces, is heat resistant, and can tolerate high salt media. The natural history of *S. aureus* infection is colonization (preferentially in the nasopharynx, occasionally the skin, and rarely vaginal/rectal/perineal areas), and when natural mechanical barriers are breached, *S. aureus* can cause direct infection with possible subsequent BSI.

Risk Factors

Certain subsets of patients are known to have high rates of *S. aureus* colonization: diabetics receiving insulin injections, chronic hemodialysis, chronic ambulatory peritoneal dialysis, dermatologic conditions, IV drug use, HIV infection, surgical patients, and patients with poor leukocyte function.

Clinical Manifestations

Most patients with *S. aureus* bacteremia present with fevers and rigors. As with GNB bacteremia, patients at risk for *S. aureus* bacteremia may have a blunted febrile response and may present with other symptoms, such as mental status changes, tachycardia, or tachypnea (see above). Although the incidence of shock with GPC bacteremia is lower than with GNB bacteremia, *S. aureus* is associated with the highest incidence of shock from GPC. Factors that put patients at an increased risk of shock with *S. aureus* bacteremia include advanced age, immunosuppression, chemotherapy, and invasive procedures. As *S. aureus* infection has a tendency toward abscess formation, it is important to identify possible primary sites of infection. *S. aureus* has a high incidence of metastatic infections, and bacteremic patients may present with osteomyelitis, septic arthritis, or endocarditis. Endocarditis should always be considered in patients with *S. aureus* bacteremia, especially if the bacteremia is community acquired.

Sources and Evaluation

As mentioned above, the natural history of *S. aureus* infection involves colonization followed by disruption of natural mechanical barriers and direct infection. Patients with *S. aureus* bacteremia should have a thorough exam of the skin, as *S. aureus* is a common cause of folliculitis, carbuncles, impetigo, hidradenitis, cellulitis, wound infections, and abscesses. All CVCs should be inspected for evidence of tunnel infections and colonization (see below). Deep infection (e.g., bursitis, arthritis, or osteomyelitis) may occur after trauma or surgery. Hospitalized patients should be evaluated for pneumonia, as *S. aureus* is the leading cause of nosocomial pneumonia. Local infections can lead to bacteremia and subsequent metastatic infections (e.g., arthritis, osteomyelitis, meningitis, endocarditis, pericarditis, lung abscess, pyomyositis).

Central Venous Catheter or Implanted Device–Associated Infection

A nontunneled CVC should be removed if suspected to be the source of S. aureus bacteremia. A tunneled CVC or implanted device should be removed if there is evidence of tunnel, pocket, or exit site infection. TEE should be strongly considered in patients without contraindications to identify patients with endocarditis (studies have shown rates of endocarditis associated with S. aureus CVC infections from 0% to 26%). If TEE is negative for endocarditis and the CVC is removed, then the patient should be treated with 14 days of parenteral antibiotics. If the patient remains febrile or has bacteremia >3 days after catheter removal or initiation of antibiotics, a longer course of antibiotics is needed (4–6 wks), and evidence of metastatic infection should be investigated. A tunneled CVC or implanted device with uncomplicated intraluminal infection should be removed or, in select cases, retained and treated with parenteral antibiotics and antibiotic lock therapy for 14 days.

Treatment

Therapy for suspected S. aureus bacteremia should be initiated promptly, as it is associated with mortality rates of 11–43%. Subsets of patients with increased mortality include patients >50 yrs, those with a nonremovable focus of infection, and those with serious underlying cardiac, neurologic, or respiratory disease. Because of increasing rates of methicillin-resistant S. aureus (MRSA) infection, initial empiric therapy with vancomycin (Vancocin) should be started while awaiting sensitivities. A minority of isolates remain susceptible to PCN, and these can be treated with such. Strains that are resistant to PCN produce a beta-lactamase. These isolates can be treated with a semisynthetic PCN (nafcillin, oxacillin), cephalosporin (cefazolin, cephalothin), or a PCN derivative with a beta-lactamase inhibitor [ampicillin (Principen, Totacillin) with sulbactam]. Vancomycin can be used, although it is not an ideal agent because it is less effective against S. aureus than beta-lactam antibiotics. MRSA infections are resistant to beta-lactam antibiotics because of a chromosomally altered PCN-binding protein (PBP-2a). Vancomycin is the drug of choice for these isolates. Sensitivity testing should be performed before alternate antibiotics are used because MRSA infection is often resistant to other antibiotics. Patients intolerant to vancomycin have been treated with fluoroquinolones, TMP-SMX (Bactrim), clindamycin, minocycline, quinupristin-dalfopristin (Synercid), and linezolid (Zyvox). Isolates with intermediate resistance to vancomycin have been reported. The mechanism of resistance is unclear. Sensitivity testing should guide therapy in these patients. All abscesses or infected devices must be drained or removed, respectively.

Organism: Coagulase-Negative *Staphylococcus*

The most common clinical isolate of CoNS is *Staphylococcus epidermidis*. It can adhere to and proliferate on prosthetic surfaces. S. epidermidis produces a slime-like substance that interferes with phagocytosis. Up to 85% of S. epidermidis–positive blood cultures are contaminates.

Risk Factors

Patients at risk for S. epidermidis bacteremia include neutropenic patients and patients with abnormal heart valves, as well as patients with prosthetic devices (e.g., prosthetic valves, CVCs, CNS shunts, vascular grafts, pacemakers, prosthetic joints).

Clinical Manifestations

Patients with CoNS bacteremia typically present with fever and chills, and they tend to have a risk factor or CoNS bacteremia as well. It is uncommon for CoNS bacteremia to cause shock.

Evaluation

As most CoNS-positive blood cultures represent contamination rather than infection, clinical judgment is necessary to determine which patients are truly infected. A single positive bottle suggests contamination. If a patient has risk factors for CoNS bacteremia, repeat cultures should be drawn. Multiple positive cultures suggest infection. Antibiograms can be compared to determine whether positive cultures represent the same or different strains. This is complicated by the fact that CoNS in nosocomial settings are often resistant to multiple antibiotics, and certain resistance patterns may be unstable within a strain. Persistent CoNS bacteremia is strong evidence for true infection. If endocarditis is suspected, TTE or TEE may be of value.

Central Venous Catheter or Implanted Device–Associated Infection

CoNS is the most common cause of CVC-related infection. If bacteremia is not persistent and there is no clinical evidence of local or metastatic complications, the CVC can be retained. Patients with retained CVCs should be treated with 10–14 days of systemic antibiotics, possibly with antibiotic lock therapy. If the CVC is removed, systemic antibiotics should be administered for 5–7 days. Persistent fevers, persistent bacteremia, or relapse of infection after antibiotics are discontinued is a clear indication for CVC removal.

Treatment

Empiric therapy with vancomycin is appropriate. If the isolate is beta-lactamase negative, PCN is the drug of choice. If it is beta-lactamase positive and methicillin sensitive, then a semisynthetic PCN can be used.

Organism: Enterococcus

Most clinical isolates of enterococci are *Enterococcus faecalis*, accounting for 80–90% of isolates. *Enterococcus faecium* accounts for 5–10% of clinical isolates, although this percentage is increasing. This is likely related to the increased prevalence of VRE because most VRE isolates are *E. faecium*.

Risk Factors

Risk factors for enterococcal bacteremia include prior GI colonization, serious underlying disease, prolonged hospital stay, surgery, end-stage renal disease, neutropenia, transplantation, HIV, IV drug use, urinary or vascular catheters, and recent ICU stay. Prior antibiotics (particularly vancomycin, cephalosporins, and aminoglycosides), hemodialysis, corticosteroids or antineoplastic agents, and surgery are risk factors for VRE bacteremia.

Presentation

Patients typically present with fever and chills. *Enterococcus* is not a very intrinsically virulent organism and is rarely associated with shock. The high mortality rates associated with enterococcal bacteremia (42–68%) are a reflection of the severely debilitated state of patients who develop it.

Source

Only 1:50 enterococcal bacteremias are associated with endocarditis (although most series report *Enterococcus* causing 10–15% of cases of endocarditis). Origins of bacteremia, in descending order, include the urinary tract, intraabdominal/pelvic infections, wounds (burns, decubitus ulcers, and diabetic foot ulcers), CVCs, and the hepatobiliary tract. There are reports of "primary enterococcal bacteremia." These tend to occur in patients with severe underlying illness and are presumed to come from a GI source.

Evaluation

Enterococcus is a common colonizing organism, particularly in hospitalized patients on broad-spectrum antibiotics. It may be difficult to determine which positive blood cultures represent true infection; thus, as with CoNS, clinical judgment is necessary (see above). Infection is more likely in patients who are at risk for enterococcal bacteremia and who also have an identified primary infection.

Central Venous Catheter or Implanted Device–Associated Infection

Although *Enterococcus* is not a virulent organism, it is prudent to remove the CVC or implanted device infected with *Enterococcus*. It is an organism that is intrinsically resistant to many antibiotics and can be difficult to eradicate. Treatment recommendations should parallel those for CVC-associated *S. aureus* infections (see above).

Treatment

Enterococci display high levels of both intrinsic and acquired antimicrobial resistance. All enterococci have relative resistance to beta-lactam antibiotics due to low affinity of the low-molecular-weight PCN-binding proteins (particularly PBP-5) of *E. faecalis* and *E. faecium*. None of the presently available cephalosporins has significant *in vivo* activity against enterococci. Further alterations in PBP-5 have led to increased resistance to the PCNs. Resistance to aminoglycosides can be overcome by addition of appropriate cell wall–active agents, although some strains have acquired resistance to aminoglycosides, which negates this synergistic combination of antibiotics. Enterococci are able to use exogenous folinic acid, dihydrofolate, and tetrahydrofolate; therefore, they are resistant to TMP-SMX.

In the late 1980s, VRE was first described. VRE now accounts for 7.9% of enterococci isolates outside of the ICU and 13.6% of isolates inside of the ICU. The van A-D genes have been described and result in variable resistances to vancomycin and teicoplanin (Targocid). These genes alter the target of glycopeptide antibiotics and have been shown to be transferable.

PCN and ampicillin are the initial antibiotics of choice even if the susceptibility report shows moderate resistance to PCN (which is "standard" for enterococci) and susceptibility to vancomycin. PCN or ampicillin alone is fine if bactericidal therapy is not needed. If bactericidal therapy is needed (e.g., endocarditis, meningitis), then an aminoglycoside should be added. Vancomycin should be used if there is a significant PCN allergy.

Treatment of VRE requires susceptibility testing. Chloramphenicol and high-dose ampicillin-sulbactam (30 g/day) have been used with some success. Dalfopristin-quinupristin is effective against some strains of *E. faecium* but not *E. faecalis*. Linezolid and daptomycin can also be used for treatment of sensitive VRE organisms.

CANDIDA SPECIES

Candida species are the most common cause of fungemia. Although *Candida albicans* remains the most common *Candida* species causing infection, the incidence of non-*albicans* species causing fungemia is increasing.

Risk Factors

Risk factors for candidemia include colonization, prolonged use of antibiotics, CVC, hyperalimentation, surgery (particularly if the GI tract wall is transected), and prolonged ICU stay.

Evaluation

Candidemia should be suspected in patients who have persistent fever and chills despite antibiotics. Neutropenic patients have approximately a 20% risk of developing overt invasive fungal infection in this setting. Candidemia can be a cause of sepsis. Use of fungal isolator blood culture bottles may be of use, but *Candida* grow on routine blood cultures. A search for a primary site of infection should commence: CVC, urine, intraabdominal process, endocarditis, and mucous membranes. Translocation across the GI tract may be a source of candidemia in neutropenic patients. If a patient has candidemia and persistent fever despite appropriate antifungals, areas of metastatic infection should be sought. All patients with candidemia should have a dilated ophthalmic exam to look for endophthalmitis.

Central Venous Catheter or Implanted Device–Associated Infection

Removal of an infected CVC or implanted device is associated with a significant reduction in candidemia. If the patient has a nontunneled catheter, it should be removed, and semiquantitative/quantitative catheter cultures should be done. If a tunneled CVC or implanted device is present during an episode of candidemia, then the likelihood of catheter-related candidemia must be determined. Predictors of tunneled CVC–related candidemia include the following:

- Isolation of *Candida parapsilosis* from the blood
- Quantitative blood cultures that suggest catheter-related candidemia (see below)
- Differential time to positivity from blood cultures drawn from a percutaneous site, compared with those drawn through the CVC
- Candidemia in a patient without neutropenia who has a CVC and no other apparent source for BSI other than a vascular catheter
- Candidemia in a patient receiving hyperalimentation through the catheter
- Persistent candidemia in a patient who is not responding to systemic antifungal therapy

All catheters should be removed with documented catheter-related candidemia because of poor response rates to salvage therapy (<30%). Amphotericin B (Amphocin, Fungizone) is recommended for suspected catheter-related candidemia in patients who are hemodynamically unstable or who have received prolonged fluconazole therapy. Fluconazole (Diflucan) can be used in patients who are hemodynamically stable and have not received prior fluconazole therapy and in whom the organism is fluconazole sensitive. Therapy should be continued for 14 days after the last positive blood culture and when signs and symptoms of infection have resolved.

Treatment

Antifungal susceptibility can be predicted once the isolate has been speciated, although if the patient does not respond appropriately, antifungal sensitivities should be considered. *C. albicans*, *Candida tropicalis*, and *C. parapsilosis* can be treated with either amphotericin B at 0.6 mg/kg/day or fluconazole at 6 mg/kg/day. *Candida glabrata* often has decreased susceptibility to both azoles and amphotericin B. Most authorities recommend amphotericin B at ≥0.7 mg/kg/day as initial therapy. Caspofungin and voriconazole would also be appropriate for empiric antifungal therapy until the species has been determined. Fluconazole at 12 mg/kg/day may be suitable in less critically ill patients. For *Candida krusei*, amphotericin B at 1 mg/kg/day is preferred. Most isolates of *Candida lusitaniae* are resistant to amphotericin B; therefore, fluconazole at 6 mg/kg/day is preferred. In a randomized trial, amphotericin B lipid complex at 5 mg/kg/day was found to be equivalent to 0.6–1.0 mg/kg/day for nosocomial candidal infections.

Empiric antifungal therapy in suspected, but not confirmed, cases of candidemia is not recommended for non-neutropenic patients. In neutropenic patients, empiric antifungal therapy is recommended because it reduces the frequency of development of clinically overt invasive fungal infections.

CENTRAL VENOUS CATHETER AND IMPLANTED DEVICE INFECTIONS

>5 million CVCs are placed each year in the United States. The majority (90%) of CVC infections occur with nontunneled CVCs.

Risk Factors

Risk factors for CVC infections include the type of catheter, hospital size/unit/service, location of CVC, duration of catheter placement, number of lumens, and number of manipulations.

Sources

The majority of nontunneled CVC infections result from extraluminal colonization, usually from skin organisms. Less common is intraluminal colonization of the hub and lumen of the CVC. With tunneled catheters, the latter is the most common cause of infection.

Organisms

A recent study showed the most common causative organism of CVC-related bacteremia is CoNS, followed by *S. aureus*, enterococci, GNB, and then fungi. The greatest mortality is associated with *S. aureus* (8.2%), which far exceeds the other organisms. The lowest mortality (0.7%) is associated with CoNS.

Evaluation

Clinical findings can be unreliable. The most sensitive sign is **fever.** Inflammation and purulence are more specific but less sensitive. **Positive blood cultures without other identifiable sources of infection** should raise the suspicion of CVC infection. Gram's stain may be helpful, but it is not as sensitive as quantitative methods. Acridine orange stain for rapid diagnosis had a positive predictive value of 91% and negative predictive value of 97% in one study.

The most reliable diagnostic methodologies are semiquantitative (roll plate) and quantitative (vortex, sonification) **catheter culture techniques.** CVC infections occurring <1 wk after insertion are most likely caused by colonizing skin organisms, and roll plate culturing is very sensitive in this situation. If the catheter has been in place for >1 wk, then intraluminal colonization is more likely, and quantitative methods are better. At least 15 colony-forming units (cfu) by roll plate method or $\geq 10^2$ cfu/mL by quantitative methods with accompanying signs of local or systemic infection are consistent with catheter-related infection. A prospective study showed that sensitivity of the flush method is 50%, roll plate 60%, and sonification 80%.

Blood cultures should be drawn in patients with suspected catheter-related infection. At least two sets should be drawn, one peripheral and one central. In patients who have not received antibiotics, the negative predictive value of cultures drawn from the catheter is 99% and from peripheral venipuncture is 98%. The positive predictive value is 63% and 73%, respectively. Therefore, negative cultures are helpful in excluding infection, but positive cultures require some interpretation.

Quantitative blood culture techniques can be used if removing the CVC is undesirable. When the colony count of the blood culture drawn from the CVC is 5–10 times greater than the colony count of the peripheral blood cultures, then it is likely the CVC is the source of bacteremia. This method is most accurate for tunneled catheters because they are more likely to have intraluminal colonization. A quantitative culture drawn from a tunneled CVC with a colony count >100 cfu/mL may be diagnostic of CVC infection without peripheral blood cultures.

Use of continuous blood culture monitoring techniques can compare the differential time to positivity for cultures drawn simultaneously from a CVC and a peripheral vein. A positive result from the CVC ≥ 2 hrs earlier than the peripheral culture becoming positive has a sensitivity of 91% and specificity of 94%.

Treatment

There are no data to support specific antibiotic therapy. Use of antibiotics depends on index of suspicion, severity of the patient's illness, risk factors for infection, and likely pathogen. Vancomycin is the antibiotic usually recommended for empiric therapy. Additional coverage of GNB should be considered in patients who are severely ill or immunocompromised. Nontunneled CVCs in patients with fever and mild to moderate disease should not be routinely removed. The CVC should be removed if the patient is seriously ill or if there is erythema overlying the catheter exit site, purulence at the catheter exit site, or clinical signs of unexplained sepsis. Tunneled catheters should be removed if there is a tunnel infection, port abscess, or evidence of a complicated CVC infection (septic thrombosis, endocarditis, and osteomyelitis). See above for management of tunneled and nontunneled infections caused by specific organisms.

SEPSIS

Sepsis is the most severe manifestation of inflammation. It occurs when proinflammatory mediators overwhelm endogenous counterregulatory mechanisms. Although mortality from sepsis has been decreasing, it still remains at >20%. Classically described with GNB, any microorganism (GPC, fungi, viruses, protozoa, and multicellular organisms) can cause sepsis. There are 400,000–500,000 cases of sepsis per year in the United States; in 1989 there were 176 cases/100,000 population accounting for 1.3% of hospital discharge diagnoses.

Risk Factors

Incidence, as well as mortality, increases with advanced age, treatment with prior antimicrobials, immunosuppression, diabetes mellitus, congestive heart failure, azotemia, or rapidly fatal illness.

Pathophysiology

Bacterial products, particularly lipopolysaccharide, activate monocytes and macrophages that in turn release tumor necrosis factor and interleukin-1. This promotes neutrophil-endothelial cell adhesion, activation of the coagulation cascade, and generation of numerous secondary mediators of inflammation (other cytokines, prostaglandins, leukotrienes, platelet-activating factor, oxygen radicals, and proteases). Counterregulatory mediators are also produced to serve as negative feedback. When the negative feedback becomes overwhelmed, sepsis ensues. The end result of sepsis involves endothelial dysfunction, microthrombosis, and tissue hypoperfusion, leading to organ ischemia and dysfunction/failure.

Definitions

There are many different overlapping terms in regard to sepsis (they are addressed in the following sections). All are used to describe the constellation of signs and symptoms related to host response to inflammation. Currently, the most commonly used definitions were derived by the American College of Chest Physicians/Society of Critical Care Medicine Conference Committee to aid in evaluations of clinical treatment trials for sepsis combined with mortality risk stratification.

Systemic Inflammatory Response Syndrome

Systemic inflammatory response syndrome is present when two or more of the following are present:

- A core temperature of $\geq 38°C$ (100.4°F) or $\leq 36°C$ (96.8°F)
- A heart rate ≥ 90 bpm
- A respiratory rate ≥ 20/min
- Partial arterial pressure of CO_2 ≤ 32 mm Hg
- A WBC count $\geq 12,000$/mm^3 or ≤ 4000/mm^3 or a differential count showing $>10\%$ immature neutrophils

It can be caused by any source of inflammation (e.g., infarction, pancreatitis, infection).

Sepsis

Sepsis is defined as systemic inflammatory response syndrome plus a focus of infection.

Multisystem Organ Failure

Multisystem organ failure is defined as systemic inflammatory response syndrome plus evidence of ≥ 1 organ not functioning properly acutely in the setting of hypoperfusion.

Severe Sepsis

Severe sepsis is defined as sepsis plus multisystem organ failure. Patients can have *hypotension*, defined as arterial BP <90 mm Hg or a mean arterial BP <70 mm Hg, but the hypotension corrects with <500 mL bolus of a crystalloid/colloid.

Septic Shock

Septic shock is defined as sepsis plus *refractory hypotension*, which is defined as requiring >500 mL of fluid or vasopressors.

Clinical Manifestations

There are many signs and symptoms of sepsis. Primary manifestations of sepsis include fever, chills, hyperventilation, hypothermia, skin lesions (see above), and mental status changes. Complications of sepsis, which may exist on presentation, include hypotension, bleeding, leukopenia, thrombocytopenia, and evidence of end-organ failure (e.g., hypoxemia, acidosis, oliguria, jaundice, heart failure).

Sources

The lung is the most common site of infection leading to sepsis (50%), followed by intraabdominal infections (20%) and the urinary tract (10%). A definite site of infection is not found in 20–30% of patients. Positive blood cultures are present in up to 30% of cases.

Treatment

Prompt antibiotic therapy is paramount to successful treatment of sepsis. Mortality rates are 10–15% higher in patients who do not receive prompt therapy against the causative pathogen. Antimicrobials can be selected to treat the most likely pathogens if the probable source of infection is known. For community-acquired sepsis with no obvious underlying disease, a first-generation cephalosporin plus an aminoglycoside covers most potential pathogens. Asplenic patients are at particular risk for fulminant sepsis with encapsulated organisms such as *Streptococcus pneumoniae, H. influenzae,* and *Neisseria meningitidis*. PCN G, 2 million units IV q2–4h, or vancomycin, 1 g IV q12h, plus a third-generation cephalosporin (e.g., ceftriaxone, 2 g IV q12h) should be promptly administered. Gram's staining of a buffy-coat specimen can subsequently be performed and sometimes reveals the pathogen. Catheter-associated nosocomial septicemia usually is due to *S. aureus,* CoNS, aerobic GNB, or enterococci. Vancomycin plus an aminoglycoside is appropriate initial therapy. Neutropenic hosts, in whom *P. aeruginosa* sepsis may be likely, usually are treated with an antipseudomonal beta-lactam antimicrobial agent plus an aminoglycoside. The addition of an antistaphylococcal agent, such as vancomycin, may be warranted in patients with indwelling CVCs.

   Supportive care is essential in septic patients, particularly those in septic shock. Supplementary O_2 should be used as needed. BP support is needed in septic shock. "Renal doses" of dopamine may increase urine output, but it does not improve renal function. A recent study showed that norepinephrine may be of benefit in patients with refractory shock. Dobutamine can be used in patients with poor cardiac inotropic function. Use of alkali for acidosis is generally not recommended unless the pH <7.2 and cardiac arrhythmias are present. Activated protein C (Xigris) may be used in severe sepsis or septic shock. Familiarity with the inclusion and exclusion criteria for this agent is crucial in treating patients with sepsis (discussion is beyond the scope of this text). Replacement corticosteroids should also be considered for patients with sepsis. A random cortisal level <25 is suggestive of a functional adrenal insufficiency and warrants short-term replacement (e.g., hydrocortisone, 50–100 mg IV q8h, tapered over approximiately 7–10 days).

Prognosis

Overall mortality for sepsis is in the range of 20–30%. The mortality increases with each organ system that fails and is >50% for septic shock. In fatal cases, approximately 50% die within the first 24 hrs, and up to 90% die within the first week. A worse prognosis is associated with a failure to mount a febrile response, lack of or inappropriate antibiotics, prior antibiotic use, prior antineoplastic chemotherapy or corticosteroids, azotemia, congestive heart failure, diabetes mellitus, neutropenia, lactic acidosis, disseminated intravascular coagulation, and ARDS.

KEY POINTS TO REMEMBER

- The greatest risk factor for GNB bacteremia is neutropenia. Other risk factors include advanced age, prior antimicrobial use, prolonged hospitalization, severe underlying disease, surgical procedures, and corticosteroid use. The most common source is the urinary tract.
- GNB bacteremia (most commonly, Enterobacteriaceae) should be suspected in any patient with fever, rigors, and a known predisposing condition. Ecthyma gangrenosum is considered the pathognomonic lesion of *Pseudomonas aeruginosa* bacteremia.

- GPCs have become the most common overall cause of bacteremia, mostly associated with intravascular devices. CVCs should be removed in the setting of *S. aureus* or *Enterococcus* bacteremia, and a TEE should be strongly considered to evaluate for endocarditis. Vancomycin may be used as initial empiric therapy for *S. aureus* while awaiting sensitivities. Ampicillin may be used as initial therapy for enterococcal infections.
- CoNS is the most common cause of CVC-related infection and may be treated with vancomycin as empiric therapy.
- Risk factors for candidemia include colonization, prolonged use of antibiotics, CVC, hyperalimentation, surgery, prolonged ICU stay, and neutropenia.
- All patients with candidemia should have a dilated eye exam to look for endophthalmitis, and all CVCs should be removed.
- Clinical findings can be unreliable in CVC infections; one peripheral and one central blood culture set should be drawn for evaluation.
- Prompt antibiotic therapy and supportive care are paramount to the success of sepsis treatment. Consider empiric antimicrobial coverage for *Pseudomonas aeruginosa* in susceptible patients.

REFERENCES AND SUGGESTED READINGS

Bernard GR, Vincent JL, Laterre PF, et al. Efficacy and safety of recombinant human activated protein C for severe sepsis. *N Engl J Med* 2001;344:699–709.

Bhavnani SM, Drake JA, Forrest A, et al. A nationwide, multicenter, case-control study comparing risk factors, treatment, and outcome for vancomycin-resistant and -susceptible enterococcal bacteremia. *Diagn Microbiol Infect Dis* 2000;36:145–158.

Edmond MB, Wallace SE, McClish DK, et al. Nosocomial bloodstream infections in United States hospitals: a three-year analysis. *Clin Infect Dis* 1999;29:239–244.

Eisenstein BI, Zaleznik DF. Enterobacteriaceae. In: Mandell GL, Bennett JE, Dolin R, eds. *Mandell, Douglas, and Bennett's principles and practice of infectious disease,* 5th ed. Philadelphia: Churchill Livingstone, 2000:2294–2309.

Kreger BE, Craven DE, Carling PC, McCabe WR. Gram-negative bacteremia III. Reassessment of etiology, epidemiology and ecology in 612 patients. *Am J Med* 1980;68:332–343.

Kreger BE, Craven DE, McCabe WR. Gram-negative bacteremia IV. Re-evaluation of clinical features and treatment in 612 patients. *Am J Med* 1980;68:344–355.

Lowy FD. *Staphylococcus aureus* infections. *N Engl J Med* 1998;339:520–532.

Martin C, Viviand X, Leone M, Thirion X. Effect of norepinephrine on the outcome of shock. *Crit Care Med* 2000;28:2758–2765.

Mermel LA, Farr BM, Sherertz RJ, et al. Guidelines for the management of intravascular catheter-related infections. *Clin Infect Dis* 2001;32:1249–1272.

Moellering R Jr. *Enterococcus* species, *Streptococcus bovis,* and *Leuconostoc* species. In: Mandell GL, Bennett JE, Dolin R, eds. *Mandell, Douglas, and Bennett's principles and practice of infectious disease,* 5th ed. Philadelphia: Churchill Livingstone, 2000:2147–2155.

Mundy L. Treatment of infectious diseases. In: Ahya SN, Flood K, Paranjothi S, eds. *The Washington manual of medical therapeutics,* 30th ed. Philadelphia: Lippincott Williams & Wilkins, 2001:294–326.

Rex JH, Walsh TJ, Sobel JD, et al. Practice guidelines for the treatment of candidiasis. *Clin Infect Dis* 2000;30:662–678.

Waldvogel FA. *Staphylococcus aureus* (including staphylococcal toxic shock). In: Mandell GL, Bennett JE, Dolin R, eds. *Mandell, Douglas, and Bennett's principles and practice of infectious disease,* 5th ed. Philadelphia: Churchill Livingstone, 2000:2069–2091.

Wheeler AP, Bernard GR. Treating patients with severe sepsis. *N Engl J Med* 1999; 340:207–214.

Young LS, Stevens P, Kaijser B. Gram-negative pathogens in septicaemic infection. *Scand J Infect Dis* 1982;31[Suppl]:78–94.

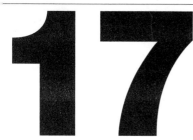

Travel Medicine

Erik Dubberke

PROPHYLAXIS

Over 30 million people from industrialized nations travel to developing countries each year. Although most travelers are concerned about illness from infectious diseases, <1% of deaths in travelers abroad are caused by infectious pathogens. As recommendations are frequently changing, one should refer to the CDC travel information Web site for specific, up-to-date information (**http://www.cdc.gov/travel/index.htm**).

Before Departure

To give advice on health maintenance, one must be familiar with health risks encountered in specific situations while traveling. Risk assessment involves knowing the patient's health status, where he or she is traveling, accommodations, purpose of travel, itinerary, duration of stay, and lifestyle while traveling.

Immunizations

Immunizations for travelers fall into three categories: routine, required, and recommended.

ROUTINE. Routine immunizations are childhood/adult boosters required regardless of travel.

Diphtheria, tetanus, and polio: Diphtheria remains a problem worldwide, particularly in the former Soviet republics. Tetanus boosters should be given if it has been >10 yrs since the last booster or if the patient is unsure when the last booster was. Approximately 10% of adult Americans are not protected against at least one serogroup of poliovirus.
Measles: Measles is still prevalent in many developing nations. Most cases in the United States are imported from these countries. Travelers born after 1956 and vaccinated before 1980 should be reimmunized.
Influenza: Influenza occurs year round in the tropics and during the summer months in the southern hemisphere (this corresponds to winter months in the northern hemisphere). Vaccination should be considered for all travelers to these areas, particularly those at high risk (see Chap. 18, Immunizations).
Pneumococcal vaccine: Pneumococcal vaccine should be administered to those at high risk (see Chap. 18, Immunizations).

REQUIRED. Required immunizations are those mandated by international regulations for entry into a country.

Yellow fever: Documentation of yellow fever vaccination may be required for entry into sub-Saharan Africa and equatorial South America where the disease is endemic. The vaccine is highly efficacious and is available only at state-authorized yellow fever centers.
Meningococcus: Meningococcal vaccine is required for entry into Saudi Arabia during the hajj.

RECOMMENDED. Recommended immunizations are those that confer protection against pathogens that travel increases the risk of contracting.

- **HAV and HBV:** The most frequently acquired vaccine-preventable disease in travelers is HAV. The incidence is 0.5% and increases sixfold for those who do not stay within the usual tourist areas. For reasons that are not entirely clear, the risk of acquiring HBV is considerable for those overseas for prolonged periods.
- **Typhoid:** The incidence of typhoid in travelers is 1/30,000/mo. The risk increases tenfold in travelers to India, Senegal, and North Africa. The efficacy of both the oral and injectable vaccine is approximately 70%, although the booster interval is 2–5 yrs.
- **Meningococcal meningitis:** Meningococcal disease is more common among those who travel to poor, overcrowded areas. Those traveling to sub-Saharan Africa during the dry season or to areas where there are epidemics should be vaccinated. The vaccine is >90% efficacious and protects against the A/C/Y/W-135 serogroups.
- **Japanese encephalitis:** In rural Asia and Southeastern Asia, the risk of Japanese encephalitis is 1/5000/mo of stay in an endemic area. Efficacy of the vaccine is >80%.
- **Cholera:** The injectable vaccine available in the United States has an efficacy of only 30–50%, and risk of acquiring cholera in an endemic area is extremely low (1/500,000). Vaccination is considered only for those who will be working as aid workers in refugee camps or in disaster/war-torn areas.
- **Rabies:** Rabies vaccination is recommended for long stays in areas where rabies is highly endemic (Mexico, the Philippines, Sri Lanka, India, Thailand, and Vietnam) or in persons who may be occupationally exposed to rabies.

Prevention of Diarrhea
Although the incidence of traveler's diarrhea is proportional to the number of dietary indiscretions, within 2 days of arrival, >95% of travelers do not adhere to dietary recommendations. In general, food should be eaten hot; foods that are raw, undercooked, or sold by street vendors should be avoided; and only boiled water or commercially carbonated beverages should be consumed. As freezing does not kill diarrhea-causing organisms, ice cubes should be avoided. The most common pathogen is enterotoxigenic *Escherichia coli*. Other common pathogens include *Campylobacter*, *Salmonella*, *Shigella*, rotavirus, and Norwalk virus. Of concern is the increase in antibiotic resistance among the bacterial pathogens. Travelers should carry medications for self-treatment (e.g., ciprofloxacin, 500 mg PO bid). For mild or moderate diarrhea, an antidiarrheal and fluid replacement is adequate. For more severe diarrhea, a 3-day course of a quinolone antibiotic may decrease the duration of illness (in areas with high rates of *Campylobacter*, a macrolide should be used). Prophylaxis with bismuth subsalicylate is 60% effective.

Prevention of Insect-Borne Diseases
Over 25,000 North American and European travelers develop malaria while abroad, although <50% of U.S. travelers adhere to recommendations for malaria prevention. The risk increases from <1/50,000 in South and Central America to 1/12,000 to 1/1000 in Haiti and the Indian subcontinent to 1/1000 to 1/50 in sub-Saharan Africa. 90% of the approximately 1000 cases of malaria that occur in the United States annually are due to *Plasmodium falciparum* acquired in Africa or Oceania. Increasing incidence of drug-resistant *P. falciparum* and *Plasmodium vivax* has made chemoprophylaxis more difficult. The drug of choice depends on the area traveled to (Table 17-1). Personal protection measures are designed to decrease the chance of being bitten by an insect. In addition to malaria prevention, they help decrease the risk of acquiring other vector-borne diseases (e.g., dengue fever, kala-azar, Chagas' disease). These include the use of DEET-containing insect repellents, permethrin-impregnated bed nets, and clothing (long sleeves, pants). For assistance with antimalarial treatment, the CDC has a malaria hotline at (770) 488-7788 [weekends and after hours: (404) 639-2888]. More information can also be found at http://www.cdc.gov/travel/diseases.htm#malaria.

Other Preventable Conditions
People traveling to areas where schistosomiasis occurs (tropical South America, Africa, Southeast Asia, and the Caribbean) should avoid swimming in lakes, rivers, and streams. Travelers should be advised to use condoms for all sexual activity. Shoes should be worn at all times to prevent hookworm, strongyloidiasis, and snake bites. Common sense precautions should be advised to prevent travel-associated injury.

TABLE 17-1. MALARIA CHEMOPROPHYLAXIS

Geographic area	Drug of choice
Thailand, Laos, and Cambodia	Doxycycline, 100 mg PO qd[a]
Central America (north of Panama), Haiti, Dominican Republic, Iraq, Egypt, Turkey, northern Argentina, and Paraguay	Chloroquine (Aralen), 500 mg PO qwk[b]; atovaquone + proguanil (Malarone), 1 PO qd[c]
South America (including Panama), Asia (excluding Southeast Asia), Africa, and Oceania	Mefloquine (Lariam), 250 mg PO qwk[d]; atovaquone + proguanil (Malarone), 1 PO qd[c]

[a]Doxycycline alone (100 mg PO qd) beginning 1–2 days before travel and for 4 wks after leaving risk area.
[b]Chloroquine alone (300 mg base) given weekly beginning 1–2 wks before travel and for 4 wks after leaving risk area.
[c]Atovaquone + proguanil (1 tablet PO qd) beginning 1–2 days before travel and for 7 days after leaving risk area.
[d]Mefloquine alone (250 mg PO) given weekly beginning 1–2 wks before travel and for 4 wks after leaving risk area.
Adapted from Keystone JS, Kozarsky PE. Health advice for international travel. In: Braunwald E, Fauci AS, Kasper DL, et al., eds. *Harrison's principles of internal medicine*, 15th ed. New York: McGraw-Hill, 2001:793–798.

On Return

The most frequent medical problems travelers have on return include diarrhea, fever, respiratory illnesses, and skin diseases. To come to a diagnosis, one must be familiar with the traveler's exact itinerary, exposure history (food, water, swimming, insect and animal bites, sexual contacts), and prophylaxis (vaccinations, chemoprophylaxis, condoms).

Diarrhea

Most cases of persistent diarrhea after travel are related to postinfectious sequelae, such as lactose intolerance and irritable bowel syndrome. The most common infectious cause of persistent diarrhea is giardiasis. Less commonly, patients may have cyclosporiasis, cryptosporidium, or amebiasis. Treatment should start with lactose avoidance, and, if unsuccessful, a trial of metronidazole (Flagyl) may be warranted.

Fever

When a patient returns from a malarious area and presents with fever, malaria should be considered first. Even when prophylaxis is taken, malaria can develop. Other causes of fever in patients returning from the tropics include viral hepatitis, bacterial enteritis, acute HIV, amebic liver abscess, arbovirus infections (dengue fever), typhoid, rickettsial infections, and leptospirosis. In up to 25% of cases, no cause is identified, and the patient improves spontaneously. Knowledge of incubation periods may aid in excluding or including diseases in the differential diagnosis. The following diagnostic tests may be of use: CBC, thick and thin blood smears, liver function tests, UA, blood cultures, and collection of acute-phase serum to be held for future testing.

Skin Diseases

The most common skin disorders in travelers returning from tropical areas include sunburn, insect bites, pyodermas, and cutaneous larval migrans. In persistent skin lesions, leishmaniasis, mycobacterial infections, and fungal infections should be considered.

KEY POINTS TO REMEMBER

- The CDC travel information Web site (http://www.cdc.gov/travel/index.htm) regarding required and recommended immunizations is a valuable resource.
- Travelers may carry a 3-day course of quinolone antibiotic to decrease duration of a severe bout of nonbloody traveler's diarrhea.
- DEET-containing insect repellent and protective clothing, in addition to chemoprophylaxis, are strongly recommended to those traveling to regions where malaria is present.
- Travelers should be advised to use condoms for all sexual activity.

REFERENCES AND SUGGESTED READINGS

Bartlett JG. *Pocket book of infectious disease therapy*. Philadelphia: Lippincott Williams & Wilkins, 2000:154–158.

Ericsson CD. Travelers' diarrhea. Epidemiology, prevention, and self-treatment. *Infect Dis Clin North Am* 1998;12:285–303.

Fradin MS. Mosquitoes and mosquito repellent: a clinician's guide. *Ann Intern Med* 1998;128:931–940.

Keystone JS, Kozarsky PE. Health advice for international travel. In: Braunwald E, Fauci AS, Kasper DL, et al., eds. *Harrison's principles of internal medicine*, 15th ed. New York: McGraw-Hill, 2001:793–798.

Magill AJ. Fever in the returned traveler. *Infect Dis Clin North Am* 1998;12:445–469.

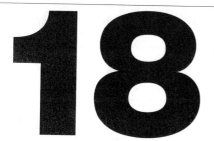

Immunizations

Bing Ho

RECOMMENDATIONS AND COMPLICATIONS

The development and introduction of vaccines have had an enormous impact on human health and have been surpassed only by access to safe water and sanitation. The goal of immunization programs is the prevention of infectious diseases and therefore the sequelae associated with these diseases. The power of immunization when coupled with appropriate resources and planning was demonstrated by the successful eradication of endogenous smallpox in 1977. Technologic advances have led to new methods of vaccine development, and the 21st century should usher in many novel vaccines and methods of delivery.

Passive vs Active Immunity

Passive immunity is the transfer of antibody to an individual, which confers short-term (a few weeks at most) protection against some infections. Active immunity refers to antigen-specific immune response and involves both humoral and cell-mediated immunity. Active immunity is based on memory B cells, which can clonally expand and produce antibodies against a previously encountered antigen. This is the principle by which most vaccines operate.

Live Attenuated and Inactivated Vaccines

Live attenuated vaccines are modified wild-type viruses that are able to replicate but cause little or minimal disease when injected into a host. Inactivated vaccines are whole, fractionated, or recombinant viruses or bacteria that are immunogenic and, because they are not able to replicate, do not produce disease even in immunocompromised individuals. Some inactivated vaccines are conjugated with another protein to enhance the immunogenicity.

The latest **recommendations for vaccinations from the CDC** can always be found on the Web site http://www.cdc.gov/nip/publications and should be referred to, as they are updated annually. See Table 18-1 for the recommended immunization schedule for adults and Table 18-2 for the recommended immunizations for adults with medical conditions.

Many vaccines require a series of injections involving ≥2 shots. In general, the recommendations focus on the **minimum** interval necessary to produce a high level of seroconversion in the general population. Decreasing the interval will have an unpredictable effect on response and effectiveness.

Adverse reactions vary from vaccine to vaccine but can be divided into three general categories: local, systemic, and allergic. Local reactions are common and involve the site of injection, such as pain, swelling, and erythema. Systemic reactions include fever, malaise, myalgias, headaches, or nausea and tend to lag behind local reactions. Allergic reactions include anaphylaxis (this is why patients should be observed for 30 mins after vaccination). The risk is low, approximately 1/500,000 doses. Patients should be screened before vaccination with detailed histories regarding any prior vaccination reactions or food and drug allergies. It is important to realize that vaccines carry not only the target for the immune response but also contain suspending solutions, preservatives, and stabilizers that may cause some of the adverse events associated with vaccine delivery.

TABLE 18-1. CDC RECOMMENDED ADULT IMMUNIZATION SCHEDULE (U.S., 2004–2005)

Vaccine	Age		
	19–49 yrs	**50–64 yrs**	**>65 yrs**
Tetanus-diphtheria[a]	1 dose booster every 10 yrs[b,c]		
Influenza	1 annual dose[d,e]	1 annual dose[d,e]	1 annual dose[b]
Pneumococcal (polysaccharide)	1 dose[d,f,g]		1 dose[b,f,g]
HBV[a]	3 doses (0, 1–2, 4–6 mos)[d,h]		
HAV[a]	2 doses (0, 6–12 mos)[d,i]		
MMR[a]	1 or 2 doses[j,k]	—	—
Varicella[a]	2 doses (0, 4–8 wks)[j,l]		
Meningococcal (polysaccharide)	1 dose[d,m]		

MMR, measles-mumps-rubella.

[a]Covered by the Vaccine Injury Compensation Program. For information on how to file a claim, call 1-800-338-2382. To file a claim for vaccine injury, write to the U.S. Court of Federal Claims, 717 Madison Place NW, Washington, DC 20005, or call 1-202-219-9657.

[b]For *all persons* in this age group.

[c]Adults, including pregnant women with uncertain history of a complete primary vaccination series, should receive a primary series of tetanus-diphtheria. A *primary series for adults* is 3 doses: Give the first 2 doses ≥4 wks apart and the third dose 6–12 mos after the second. Administer 1 dose if the patient had received the primary series and the last vaccination was ≥10 yrs ago [1]. The ACP Task Force on Adult Immunization supports a second option: a single tetanus and diphtheria booster at age 50 yrs for persons who have completed the full pediatric series, including the teen-age/young adult booster [2].

[d]For persons at risk (i.e., with medical or exposure indications).

[e]The Advisory Committee on Immunization Practices recommends inactivated influenza vaccination for the following indications, when vaccine is available. *Medical indications:* chronic disorders of the cardiovascular or pulmonary systems, including asthma; chronic metabolic diseases, including diabetes mellitus, renal dysfunction, hemoglobinopathies, immunosuppression (including immunosuppression caused by medications or by HIV); and pregnancy during the influenza season. *Occupational indications:* health care workers and employees of long-term care and assisted living facilities. *Other indications:* residents of nursing homes and other long-term care facilities; persons likely to transmit influenza to persons at high risk (in-home caregivers to persons with medical indications, household/close contacts and out-of-home caregivers of children aged birth to 23 mos, household members and caregivers of elderly and adults with high-risk conditions); and anyone who wishes to be vaccinated. For healthy persons aged 5–49 yrs without high-risk conditions who are not contacts of severely immunocompromised persons in special care units, either the inactivated vaccine or the intranasally administered influenza vaccine (FluMist) may be administered [3]. **Note:** Because of the vaccine shortage for the 2004–2005 influenza season, CDC has recommended that vaccination be restricted to the following priority groups, which are considered to be of equal importance: all children aged 6–23 mos; adults aged ≥65 yrs; persons aged 2–64 yrs with underlying chronic medical conditions; all women who will be pregnant during the influenza season; residents of nursing homes and long-term care facilities; children aged 6 mos to 18 yrs on chronic aspirin therapy; health care workers involved in direct patient care; and out-of-home caregivers and household contacts of children aged <6 mos. For the 2004–2005 season, intranasally administered, live, attenuated influenza vaccine, if available, should be encouraged for healthy persons aged 5–49 yrs who are not pregnant, including health care workers (except those who care for severely immunocompromised patients in special care units) and persons caring for children aged <6 mos [4].

[f]*Medical indications:* chronic disorders of the pulmonary system (excluding asthma); cardiovascular diseases; diabetes mellitus; chronic liver diseases, including liver disease as a result of alcohol abuse (e.g., cirrhosis); chronic renal failure or nephrotic syndrome; functional or anatomic asplenia (e.g., sickle cell disease or splenectomy); immunosuppressive conditions (e.g., congenital immunodeficiency, HIV infection, leukemia, lymphoma, multiple myeloma, Hodgkin's disease, generalized malignancy, organ or bone marrow transplantation); chemotherapy with alkylating agents, antimetabolites, or long-term systemic corticosteroids; or cochlear implants. *Geographic/other indications:* Alaskan natives and certain Native American populations. *Other indications:* residents of nursing homes and other long-term care facilities [5,6].

[g]*Revaccination* with pneumococcal polysaccharide vaccine: one-time revaccination after 5 yrs for persons with chronic renal failure or nephrotic syndrome; functional or anatomic asplenia (e.g., sickle cell disease or splenectomy); immunosuppressive conditions (e.g., congenital immunodeficiency, HIV infection, leukemia, lymphoma, multiple myeloma, Hodgkin's disease, generalized malignancy, organ or bone marrow transplantation); chemotherapy with alkylating agents, antimetabolites, or long-term systemic corticosteroids. For persons ≥65, one-time revaccination if they were vaccinated ≥5 yrs previously and were <65 yrs of age at the time of primary vaccination [5].

[h]*Medical indications:* hemodialysis patients, patients who receive clotting-factor concentrates. *Occupational indications:* health care workers and public safety workers who have exposure to blood in the workplace; persons in training in schools of medicine, dentistry, nursing, lab technology, and other allied health professions. *Behavioral indications:* IV drug users, persons with more than one sex partner in the previous 6 mos, persons with a recently acquired STD, all clients in STD clinics, men who have sex with men. *Other indications:* household contacts and sex partners of persons with chronic HBV infection, clients and staff of institutions for the developmentally disabled, international travelers who will be in countries with high or intermediate prevalence of chronic HBV infection for >6 mos, inmates of correctional facilities [7,8].

[i]*For the combined HAV-HBV vaccine,* use 3 doses at 0, 1, and 6 mos. *Medical indications:* persons with clotting-factor disorders or chronic liver disease. *Behavioral indications:* men who have sex with men, users of illegal drugs. *Occupational indications:* persons working with HAV-infected primates or with HAV in a research lab setting. *Other indications:* persons traveling to or working in countries that have high or intermediate endemicity of HAV [9,10].

[j]For persons lacking documentation of vaccination or evidence of disease.

[k]**Measles component:** Adults born before 1957 may be considered immune to measles. Adults born in or after 1957 should receive at least 1 dose of MMR unless they have a medical contraindication, documentation of at least 1 dose, or other acceptable evidence of immunity. A second dose of MMR is recommended for adults who (a) have recently been exposed to measles or were in an outbreak setting, (b) were previously vaccinated with killed measles vaccine, (c) were vaccinated with an unknown vaccine between 1963 and 1967, (d) are students in postsecondary educational institutions, (e) work in health care facilities, or (f) plan to travel internationally. **Mumps component:** One dose of MMR should be adequate for protection. **Rubella component:** Give 1 dose of MMR to women whose rubella vaccination history is unreliable and counsel women to avoid becoming pregnant for 4 wks after vaccination. For women of child-bearing age, regardless of birth year, routinely determine rubella immunity and counsel women regarding congenital rubella syndrome. Do not vaccinate pregnant women or those planning to become pregnant in the next 4 wks. If pregnant and susceptible, vaccinate as early in postpartum period as possible [11,12].

[l]*Recommended* for all persons who do not have reliable clinical history of varicella infection or serologic evidence of VZV infection who might be at high risk for exposure or transmission. This includes health care workers and family contacts of immunocompromised persons; those who live or work in environments where transmission is likely (e.g., teachers of young children, day care employees, and residents and staff members in institutional settings); persons who live or work in environments where VZV transmission can occur (e.g., college students, inmates and staff members of correctional institutions, and military personnel); adolescents aged 11–18 yrs and adults living in households with children; women who are not pregnant but who may become pregnant in the future; international travelers who are not immune to infection. **Approximately 95% of U.S.-born adults are immune to VZV.** Do not vaccinate pregnant women or those planning to become pregnant in the next 4 wks. If pregnant and susceptible, vaccinate as early in postpartum period as possible [13].

[m]*Meningococcal vaccine* (quadrivalent polysaccharide for serogroups A, C, Y, and W-135). *Medical indications:* adults with terminal complement component deficiencies, with anatomic or functional asplenia. *Other indications:* travelers to countries in which disease is hyperendemic or epidemic (e.g., "meningitis belt" of sub-Saharan Africa; Mecca, Saudi Arabia). Revaccination at 3–5 yrs may be indicated for persons at high risk for infection (e.g., persons residing in areas in which disease is epidemic). Counsel college freshmen, especially those who live in dormitories, regarding meningococcal disease and the vaccine so that they can make an educated decision about receiving the vaccination [14]. The American Academy of Family Physicians recommends that colleges should take the lead on providing education on meningococcal infection and vaccination and offer it to those who are interested. Physicians need not initiate discussion of the meningococcal quadrivalent polysaccharide vaccine as part of routine medical care.

TABLE 18-2. CDC RECOMMENDED IMMUNIZATIONS FOR ADULTS WITH MEDICAL CONDITIONS (U.S., 2004–2005)

Medical conditions	Tetanus-diphtheria[a]	Influenza	Pneumococcal (polysaccharide)	HBV[a]	HAV[a]	Measles-mumps-rubella[a]	Varicella[a]
Pregnancy	b	b	c	c	c	d	d
Diabetes; heart disease; chronic pulmonary disease; chronic liver disease, including chronic alcoholism	b	b,e,f	b,f	c	c,g	h	h
Congenital immunodeficiency; cochlear implants; leukemia; lymphoma; generalized malignancy; therapy with alkylating agents, antimetabolites, CSF leaks, radiation, or large amounts of corticosteroids	b	b	b,i	c	c	d	d,j
Renal failure/end-stage renal disease, recipients of hemodialysis or clotting-factor concentrates	b	b	b,i	b,k	c	h	h
Asplenia, including elective splenectomy and terminal complement component deficiencies	b	l	b,i,m,n	c	c	h	h
HIV infection	b	b	b,i,o	b	c	h,p	d

[a]Covered by the Vaccination Injury Compensation Program.
[b]For all persons in this group.
[c]For persons at risk (i.e., with medical/exposure indications).
[d]Contraindicated.
[e]Although chronic liver disease and alcoholism are not indications for influenza vaccination, give 1 dose annually if the patient is ≥50 yrs, has other indications for influenza vaccine, or requests vaccination.
[f]Asthma is an indicator condition for influenza vaccine but not for pneumococcal vaccination.
[g]For all persons with chronic liver disease.
[h]For persons lacking documentation of vaccination or evidence of disease.
[i]For persons aged <65 years, revaccinate once after ≥5 yrs have elapsed since initial vaccination [13].
[j]Persons with impaired humoral but not cellular immunity may be vaccinated [13].
[k]For hemodialysis patients, use special formulation of vaccine (40 μg/mL) or two 20-μg/mL doses at one body site. Vaccinate early in the course of renal disease. Assess antibody titer to HBV surface antigen (anti-HBVs) levels annually. Administer additional dose if anti-HBV levels decline to <10 mIU/mL.
[l]No data exist specifically on the risk for severe or complicated influenza infections among persons with asplenia. However, influenza is a risk factor for secondary bacterial infections that can cause severe disease among persons with asplenia.
[m]Administer meningococcal vaccine and consider *Haemophilus influenzae* type B vaccine.
[n]For elective splenectomy, vaccinate ≥2 wks before surgery.
[o]Vaccinate as close to diagnosis as possible.
[p]Withhold measles-mumps-rubella or other measles-containing vaccines from HIV-infected persons with evidence of severe immunosuppression [11,15].

Please see the CDC Web site for complete lists of **contraindications** and **precautions** that should be considered before administering immunizations.

Complications Associated with Adult Vaccinations

There have been many reported adverse events associated with immunizations. Many of these have little or no causal relationship to the vaccine. The known associations are listed below, and further details can be obtained from the CDC Web site.

- Diptheria taxoid, tetanus-diphtheria, or tetanus toxoid has been implicated in anaphylactic reactions.
- HBV recombinant vaccine has been implicated in anaphylactic reactions. It has also been associated with Guillain-Barré syndrome; however, in wide practice, there appears to be no relationship between the two.
- Oral polio vaccine has been shown to be associated with a greatly increased risk for vaccine-associated disease in immunocompromised individuals. In these populations, injectable polio vaccine is recommended for immunocompromised individuals and people living in their household. There is a low rate of paralytic poliomyelitis even in immunocompetent patients receiving oral polio vaccine.
- Live measles vaccine is *not* associated with subacute sclerosing panencephalitis. The measles-mumps-rubella vaccine is associated with clinically apparent thrombocytopenia that may last for up to 2 mos after vaccination, as well as anaphylaxis.

Special Populations

Health care workers are a particularly high-risk population because of their contact with patients and infective material. It is particularly recommended that all health care workers be immunized for HBV, measles-mumps-rubella, varicella, and an annual influenza vaccination. Please refer to CDC guidelines for further specific recommendations.

Immunocompromised patients, including HIV-infected patients, are at considerable risk of severe reactions to live vaccines. Furthermore, oral polio vaccine should not be given to patients living in a household with immunocompromised individuals. Other live vaccines should be safe for household contacts.

Pregnant women are not recommended to be vaccinated with live vaccines due to a theoretic risk of infection to the fetus. Inactivated vaccines appear safe.

International travelers should be assessed well before any planned travel, as many vaccination series require multiple shots. Recommendations are based on specific travel destinations and duration of stay. Please refer to http://www.cdc.gov/nip/webutil/menu-travelers.htm for further information. A referral to a travel clinic may be advisable especially when time is available or when traveling in large parties.

KEY POINTS TO REMEMBER

- The Web site http://www.cdc.gov/nip/publications contains the latest vaccination recommendations from the CDC.
- Adverse reactions can be categorized as local, systemic, or allergic. Patients should be asked about other allergies or prior reactions.
- Although the risk for anaphylaxis is low, patients should be observed for at least 30 mins after vaccination.
- Health care workers and international travelers may require additional vaccinations.
- Vaccinations given to immunocompromised patients and pregnant women need to be considered carefully as these patients may be at greater risk of having an adverse reaction.

SUGGESTED READING

Immunization of health-care workers: recommendations of the Advisory Committee on Immunization Practices (ACIP) and the Hospital Infection Control Practices Advisory Committee (HICPAC). *MMWR Recomm Rep* 1997;46(RR-18):1–42.

CDC Web site (travel): http://www.cdc.gov/nip/webutil/menu-travelers.htm. Accessed October 11, 2003.

CDC Web site (vaccinations): http://www.cdc.gov/nip/publications/. Accessed October 11, 2003.

REFERENCES

1. Diphtheria, tetanus, and pertussis: recommendations for vaccine use and other preventive measures. Recommendations of the Immunization Practices Advisory committee (ACIP). *MMWR Recomm Rep* 1991;40(RR-10):1–28.
2. ACP Task Force on Adult Immunization and Infectious Diseases Society of America. *Guide for adult immunization*, 3rd ed. Philadelphia: American College of Physicians, 1994:20.
3. Harper SA, Fukuda K, Uyeki TM, et al.; Centers for Disease Control and Prevention (CDC) Advisory Committee on Immunization Practices (ACIP). Prevention and control of influenza: recommendations of the Advisory Committee on Immunization Practices (ACIP). *MMWR Recomm Rep* 2004;53(RR-6):1–40.
4. Interim influenza vaccination recommendations, 2004–2005 influenza season. *MMWR* 2004;53:923–924.
5. Prevention of pneumococcal disease: recommendations of the Advisory Committee on Immunization Practices (ACIP). *MMWR Recomm Rep* 1997;46(RR-8):1–24.
6. Pneumococcal vaccination for cochlear implant candidates and recipients: updated recommendations of the Advisory Committee on Immunization Practices. *MMWR* 2003;52:739.
7. Hepatitis B virus: a comprehensive strategy for eliminating transmission in the United States through universal childhood vaccination. Recommendations of the Immunization Practices Advisory Committee (ACIP). *MMWR Recomm Rep* 1991;40(RR-13):1–25.
8. Alter M, Bell B, Fiore A, et al. CDC Travelers' Health Information on Hepatitis, Viral, Type B. http://www.cdc.gov/travel/diseases/hbv.htm. Accessed March 17, 2005.
9. Alter M, Bell B, Fiore A, et al. CDC Travelers' Health Information on Hepatitis, Viral, Type A. http://www.cdc.gov/travel/diseases/hav.htm. Accessed March 17, 2005.
10. Prevention of hepatitis A through active or passive immunization: Recommendations of the Advisory Committee on Immunization Practices (ACIP). *MMWR Recomm Rep* 1999;48(RR-12):1–37.
11. Watson JC, Hadler SC, Dykewicz CA, et al. Measles, mumps, and rubella—vaccine use and strategies for elimination of measles, rubella, and congenital rubella syndrome and control of mumps: recommendations of the Advisory Committee on Immunization Practices (ACIP). *MMWR Recomm Rep* 1998;47(RR-8):1–57.
12. Revised ACIP recommendation for avoiding pregnancy after receiving a rubella-containing vaccine. *MMWR Morb Mortal Wkly Rep* 2001;50(49):1117.
13. Prevention of varicella. Update recommendations of the Advisory Committee on Immunization Practices (ACIP). *MMWR Recomm Rep* 1999;48(RR-6):1–5.
14. Meningococcal disease and college students. Recommendations of the Advisory Committee on Immunization Practices (ACIP). *MMWR Recomm Rep* 2000;49(RR-7):13–20.
15. Atkinson WL, Pickering LK, Schwartz B, et al. General recommendations on immunization. Recommendations of the Advisory Committee on Immunization Practices (ACIP) and the American Academy of Family Physicians (AAFP). *MMWR Recomm Rep* 2002;51(RR-2):1–35.

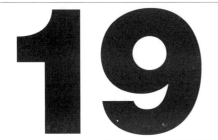

Immune Deficiency Disorders

Maria B. Ristig

IMMUNE DEFICIENCIES: PRIMARY AND SECONDARY

It is important to suspect immune deficiency disorders in patients presenting with recurrent, persistent, or unusual infections. If diagnosis is made early in the course of disease, it will prevent or at least decrease frequency plus severity of subsequent infections and improve the patient's quality of life. Complications of infections in immunosuppressed hosts include, in particular, chronic respiratory tract diseases, localized purulent infections, and sepsis syndromes. See Table 19-1 for common infections associated with primary immune deficiency disorders. In this chapter, we focus on primary and secondary immune deficiency disorders in adults who are not suffering from HIV or undergoing cytotoxic chemotherapy with subsequent neutropenia or transplantation.

Primary Immune Deficiencies

Primary immune deficiencies can be divided into four subgroups depending on specific or innate immune system defects and humoral, antibody, or cellular deficiency states:

- B-cell associated disorders
- T-cell linked defects
- Complement deficiencies
- Phagocytic disorders, including chemotactic or microbicidal disorders

Two or more defects can be combined in certain immune deficiency states. Most common are B-cell or antibody defects. The overall incidence of primary immune deficiencies is approximately 1/10,000, with selective IgA deficiency in up to 1/400 adults. Of note, most of the inherited immune disorders are diagnosed during the first 5 yrs of life, but in some cases, they manifest later in adulthood. Common variable immune deficiency usually becomes apparent in the second or third decade of life. It is a heterogenous disorder with case presentations that appear less obviously inherited and perhaps acquired in certain cases. Causes of defects are often unknown but are sometimes linked with viral infections. Patients with selective IgA deficiency, chronic mucocutaneous candidiasis, or IgG subclass or complement deficiencies have a good prognosis and may even have a normal lifespan with optimal therapy.

Secondary Immune Deficiencies

Secondary immune deficiencies are usually acquired and occur in individuals who had previously normally functioning immune systems. Impairment can be temporary and reversible or persistent. Special populations at increased risk of host defense defects include particular diabetics, patients with protein-losing states, and malnourished individuals. Often, several factors of the host defense system are impaired: loss of integrity of surface plus mucosal barriers, phagocytosis, proinflammatory cytokines, and T-cells, as is the case in steroid-dependent subjects. In other states, function of complement cascade, antibodies, B-cell system, or natural killer cells can be abnormal.

**TABLE 19-1. COMMON INFECTIONS ASSOCIATED WITH
PRIMARY IMMUNE DEFICIENCY DISORDERS**

Primary immune deficiency disorders	Bacterial infections	Fungal and parasitic infections	Viral infections
B-lymphocyte defects	*Streptococcus* species	*Giardia lamblia*	Rotavirus
Selective IgA deficiency or selective IgM deficiency	Pneumococci	*Cryptosporidium* species	RSV
Hyper-IgM syndrome	*Haemophilus influenzae*		*Enterovirus* species
Common variable immune deficiency	*Neisseria*		Echo/coxsackie/ polioviruses
Transient or X-linked hypogammaglobulinemia	*Pseudomonas aeruginosa*		
	Klebsiella		
	Escherichia coli		
T-lymphocyte defects	*Listeria*	*Aspergillus* species	RSV
Chronic mucocutaneous candidiasis	*Salmonella*	*Candida* species	Parainfluenza
DiGeorge syndrome/thymic hypoplasia	*Mycobacteria*	*Pneumocystis jiroveci*	Herpesviruses: Epstein-Barr virus, CMV, HSV
			Enterovirus species
Phagocytic disorders	*Staphylococcus* species	*Aspergillus* species	
Hyper-IgE/Job's syndrome	*P. aeruginosa*	*Candida* species	
Chronic granulomatous disease	*Nocardia*		
Leukocyte adhesion deficiency			
Chronic benign neutropenia or lethal agranulocytosis			
Complement disorders	*Neisseria* species	—	—
Classic pathway defects	*H. influenzae*		
Deficiency of C5 and C3	Pneumococci		
Alternative pathway defects			
Combined disorders	Similar to B- and T-lymphocyte defects	Similar to B- and T-lymphocyte defects	Similar to B- and T-lymphocyte defects
Severe combined immune deficiency			
Ataxia telangiectasia			
Wiskott-Aldrich syndrome			

RSV, respiratory syncytial virus.

Secondary immune deficiency disorders linked with certain risk groups

I. Age-dependent populations
   A. Premature or newborns
   B. Elderly population
II. Patients with metabolic diseases and organ failures
   A. Chronic renal failure/uremia
   B. Liver cirrhosis
   C. Diabetes mellitus
   D. Malnutrition (e.g., Kwashiorkor, vitamin A deficiency)
III. Patients with other protein-losing diseases
   A. GI: chronic protein-losing enteropathies, chronic inflammatory bowel syndrome
   B. Renal: nephrotic syndrome
   C. Skin: burns and large pressure ulcers and other skin defects
IV. Patients on immunosuppressive agents and with other secondary immune deficiency disorders
   A. Steroids
   B. Chemotherapy and immune modulatory agents
   C. Graft-vs-host disease
   D. Organ transplant, bone marrow transplant
   E. Radiation therapy
V. Patients who have undergone radiation therapy
VI. Subjects with malignant hematologic diseases and other infiltrative diseases
   A. Lymphoma, non-Hodgkin's lymphoma, neoplastic disease
   B. Leukemia
   C. Aplastic anemia
   D. Sarcoidosis
VII. Individuals with other systemic disorders and hereditary diseases
   A. Vasculitis
   B. Collagenosis
   C. Sickle cell disease and other diseases with functional splenectomy
VIII. Patients who have undergone surgery or trauma, including splenectomy
IX. Individuals with infectious diseases
   A. Viral infections (e.g., CMV, Epstein-Barr virus, HIV)
   B. Bacterial infections (e.g., mycobacterial)
   C. Fungal infections
X. Patients with autoimmune diseases
   A. SLE
   B. Polymyositis
   C. Rheumatoid arthritis

History and Physical Exam

Most patients with immune deficiencies are suffering from recurrent infections. Frequent complaints are upper respiratory, throat, sinus, ear, or pulmonary infections. Pneumonia is a common diagnosis in this patient population. Bronchitis can progress to bronchiectasis, chronic lung disease, and eventually respiratory failure. Moreover, other organ systems are involved, in particular, GI tract and skin plus mucosal surfaces. Frequent symptoms are diarrhea and skin infections or mucocutaneous candidiasis.

Furthermore, immune deficiency disorders can be linked with characteristic clinical patterns. Ataxia telangiectasis presents with neurologic deterioration, telangiectasia, and sinopulmonary infections. Complement disorders can resemble collagen vascular disorders. During the physical exam, it is essential to detect skin, hair, or skeletal abnormalities (e.g., dysmorphic body or facial abnormalities). Moreover, organ dysfunction and endocrinopathies can be associated with immune disorders. Patients often appear chronically ill and are malnourished with muscle dystrophy. In the case of B- or T-cell defects, lymphoid tissue is diminished or absent. Despite recurrent upper respiratory tract infections, there may be decreased or no lymphadenopathy or adenoidal tissue. Primary immune defects can be autosomal or, in particular, X-linked with predominance in males. Therefore, a family history is helpful for diagnosis as well as the age of onset.

Diagnosis

Specific defects are associated with certain pathogens plus typical clinical features and therefore can suggest an underlying immune deficiency. **B-cell and antibody deficiencies** are typically linked with infections caused by gram-positive organisms. The antibody-deficient host is at risk for infection by encapsulated bacteria (e.g., *Pneumococci*, *Haemophilus influenzae*, *Neisseria* species plus some gram-negatives, in particular *Escherichia coli* or *Klebsiella pneumoniae*). Viruses such as adenovirus or respiratory syncytial virus and enteroviruses are other important pathogens. Clinical presentation in general is associated with symptoms of the sinopulmonary system and GI tract. **T-cell–mediated defects** are typically linked with infections from fungi; viruses, such as rotavirus, RSV, and herpes; and other opportunistic pathogens, such as *Toxoplasma gondii*, *Pneumocystis jiroveci*, and *Cryptosporidium*. Concerning phagocytic syndromes, staphylococcal and gram-negative infections such as those seen with *Pseudomonas* are characteristic. Clinical manifestations result in recurrent cutaneous or deeper tissue and organ abscesses, cervical lymphadenitis, or fungal infections (e.g., *Aspergillus* and *Burkholderia*). Infections in patients with underlying complement defects can vary according to the nature of the deficient component. Infections with *Neisseria* species are common in individuals with complement deficiencies or sepsis with encapsulated bacteria and can be similar to antibody-deficient states (Table 19-1).

Microbiology Lab Evaluation

Specimen for culture and susceptibility testing is essential (e.g., blood, other sterile body fluids, and in particular CSF). Culture should include routine bacterial and fungal culture and, in certain cases, viral and mycobacterial culture. Direct fluorescent antibody stains and polymerase chain reaction (PCR) are available for diagnostic modalities for adenovirus, respiratory syncytial virus, and enteroviruses. In addition, serology for antigen detection (*Histoplasma*, *Cryptococcus*) may be helpful.

Lab Evaluation

Antibody deficiency syndromes are a major group of immune defects. Diagnosis is supported by lab tests—in particular, qualitative and quantitative immunoglobulin levels, especially hypogammaglobulinemia and diminished response to vaccination (e.g., tetanus, diphtheria, or rubeola). Table 19-2 categorizes some screening tests.

Treatment and Prophylaxis

Symptomatic immunodeficient patients with fever need **immediate medical care;** cultures and empiric antibiotic regimen based on the above considerations should be implemented. Treatment may require prolonged courses. Antibiotics with intracellular activity should be used in patients with phagocytic disorders.

   Prevention of recurrent infections is a primary goal. A variety of vaccines may be of benefit (e.g., pneumococcal conjugate, *H. influenzae* conjugate, the meningococcal vaccine, and especially diphtheria, tetanus, and influenza vaccines). Live vaccines, such as measles-mumps-rubella and polio, bear the risk of vaccine-induced illness. Antimicrobial prophylaxis may be started if the benefit outweighs the risk for selection of resistant organisms, such as for *P. jiroveci* with co-trimoxazole (Bactrim, Septra). Parenteral immunoglobulins are important in cases of antibody deficiency syndromes.

TABLE 19-2. IMMUNOLOGIC SCREENING TESTS FOR PRIMARY IMMUNE DEFICIENCIES

Expected immune deficiency defect	Immunologic tests
Antibody-mediated	Qualitative and quantitative serum immunoglobulin levels for IgA, IgG, IgM
	IgG subclass levels
	IgG response to vaccine proteins (e.g., diphtheria and tetanus) and polysaccharides (e.g., pneumococcal and meningococcal)
	Isohemagglutinin titers (e.g., anti-A, anti-B)
Cell-mediated	Total lymphocyte count compared with CBC and differential
	Delayed hypersensitivity skin tests (e.g., *Candida albicans*, tetanus, diphtheria, trichophyton)
	Antigen proliferation responses and mitogen
Phagocytic function	Baseline: CBC and differential count
	Quantitative nitroblue tetrazolium test or chemiluminescence assay for respiratory burst activity
	Serum IgE level
	Chemotaxis assay
	Flow cytometric analysis of CD11–18
Complement	Qualitative and quantitative serum complement components (e.g., C2, C3, C4, C6) or other components
	Total hemolytic activity (CH50)

Adapted from Armstrong D, Cohen J. *Infectious diseases*, Vol. 1. St. Louis: Mosby, 1999.

Of note, anaphylactic reactions can occur in individuals with IgA deficiency. Only if absolutely indicated should these patients be provided with IgA-depleted IV Ig, 300–400 mg/kg (increases blood levels only by 100 mg/dL). In selected case scenarios, doses up to 1000 mg/kg IV immunoglobulin are given monthly. Supportive therapy may prevent adverse reactions, including fevers, headaches, rash, and, in rare cases, aseptic meningitis. It should be mentioned that IgG immunoglobulins do not replace IgA or IgM deficiencies.

For more details regarding the treatment and prevention of a specific infection, please refer to the appropriate section elsewhere in this manual.

KEY POINTS TO REMEMBER

- Any patient with recurrent, persistent, or unusual infections should have an immunodeficiency workup.
- Initial screening tests for primary immunodeficiencies should probably include quantitative immunoglobulins, immune competency panel (T-cell counts), CBC with differential, and complement profile. An HIV test is also recommended.
- Performing a careful medical history is important in ruling out secondary immune deficiency. Family history is also important to rule out hereditary causes.

REFERENCES AND SUGGESTED READINGS

Armstrong D, Cohen J. *Infectious diseases,* Vol. 1. St. Louis: Mosby, 1999.
Buckley RH. Immunodeficiency diseases. *JAMA* 1992;268:2797–2806.

Delves P, Roitt IM. The immune system. Review. First part. *N Engl J Med* 2000;343:
  37–49.
Delves P, Roitt IM. The immune system. Review. Second part. *N Engl J Med* 2000;343:
  108–117.
Stiehm ER. *Immunologic disorders in infants and children,* 4th ed. Philadelphia: WB
  Saunders, 1996.

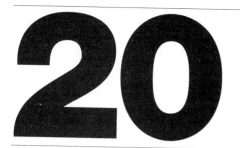

Human and
Animal Bites

Erin K. Quirk

INFECTIONS FROM HUMAN AND ANIMAL BITES

Approximately 50% of Americans will suffer a bite wound at least once in their lives; 80% do not require treatment. Those who do receive treatment account for 300,000 ER visits, 10,000 hospitalizations (1% of all admissions originating within the ER), and approximately 20 deaths annually. Infection is the most common complication of bites.

The microbiology of human bite infections is complex, and studies published to date are problematic in terms of small numbers of patients and poor culture technique. The best data indicate that most infections are polymicrobial (five organisms are cultured on average) and usually involve anaerobes that are commonly beta-lactamase producers and penicillin resistant. *Streptococcus viridans* is usually the most frequent organism reported. *Staphylococcus aureus* has also been reported in up to 40% of wounds and may have a particular association with a patient's attempts at self-débridement. Other "commonly reported" organisms vary with widely contradictory bacteriologic reports depending on the study.

Clinical Manifestations

In the early period (approximately up to 8 hrs) after a bite, the primary concern is that of crush injury. It is more common with bites induced by animals with teeth designed for grinding (e.g., dogs). After this period, the concern for infectious complications arises. Complications include cellulitis, tenosynovitis, local abscess formation, septic arthritis, osteomyelitis, and occasionally sepsis, endocarditis, meningitis, and brain abscess. Concerning symptoms include fever, lymphangitis, lymphadenopathy, and decreased range of motion in or tenderness over a joint, tendon, or muscle in the proximity of the bite.

Dog bites are the most common of animal bites, accounting for 80–90% of cases. Half of patients are bitten on the hand. Although previously underrecognized, *Pasteurella* species are the most common pathogens associated with dog bite infections—25% according to recent study by Talan et al. [1]. Accounting for 5–15% of bite wound injuries are cat bites, which occur on the upper extremity in approximately two-thirds of cases. *Pasteurella multocida* is the organism classically associated with cat bites and has been reported in 50–80% of patients—43% in the study by Talan et al. [1]. The next most common bacteria causing infection associated with both cat and dog bites are *Streptococcus*, *Staphylococcus*, *Moraxella*, *Corynebacterium*, and *Neisseria*. A multitude of other organisms have been found to cause infection following animal bite, and polymicrobial infection is common. In fact, most anaerobic infections are polymicrobial.

Humans are the third most common source of bite wounds. These bites more frequently develop infection than do animal bites and are best divided into two categories. **Occlusive bite wounds** are those that occur when the teeth are closed forcibly and break the skin. The affected anatomic site varies by gender: In men, human bites typically occur on the hand, arm, and shoulder, whereas women are more often bitten on the breast, genitals, leg, and arm. Complications arise more frequently after occlusive bites to the hand than to any other site. In fact, a 1987 study by Lindsay et al. [2]

compared human occlusive bites to lacerations not associated with bites and found incidences of infection of 17.7% and 13.4%, respectively. Bite wounds of the hand had a twofold greater risk of infection than did human bites at any other site.

Clenched-fist injuries account for the remainder of human bite wounds. These result when one person hits another person in the mouth, typically causing a break in the skin overlying the third metacarpal joint. This is the most serious type of human bite infection, as the metacarpal joint capsule is frequently perforated and often becomes involved in a septic arthritis. Cellulitis, tendonitis, and, rarely, nerve laceration or bone fracture are other possible complications of clenched-fist injuries.

Special Considerations for Animal Bites

When determining which antibiotic therapies to use when prophylactically or empirically treating infection associated with **dog or cat bites,** special consideration should be given to *Pasteurella* species, *Staphylococcus*, and beta-lactamase–producing anaerobes. Such anaerobes must be taken into consideration for the treatment of human bites as well. It must also be remembered that any number of unusual organisms have been reported in association with animal bite wound infections. In fact, enteric gram-negatives must be considered when evaluating the patient with an infection secondary to snake bite, as the prey of snakes often defecate in their mouths during ingestion. Indeed, infections with *Pseudomonas aeruginosa*, *Proteus*, *Clostridium*, *Bacteroides fragilis*, and *Salmonella* groups IIIa and IIIb have all been reported in association with snake bites. Most infections after venomous snake bites, however, are caused by organisms that colonize the devitalized tissue that results from local envenomation.

A rare but well-described complication of rat bites known as **rat-bite fever** results from inoculation and then hematogenous spread of *Streptobacillus moniliformis*. (See also Rat-Bite Fever in Chap. 22, Spirochetes.) Approximately 10 days after a bite from a rat or other rodent, the acute onset of fever, headache, and severe migratory arthralgias occurs. Within a few days, most patients experience the onset of a morbilliform rash that begins as either papules or macules and progresses to pustules over the palms, soles, and extremities; it can spread centripetally and desquamate in some cases. At least half of patients develop a polyarthritis of the large and medium joints. Most cases occur in children or lab workers who handle rats and are successfully treated with 1 wk of IV penicillin. It is interesting to note that rat-bite fever that occurs outside of the United States is usually attributed to *Spirillum minus* and lacks the polyarthritis seen in *S. moniliformis* infection.

Treatment

The treatment of bite wounds centers on débridement of devitalized tissue, local wound care, and antibiotic therapy, if appropriate. **Prophylactic antibiotics** should be given to all patients who present in the short term with a bite that penetrates the skin of the hand or in close proximity to bone, tendon, or muscle. All clenched-fist injuries should receive prophylaxis. Occlusive human bite injuries to any area other than the hand probably do not require prophylaxis. When patients present with an infected bite wound or any associated infectious complication, data obtained from culture of the blood and affected sites should be used to guide the choice of antimicrobial agents. Length of therapy depends on the infectious complications. Patients should be evaluated for need for anti–tetanus or rabies postexposure prophylaxis.

Preventive Measures

When any patient presents with a history of mammalian bite injury, the possibility of rabies transmission must be considered given the uniformly fatal prognosis after the symptoms of human rabies develop. The disease is rare in the United States, with 32 lab-confirmed cases between 1980 and 1996. Notably, in 25 of these 32 cases, no history of animal bite or other high-risk exposure could be elicited. Rabies virus variants associated with bats were the most common (53% of cases). Other variants included those found in domestic dogs outside of the United States (38%), domestic dogs within the United States (6%), and indigenous skunks (3%). Based on these findings, it is currently recommended that postexposure prophylaxis should be given to any person who reports a scratch, bite, or contact with mucous membranes of bats and skunks. In addition, all patients presenting with nondomestic dog bites should receive prophylaxis, as well as those with a history of close physical proximity to a bat even if contact with the animal cannot be determined. Patients with routine domestic dog and cat bites should not automatically receive rabies prophylaxis unless the animal was displaying unusual behavior or signs of hydrophobia. Instead, it is recommended that the local health department be contacted about ruling out rabies infection in the offending animal.

Rabies prophylaxis entails passive immunization with human rabies Ig and active immunization with either rabies vaccine adsorbed or human diploid cell vaccine. Typically, 10 IU/kg is injected around the exposure site, and another 10 IU/kg is given IM. A series of five 1-mL IM injections of either human diploid cell vaccine or rabies vaccine adsorbed should be given at days 0, 3, 7, 14, and 28. Of note, immunizations administered to the gluteal regions have been associated with treatment failure; therefore, injection into the deltoid or thigh is recommended.

KEY POINTS TO REMEMBER

- Cellulitis occurring within 24 hrs after a dog or cat bite is likely to be secondary to *Pasteurella multocida*.
- Empiric treatment with amoxicillin plus clavulanate potassium (Augmentin) or ampicillin plus sulbactam (Unasyn) is usually indicated for infected bite wounds or any bite that perforates the skin of the hand or is in close proximity to bone, tendon, or muscle.
- Human bites more frequently develop infections than animal bites, particularly those involving the hand. Most infections are polymicrobial and usually involve anaerobes.
- Patients are at risk for tetanus and rabies, so appropriate prophylactic measures should be strongly considered in bites from humans or animals.

SUGGESTED READING

Goldstein EJC. Bites. In: Mandell GL, Bennett JE, Dolin R, eds. *Principles and practice of infectious diseases,* 5th ed. Philadelphia: Churchill Livingstone, 2000:3202–3206.

Noah DL, Drenzek CL, Smith JS, et al. Epidemiology of human rabies in the United States, 1980 to 1996. *Ann Intern Med* 1998;128:922–930.

Pretty IA, Anderson GS, Sweet DJ. Human bites and the risk of human immunodeficiency virus transmission. *Am J Forensic Med Pathol* 1999;20:232–239.

Washburn RG. *Streptobacillus moniliformis* (rat-bite fever). In: Mandell GL, Bennett JE, Dolin R, eds. *Principles and practice of infectious diseases,* 5th ed. Philadelphia: Churchill Livingstone, 2000:2422–2424.

REFERENCES

1. Talan DA, Citron DM, Abrahamian FM, et al. Bacteriologic analysis of infected dog and cat bites. *N Engl J Med* 1999;340:85–92.
2. Lindsay D, Christopher M, Hollenback J, et al. Natural course of the human bite wound: incidence of infection and complications in 434 bites and 803 lacerations in the same group of patient. *J Trauma* 1987;27:45–48.

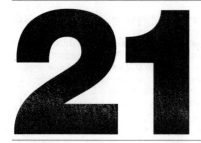

Tick-Borne Illnesses

Erin K. Quirk
Nicholas Haddad

INTRODUCTION

Ticks, along with spiders, mites, and scorpions, are noninsect members of the class Arachnida that rely on blood as a food source. The ticks are further subdivided into three families, two of which contain species that can transmit human disease. There are 3 of the 13 genera of the family Ixodidae (hard ticks) that carry human disease: *Ixodes* species, *Amblyomma* species, and *Dermacentor* species. Among the five genera of the family Argasidae (soft ticks), only the *Ornithodoros* genus contains members that can transmit disease to humans. All of these tick species have complex life cycles that involve progression from eggs to larvae (commonly known as *seed ticks*) to nymphs to adults. Blood meals are required for progression from stage to stage. Larvae, nymphs, and adults can all serve as vectors of infection while feeding on mammals, including humans. Of note, the soft ticks can survive for years in the adult form without taking blood meals and harboring human pathogens.

There are multiple human diseases carried or caused by ticks. Although the history of tick bite can be crucial to diagnosis, it is important to stress that, on average, <50% of the patients who are diagnosed with tick-borne illnesses recall having been bitten by a tick.

LYME DISEASE

Lyme disease is the most frequent **vector-borne disease** in the United States, with 15,000 cases reported yearly. It is caused by the spirochete *Borrelia burgdorferi*, which is endemic in >15 states but mostly occurs in three foci in the United States: the Northeast, upper Midwest (Wisconsin and Minnesota), and the West (California and Oregon). It is also endemic in Eurasia. The vector in the United States is *Ixodes scapularis* (also called *Ixodes dammini*), which belongs to the *Ixodes ricinus* complex. Lyme disease has a seasonal onset; most cases are reported between May and October. In Eurasia, Lyme disease is caused by one of two species, *Borrelia afzelii* and *Borrelia garinii*, that are closely related to *B. burgdorferi*.

The infection is usually **transmitted** by the nymph, which is very small and consequently often unnoticed, even on prolonged attachment. In each of its maturation stages, the tick feeds only once. Consequently, a larva that feeds on an animal reservoir (usually specific rodent species) can become infected, molt to become an infected nymph, and then infect a human. Likewise, a nymph can become infected by feeding on the animal reservoir, become an adult, and then transmit the infection to humans. If any of those steps does not occur [e.g., as in the southeastern United States, where *I. scapularis* feeds on lizards, not rodents (lizards are not reservoirs)], then the infection rarely occurs. This phenomenon explains the low prevalence of infection in the western United States, where the tick (*Ixodes neotomae*) that feeds on the infected dusky-footed woodrat rarely bites humans; crossover occurs when another tick (*Ixodes pacificus*), which prefers lizards but also bites humans, carries the spirochete from rodents on occasional exposure. Lyme disease was recognized as a distinct entity in 1975 after an outbreak in Old Lyme, Connecticut. However, the causative agent was isolated in 1982. Many aspects of the disease had been described previously in Europe and Asia in the early and mid-20th century.

Despite minor variations between the disease in the United States and Eurasia, the basic disease outline is comparable. The major differences between Lyme disease in the United States compared to its counterparts in Europe and Asia are the following:

- Erythema migrans (EM) is more intense but rarely progresses to acrodermatitis chronica atrophicans.
- Meningitic symptoms are more prominent acutely but tend to be subtle in the chronic phase.
- Dilated cardiomyopathy has not been reported in the United States.
- Arthritis is more prominent in both acute and chronic phases, with 10% treatment resistance due to autoimmune mechanisms.

Of note is that in some midwestern states, a syndrome resembling Lyme has been noted after bite of the Lone Star tick (*Amblyomma americanum*), but *B. burgdorferi* was not the causative agent. This syndrome is now being called *STARI* (southern tick-associated rash illness). The following discussion focuses on Lyme disease in the United States unless otherwise specified.

Clinical Manifestations

B. burgdorferi produces infection by having surface proteins that bind to mammalian cells, a scheme common in most spirochetal diseases. After injection into the skin, *B. burgdorferi* incubates between 3 and 32 days. Initially, it multiplies locally, then spreads to distant skin sites, and eventually disseminates to all other organ systems. Despite immune mechanisms, this spirochete may survive for years in untreated patients, especially in the skin, joints, and nervous system.

Stage I: Early Localized Infection

EM occurs at the tick bite site in ≥80% of patients. It starts as a red macule or papule, which slowly expands to a final median diameter of 15 cm, although there is a lot of variation in the final size of EM in different patients. Most lesions eventually become clear in the center, although some persist to be inflamed, red, and occasionally blue, vesicular, or necrotic. EM is usually not painful but is frequently accompanied by flu-like symptoms, regional lymphadenopathy, and occasional meningismus. Most common sites are the thighs, groin, and axilla. Spirochetes can be cultured from EM biopsy specimens. Within 3–4 wks, EM eventually resolves (range, 1–14 mos); however, in Europe, a chronic form—acrodermatitis chronica atrophicans—may develop (see below), and the organism has been cultured from these lesions up to 10 yrs later.

Stage II: Disseminated Infection

The disseminated infection stage manifests as multiple annular EM-like lesions, possibly malar rash, conjunctivitis, hepatitis, and migratory musculoskeletal pains, but not joint swelling. Most prominent systems involved are the CNS and cardiovascular system.

NEUROLOGIC INVOLVEMENT. Neurologic involvement occurs in 15% of untreated patients any time after infection up to several weeks later but typically resolves or improves within weeks to months, even in untreated patients (except in 5% who progress to develop chronic neuroborreliosis, as discussed below). Clinical symptoms include cranial neuritis (most commonly manifesting as bilateral facial palsy), meningitis, encephalitis, mononeuritis multiplex, motor and sensory radiculoneuritis, myositis, and cerebellar ataxia. A syndrome resembling pseudotumor cerebri has been described in children. These symptoms occur in various combinations, are usually fluctuating, and are accompanied by CSF lymphocytic pleocytosis and increased proteins.

CARDIAC INVOLVEMENT. Cardiac involvement occurs in approximately 5% of untreated patients within several weeks after infection. The most common abnormality is fluctuating degrees of atrioventricular block (first-degree, Wenckebach, or even transient complete heart block requiring only temporary pacemaking); rarely, diffuse myocardial involvement consistent with myopericarditis (causing mild left ventricular dysfunction) occurs, which is very rarely fatal.

Stage III: Late Persistent Infection

Late persistent infection is most prominent in three organ systems.

SKIN. Acrodermatitis chronica atrophicans has been seen in Europe but has not been described in United States Lyme disease.

NEUROLOGIC MANIFESTATIONS. 5% of untreated patients progress to develop chronic neuroborreliosis. Chronic axonal polyneuropathy manifests as spinal radicular pain or distal paresthesias. Lyme encephalopathy manifests as subtle cognitive defects and problems in mood, memory, or sleep. Immune-mediated mechanisms may play a role in its pathogenesis, which is likely due to intrathecal production of antibodies against spirochetes without CSF inflammation. Unlike Lyme arthritis, chronic neurologic Lyme can persist for >10 yrs.

LYME ARTHRITIS. Lyme arthritis occurs in approximately 60% of untreated patients, months after the onset of illness in the context of strong cellular and humoral immune responses to *B. burgdorferi*. Patients may experience intermittent attacks of oligoarticular joint swelling especially involving the knee. Attacks of arthritis last from a few weeks to months, with periods of remission between episodes. Joint fluid WBC range from 50,000–110,000 and are predominantly polymorphonuclear. *B. burgdorferi* PCR is positive in the synovial fluid or tissue. In the United States, approximately 10% of treated patients persist to have chronic arthritis (defined as ≥1 yr of continuous joint inflammation) despite an adequate course of therapy. This is believed to be secondary to an autoimmune mechanism due to molecular mimicry between *Borrelia* surface epitopes and human T-cell protein abundant in the synovium. Additional evidence for immune mechanisms is the predominance of chronic Lyme arthritis in association with certain immunogenetic and immune markers (HLA-DR4). In support of this theory, the polymerase chain reaction (PCR) for *B. burgdorferi* is negative in joint fluid of those patients after treatment despite persistence of arthritis. Chronic Lyme arthritis generally resolves spontaneously within several years; permanent joint damage is uncommon.

Diagnosis

Diagnosis of Lyme disease is difficult because of lack of tests that have a high sensitivity and specificity and that reflect active disease.

Culture of spirochetes from EM or serum during the acute phase is the gold standard for diagnosis. This test is most likely to be positive in patients with EM, in which saline-lavage needle aspiration and 2-mm punch biopsies of the leading edge successfully obtain organisms in 60–80% of cases. Although *B. burgdorferi* grows well in the lab, it is not easily recovered from clinical specimens other than biopsy samples of EM lesions. Moreover, many labs are not equipped to perform *Borrelia* cultures.

PCR is increasingly used to detect DNA mainly from joint fluid; it is more sensitive than culture but is only occasionally positive from CSF of patients with meningitis. A recent review summarizes published assays for Lyme disease diagnosis using skin, plasma, synovial fluid, CSF, and urine. Overall, assays for skin and synovial fluid have high sensitivity and uniformity (68% and 73%, respectively). The low test sensitivity of CSF (18%) and plasma (29%), variable sensitivities among CSF and urine assays, and persistence of *B. burgdorferi* DNA in urine and synovial fluid even with therapy and convalescence make these unsuitable for primary diagnosis. Molecular assays for Lyme disease are best used with other diagnostic methods and only in situations in which the clinical probability is high.

Lyme urine antigen has no role in diagnosis due to unreliable results.

Serology is the most commonly used diagnostic approach. It is insensitive during the first month after infection because only 20–30% of patients develop an IgM response during this period. By convalescence, 70–80% are seropositive even after treatment. After 1 mo, most patients have developed an IgG response. IgM after 1 mo of symptoms should not be performed, as a positive test would likely represent a false-positive result. An important consideration in interpreting ELISA results is the *pretest probability* of Lyme disease. This can be based on a thorough clinical exam and knowledge of the incidence of Lyme disease in the particular patient's population.

ELISA has a sensitivity of 89% and a specificity of 72%. If the pretest probability is low, a positive ELISA test is more likely to be false-positive. A negative test in a low-prevalence situation effectively rules out Lyme disease and may help the clinician to avoid inappropriate empiric therapy. The CDC recommends a **two-test approach** for serologic diagnosis. Samples are first tested by ELISA, and those with equivocal or positive results are further tested by Western blotting. This approach markedly improves the specificity and positive predictive value of a positive ELISA. On the other hand, for a patient who has a high clinical likelihood of having Lyme disease (rash resembling EM, arthritis, and history of recent tick bite), empiric therapy without testing is recommended. During the first month of infection, the patient should be tested for both IgM and IgG antibodies. After that time, testing only for IgG is recommended. Western blotting can differentiate infection-induced antibody response from vaccine-induced response. This is due to the nature of infection in which multiple antigenic proteins can be detected in the patient's serum, whereas after vaccination, only antibodies to the vaccine protein can be detected by Western blotting. In patients with symptoms of acute neuroborreliosis, intrathecal antibody production can aid in diagnosis if positive. However, this is a complicated test that can be performed only in reference labs.

Treatment

In June 2000, the Infectious Disease Society of America published evidence-based practice guidelines for the treatment of Lyme disease (Table 21-1). Key points can be summarized as follows:

- Doxycycline is the agent of first choice in adults, except pregnant women, for treatment of most stages except neuroborreliosis and high-degree atrioventricular block (for which ceftriaxone is preferred).
- Alternatives to doxycycline (in decreasing order of preference) are amoxicillin (Amoxil), cefuroxime (Ceftin), and erythromycin (E-Mycin).
- Prognosis is usually excellent in treated patients. As mentioned earlier, 10% of patients who develop arthritis (60% of all patients) progress to develop chronic Lyme arthritis with negative PCR, which may be treated with antiinflammatory agents or arthroscopic synovectomy. Another small subset of patients continues to have subjective symptoms—mainly musculoskeletal pain, fatigue and cognitive difficulties—which is referred to as *post–Lyme disease syndrome*. It has recently been shown that patients with chronic symptoms attributed to Lyme disease do not improve after antibiotic therapy as compared to placebo. Hence, the study concluded that these patients should be treated symptomatically rather than with prolonged courses of antibiotics.

Prevention

Protective Measures and Avoidance of Tick Exposure
There are efficient and simple ways to prevent infection. It is noteworthy to mention that the overall risk of Lyme disease after a deer tick bite is 3.2% even in areas of highest prevalence, such as northern Westchester County in New York, where disease incidence is 0.5–1/1000 persons/yr. Lyme disease develops after bite of the nymphal tick or, occasionally, the adult. Moreover, ticks must become at least partially engorged with blood after ≥36 hrs of attachment to the body for transmission to occur.

TABLE 21-1. TREATMENT REGIMENS FOR LYME DISEASE

Patient population	Regimen
Early infection (local or disseminated)	
Adults	Doxycycline, 100 mg PO q12h for 14–21 d
	Amoxicillin, 500 mg PO q8h for 14–21 d
	Cefuroxime axetil, 500 mg PO q12h for 14–21 d (for doxycycline or amoxicillin allergy)
	Erythromycin, 250 mg PO q6h for 14–21 d (for doxycycline or amoxicillin allergy)
Children	Amoxicillin, 250 PO q8h or 50 mg/kg/d divided q8h for 14–21 d
	Cefuroxime, 125 mg PO q12h or 30 mg/kg/d divided q12h for 14–21 d (for PCN allergy)
	Erythromycin, 250 mg PO q8h or 30 mg/kg/d divided q8h for 14–21 d (for PCN allergy)
Patients with neurologic abnormalities (early or late)	
Adults	Ceftriaxone, 2 g IV qd for 14–28 d
	Cefotaxime, 2 g IV q8h for 14–28 d
	PCN G sodium, 3.3 million U IV q4h [20 million U IV per d (in divided doses)] for 14–28 d
	Doxycycline, 100 mg PO q8h for 30 d (in case of ceftriaxone or PCN allergy); may be ineffective for late neuroborreliosis
	PO regimens may be adequate for facial nerve palsy
Children	Ceftriaxone, 75–100 mg/kg/d (maximum, 2 g) IV qd for 14–28 d
	Cefotaxime, 150 mg/kg/d q8h or q6h (maximum, 6 g) for 14–28 d
	PCN G sodium, 200,000–400,000 U/kg/d divided q4h for 14–28 d
Patients with arthritis (intermittent or chronic)	PO regimens listed above for 30–60 d or IV regimens listed above for 14–28 d
Patients with cardiac abnormalities	
First-degree AVB	PO regimens listed above for 14–21 d
High-degree AVB (PR >0.3)	IV regimens listed above and cardiac monitoring[a]
Pregnant women	Standard therapy for manifestation of the illness; avoid doxycycline

AVB, atrioventricular block.
Note: The recommendations for antibiotics are based on the guidelines of the Infectious Disease Society of America.
[a]Once the patient's condition has stabilized, the course may be completed with PO therapy.

Chemoprophylaxis
A recent study showed that a single dose of doxycycline was 87% effective in prevention of Lyme disease in hyperendemic areas. However, this preventive approach has the limitation of being beneficial in those areas only, necessitating the stratification of potential subjects according to their risk of Lyme disease.

Vaccination
The Lyme disease vaccine, Lymerix, was voluntarily withdrawn from the market in February 2002 by the manufacturer.

ROCKY MOUNTAIN SPOTTED FEVER

The most common rickettsial disease in the United States, Rocky Mountain spotted fever is caused by *Rickettsia rickettsii*, which is transmitted by dog ticks (*Dermacentor variabilis*) in the eastern states and by wood ticks (*Dermacentor andersoni*) in the western states. 600–1200 cases occur throughout the United States each year, with peak incidence in April through September, although fatal cases have been reported during the winter months as well.

The **classic triad** of Rocky Mountain spotted fever—fever, rash, and history of a tick bite—is described in only two-thirds of confirmed cases. The disease manifests itself as a diffuse vasculitis. 2–7 days after the rickettsial organisms are released from the salivary glands of the feeding tick, the characteristic rash begins as red macules. At first, the rash typically involves the extremities, including the palms of the hands and soles of the feet. The rash then spreads centrally, and the macules can fuse to form petechiae or purpura. The most common accompanying symptoms are malaise, headache, myalgias, nausea, vomiting, and diarrhea. Conjunctivitis is present in most cases. Lymphadenopathy, hepatosplenomegaly, leukopenia, thrombocytopenia, and anemia are common findings. In more severe cases, the vasculitis may manifest itself as mental status changes, renal failure, myocarditis, and pulmonary vasculitis leading to pneumonia and respiratory failure. Those at higher risk for these complications include men, the elderly, alcoholics, and patients with glucose-6-phosphate dehydrogenase deficiency. Of note, up to 10% of cases can occur without rash.

The **diagnosis** of Rocky Mountain spotted fever is typically made serologically, with demonstration of a fourfold convalescent rise in antibodies against the rickettsial organisms as detected by latex agglutination or immunofluorescence. The diagnosis can also be made pathologically from skin biopsies. The most successful mode of **treatment** is doxycycline, 100 mg PO twice daily for 7 days. Because tetracyclines are generally not recommended for children, mild pediatric cases are often treated with chloramphenicol. However, more severe cases in children should be treated with doxycycline.

TICK-BORNE RELAPSING FEVER

Tick-borne relapsing fever is caused by many species of the spirochete *Borrelia* transmitted in remote areas of the western United States by members of the soft tick genus *Ornithodoros*. Cases generally occur sporadically in patients who are often unaware of a history of tick bite. A 2- to 3-mm **eschar** develops at the site of the tick bite, and **high fever** begins after an incubation period of approximately 1 wk. Common associated symptoms include chills, tachycardia, myalgias, arthralgias, headache, abdominal pain, and malaise. The febrile period lasts 3–6 days and is followed by a rapid defervescence. Rash develops as the fever resolves in up to half of patients. If untreated, patients will relapse after an afebrile period of approximately 8 days. Typically, three to five relapses occur. Symptoms usually decrease in severity with each relapse. Tick-borne relapsing fever is rarely fatal. Spontaneous abortion can occur in pregnant patients.

The definitive **diagnosis** of tick-borne relapsing fever is made by isolation of *Borrelia* spirochetes from blood cultures taken from febrile patients. The diagnosis can also be made by dark-field microscopy of blood wet mounts or by thick and thin blood smears stained with Wright's or Giemsa stain (70% sensitivity). Serologic antibody testing is available, but it is not common and is limited by the extreme antigenic variation of *Borrelia* organisms.

Tick-borne relapsing fever is typically **treated** with tetracycline (Achromycin) or erythromycin for 10 days. Associated meningitis or encephalitis should be treated with parenteral PCN, cefotaxime (Claforan), or ceftriaxone for ≥2 wks.

The **Jarisch-Herxheimer reaction** occurs in up to 30% of patients with tick-borne relapsing fever within 3 hrs after initiation of antibiotic therapy. The symptoms are fever, chills, tachycardia, hypotension, and leukopenia. The reaction, which can be fatal, can be prevented by the administration of anti–tumor necrosis factor-alpha antibodies before administration of antibiotics. Glucocorticoid therapy is ineffective in Jarisch-Herxheimer reaction.

TULAREMIA

The small gram-negative coccobacillus *Francisella tularensis* can be **transmitted** to humans in a variety of ways: contact with infected animal tissues (e.g., skinning rabbits); inhalation of aerosolized particles; contact with contaminated food or water; and bites of infected ticks, mammals, mosquitoes, or deer flies. Reservoirs in nature include rabbits, other small rodents, and ticks. Approximately 50% of cases are attributed to the bite of the *A. americanum*, *D. andersoni*, and *D. variabilis* ticks. Most cases are reported in the midwestern United States, particularly Oklahoma, Missouri, and Arkansas.

Tularemia can manifest itself in **seven different forms,** depending on the route of inoculation of the organism.

- Ulceroglandular (up to 87% of cases): Regional lymphadenopathy and necrotic, painful, erythematous ulcers occur at the site of inoculation.
- Glandular (up to 20% of cases): Tender, localized lymphadenopathy without skin or mucosal involvement.
- Oculoglandular (up to 5% of cases): Painful conjunctivitis with preauricular, submandibular, or cervical lymphadenopathy secondary to conjunctival inoculation by contaminated fingers, splashes, or aerosols. Vision loss is rare.
- Pharyngeal (up to 12% of cases): Sore throat, cervical and retropharyngeal lymphadenopathy, and, rarely, a mild pseudomembranous pharyngitis result from direct pharyngeal contact with contaminated food, water, or droplets.
- GI (rare): Persistent, fulminant diarrhea secondary to consumption of contaminated food or water; can be fatal.
- Pneumonic: Lobar or diffuse pneumonia secondary to inhalation of the organism or hematologic spread of any of the above forms.
- Typhoidal/systemic (up to 30% of cases): A more severe febrile illness that can be manifested with chills, headache, myalgias, sore throat, anorexia, nausea, vomiting, diarrhea, abdominal pain, and cough. Pulmonary involvement is common. Severe cases can progress to hyponatremia, rhabdomyolysis, renal failure, and sepsis. Lymphadenopathy and skin involvement are absent.

Diagnosis is usually made serologically, with any one titer of >1:160 or a fourfold increase in convalescent titers. *F. tularensis* can be grown from a number of different specimens but is difficult to culture. Moreover, the lab should be forewarned when tularemia is suspected, as the organism can be transmitted to lab workers from actively growing cultures. The coccobacilli are rarely seen on Gram's stain.

The **treatment** of choice is streptomycin, 15 mg/kg IV bid for 10 days. Other aminoglycosides are also excellent therapeutic choices. Fluoroquinolones are rapidly being accepted as good alternative therapies. Relapses are more common after treatment with tetracyclines, beta-lactams, and chloramphenicol. Erythromycins have *in vitro* activity, but little clinical data exist to support their use. Tularemic meningitis should be treated with an aminoglycoside plus IV chloramphenicol.

HUMAN EHRLICHIOSIS: MONOCYTIC AND GRANULOCYTIC

All human ehrlichioses are bacterial diseases that have been described only in the United States and are caused by small, intracellular gram-negative rods of the genus *Ehrlichia*. **Human monocytic ehrlichiosis (HME)** and **human granulocytic ehrlichiosis (HGE)** are nearly identical in their clinical presentation: fever, myalgias, headache, thrombocytopenia, leukopenia, conjunctivitis, and abnormal liver function tests. Most cases are mild, but more severe presentations can include renal failure, mental status changes, encephalitis, and disseminated intravascular coagulation. All pathogenic *Ehrlichia* species described to date are transmitted to humans through a tick bite. After inoculation into the bloodstream, the organisms infect WBCs and become enclosed in membrane-bound structures where they replicate to form morulae. In rare cases, these membrane-enclosed morulae can be seen on Wright's stain of a peripheral blood smear. The causative agent of HME is *Ehrlichia chaffeensis*, which infects monocytes and is carried by the Lone Star tick (*A. americanum*). HGE is caused by *Anaplasma phagocytophilum,* which forms morulae in granulocytes. The agent of HGE is transmitted by black-legged ticks, *I. scapularis* in the Northeast and *I. pacificus* in the western United States. Dogs, deer, and small mammals appear to be the reservoirs of pathogenic *Ehrlichia* species.

The **diagnoses** of the ehrlichioses are evolving. PCR of bacterial DNA is probably the most sensitive and specific method currently available. PCR is only being performed at a few centers, however, which limits its usefulness. A serum antibody titer of >1:64, a fourfold increase in convalescent titers after 5 wks, and demonstration of morulae on the blood smear are also considered diagnostic criteria in combination with an appropriate clinical scenario. In **treating** patients, all species are readily susceptible to the tetracyclines (e.g., doxycycline, 100 mg PO or IV bid for 7–14 days).

COLORADO TICK FEVER

Colorado tick fever is an **acute viral illness** caused by an RNA coltivirus primarily transmitted by *D. andersoni*, although seven other tick species have been found to carry the virus. Ground squirrels and other rodents are the viral reservoirs in nature. There are case reports of Colorado tick fever transmitted by blood transfusion. The disease is limited to the mountainous regions of Washington, Oregon, California, New Mexico, Nevada, Wyoming, Idaho, Montana, South Dakota, and Colorado. There are 200–300 reported cases each year, occurring mostly in May, June, and July. The disease is **largely benign,** with the acute onset of fever, chills, headache, photophobia, and myalgias after an incubation period of 3–6 days. Symptoms resolve spontaneously after approximately 1 wk and then recur typically 3 days later in approximately half of cases. The relapse typically lasts 2–4 days and can be accompanied by rash, leukopenia, and thrombocytopenia. The prognosis for recovery is usually excellent, although encephalitis, aseptic meningitis, hemorrhage, pericarditis, orchitis, pneumonitis, and hepatitis have all been described in rare cases.

The **diagnosis** of Colorado tick fever is made by serum antibody testing or by isolation of the virus after inoculation of the patient's blood or CSF into suckling mice. No antiviral therapy has been described for the coltivirus, and **treatment** is currently supportive for this self-limited illness.

TICK PARALYSIS

Noninfectious, rapidly ascending paralysis is caused by a neurotoxin that affects acetylcholine transmission at the neuromuscular junction and that is secreted into the bloodstream by an actively feeding, engorged tick. The illness is characterized by a **symmetric ascending paralysis** that is rapid in onset—within hours of the first tick exposure. Additional symptoms include ataxia; loss of tendon reflexes; and late-stage cranial nerve and diaphragmatic muscle weakness. Mortality is approximately 10%, and children are more often and more severely affected. Tick paralysis is often confused with Guillain-Barré syndrome; however, the rapid course of the paralysis and the concomitant ataxia differentiate it from Guillain-Barré syndrome and other acute paralytic illnesses. Multiple *Dermacentor* species have been shown to transmit the neurotoxin in North America. The potentially fatal illness can be completely cured and the patient restored to normalcy within hours by **removal of the offending tick.** The exception to this is the tick paralysis caused by *Ixodes holocyclus* in Australia. The neurotoxin produced by this tick acts similarly to botulinum toxin and produces a more profound paralysis. Removal of the tick actually causes a transient worsening of symptoms. Therefore, it is recommended that the antitoxin to *I. holocyclus* neurotoxin be administered before removal of the tick.

KEY POINTS TO REMEMBER

- Patients with chronic Lyme arthritis should not be given repeated courses of antibiotic therapy; treatment is supportive only.
- A careful exposure history and a clinical exam are important in making the diagnosis, as routine cultures are usually negative.
- If an acute tick-borne illness is suspected, it is reasonable to start empiric doxycycline pending diagnostic test results.

REFERENCES AND SUGGESTED READINGS

Asbrink E, Hovmark A. Successful cultivation of spirochetes from skin lesions of patients with erythema chronicum migrans Afzelius and acrodermatitis chronica atrophicans. *Acta Pathol Microbiol Immunol Scand [B]* 1985;93:161–163.

Cross JT Jr, Penn RL. *Francisella tularensis* tularemia. In: Mandell GL, Bennett JE, Dolin R, eds. *Principles and practice of infectious diseases,* 5th ed. Philadelphia: Churchill Livingstone, 2000:2393–2402.

Felz, MW, Smith CD, Swift TR. A six-year-old girl with tick paralysis. *N Engl J Med* 2000;342:90–104.

Goodman LT, Lazarus AA, Martin GJ. Manifestations of tick-borne illness: incidence and variety are increasing worldwide. *Postgrad Med* 2001;109:43–58.

Isada CM, Kasten BL Jr, Goldman MP, et al. *Infectious diseases handbook,* 4th ed. Hudson, OH: Lexi-Comp, 2001.

Johnson WD, Golightly LM. *Borrelia* species (relapsing fever). In: Mandell GL, Bennett JE, Dolin R, eds. *Principles and practice of infectious diseases,* 5th ed. Philadelphia: Churchill Livingstone, 2000:2502–2504.

Kan L, Sood SK, Maytal J. Pseudotumor cerebri in Lyme disease: a case report and literature review. *Pediatr Neurol* 1998;18:439–441.

Krause PJ, Lepore T, Sikand VK, et al. Atovaquone and azithromycin for the treatment of babesiosis. *N Engl J Med* 2000;343:1454–1458.

McQuiston JH, Paddock CD, Holman RC, et al. The human ehrlichioses in the United States. *Emerg Infect Dis* 1999;5:635–642.

Spach DH, Liles WC, Campbell GL, et al. Tick-borne diseases in the United States. *N Engl J Med* 1993;329:936–947.

Steer AD, Sikand VK, Merice F, et al. Vaccination against Lyme disease with recombinant *Borrelia burgdorferi* outer surface lipoprotein A with adjuvant. *N Engl J Med* 1998;339:209–215.

Steere, AC. Lyme disease. *N Engl J Med* 2001;345:115–125.

Steere AC, Malawista SE, Snydman DR, et al. Lyme arthritis: an epidemic of oligoarticular arthritis in children and adults in three Connecticut communities. *Arthritis Rheum* 1977;20:7–17.

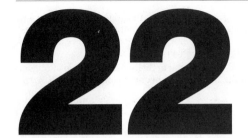

Spirochetes

Nicholas Haddad

LEPTOSPIROSIS

Leptospirosis is presumed to be the most ubiquitous zoonosis in the world and is caused by spirochetes of the genus *Leptospira*. Leptospires are thin, coiled, gram-negative bacteria, with one axial flagellum at each end conferring motility. This genus has two species: *Leptospira interrogans* (pathogenic to mammals, reptiles, and amphibians) and *Leptospira biflexa* (saprophytic, free-living, and nonpathogenic). Both species are further subclassified into multiple serovars and serogroups.

Weil's disease, a severe form of leptospirosis, was first described in 1886. The etiologic agent was described in 1915 independently in Japan and Germany. With hindsight, descriptions of different leptospira syndromes were recognized in the literature as early as the 19th century. Historically, leptospirosis was often misdiagnosed as yellow fever, malaria, dengue fever, and even influenza. It has multiple historical nomenclatures: French disease; autumnal fever; 7-day fever; Canfield fever; swineherd's disease; swamp, marsh, or mud fever; and Fort Bragg fever.

Epidemiology and Transmission

Worldwide, most human cases of leptospirosis are attributed to rodents. In the United States, most human infections result from direct or indirect contact with infected dogs or livestock. The state of Hawaii is disproportionately affected. Pathogenic *Leptospira* species infect a variety of domestic and wild mammals (up to 50% of opossums, skunks, raccoons, and foxes shed leptospires in their urine). Infected animals may become reservoirs when leptospires persist in immunologically privileged sites, especially the renal tubule and tissues of parturition. On excretion into the soil, these organisms survive for weeks to months, especially in warm climates with humid conditions. This explains epidemics after floods and tropical storms, as well as sporadic and clustered acquisition of infection after recreational exposures (e.g., wading, swimming, white-water rafting, canoeing, kayaking). Historically, those who acquired leptospirosis most commonly did so through their occupation (e.g., animal trappers, hunters, dairy and livestock farmers, abattoir workers, veterinarians, rice farmers, rodent control workers, military personnel, and sewer workers). The most recently reported outbreak occurred among participants of a triathlon competition in Illinois and Wisconsin in 1998.

Pathophysiology

The usual portals of entry are through abrasions in the skin, especially after prolonged immersion in water; via the conjunctivae; and even via respiratory droplets. Human-to-human transmission is not an important mode of transmission. However, excretion of leptospires has been recorded in human urine for months after recovery. After infection, leptospires disseminate throughout the body but localize mostly in the kidney and are excreted intermittently. Invasion of the CSF and aqueous humor may be possible due to the burrowing flagellar action and release of hyaluronidase. This explains its "protean manifestations," a description that has become a cliché. Humoral immune mechanisms respond by producing antibodies directed against the outer envelope lipopolysaccharide, the same epitopes used to serotype this organism. After opsonization and phagocytosis in the lung and liver, the leptospires are cleared from the circulation by the reticuloendothelial system, but chronic manifestations may follow and are believed to be mediated by antigen-antibody complexes in the apparent absence of organisms.

Clinical Manifestations

The incubation period is usually 5–14 days. Leptospirosis ranges from a subclinical illness detected by seroconversion in persons with frequent exposures to sources to two clinically recognizable syndromes.

Anicteric Leptospirosis

Anicteric leptospirosis is a self-limited disease that occurs in 90% of infections. It presents with fever of abrupt onset, headache with retroorbital pain and photophobia, myalgias (especially in the lower back, thighs, and calves), abdominal pain, conjunctival suffusion, and, less often, a skin rash. This syndrome lasts almost 1 wk, resolving on appearance of antibodies. Fever may recur after a remission of 3–4 days. Aseptic meningitis may occur in <25% of cases, especially in children <14. Other manifestations include respiratory involvement in 50–70% of cases and ECG abnormalities. Mortality is very low, although death can occur from massive pulmonary hemorrhage. Differential diagnosis is wide and includes viral infections (influenza, acute HIV, infectious mononucleosis, hepatitis, hantavirus, and dengue in the tropics) and bacterial infections (typhoid, rickettsiosis, brucellosis, and malaria).

Icteric Leptospirosis

Approximately 10% of cases progress rapidly to develop jaundice, acute renal failure, and sometimes pulmonary involvement. Hepatic failure is due to vascular injury to hepatic capillaries rather than hepatocellular necrosis; total bilirubin is usually <20 mg/dL, serum transaminases <200 IU/L, and alkaline phosphatase mildly elevated. These numbers return to normal if recovery occurs. Renal failure occurs in 16–40% of cases. Pulmonary symptoms range from cough to ARDS. Pulmonary hemorrhage may be severe enough to cause death.

Other manifestations include transient thrombocytopenia, pancreatitis, aseptic meningitis, and cardiac involvement. Aseptic meningitis is characteristic of the immune phase (see below), occurring in up to 80% of patients and presenting as intense, throbbing headache. CSF shows lymphocytic pleocytosis with <500 cells/mL; protein, 50–100 mg/mL; and normal glucose. Cardiac involvement ranges from abnormal T waves to myocarditis. Death occurs in 5–15% of those patients and is usually caused by pulmonary or cardiac involvement.

Presentation

The clinical presentation of leptospirosis is **biphasic.** The initial phase is termed as *acute* or *septicemic*, lasts approximately 1 wk, and manifests as those symptoms already described above. Leptospires can be recovered from most tissues during this phase. Further progression of disease during this phase produces icteric leptospirosis, of which Weil's disease is a severe form due to renal and hepatic dysfunction. Defervescence heralds the immune phase of illness, which generally lasts 4–30 days. The hallmark of this phase is antibody production, clearance of leptospiremia, and localization in the kidney. This is accompanied by initial defervescence (1–3 days) on production of opsonic IgM. Leptospires, however, remain detectable by culture and PCR in the kidney, urine, and aqueous humor for several weeks. Clinical symptoms include conjunctival suffusion, photophobia, eye pain, and muscle tenderness. Circulating antibodies likely play a role in the development of aseptic meningitis, cutaneous purpura, uveitis, and iridocyclitis.

Diagnosis

Culture of clinical specimens (blood, CSF, and urine) during the first 7–10 days of the illness is the gold standard of diagnosis. This is difficult, requires ≥16 wks even in experienced labs, and has a low sensitivity. Cultures should be checked weekly by dark-field microscopy and held up to 4 mos before discarding as negative.

Serologic diagnosis is commonly used to show a fourfold or greater rise in antibody titer between paired sera obtained ≥2 wks apart. The standard test is the microscopic agglutination test, in which patient sera are reacted with live antigen suspensions of leptospira serovars. However, this is a complex test to control, perform, and interpret, requiring live cultures of all serovars for use as antigens. Cross-reaction of different serogroups may occur, as well as with syphilis, relapsing fever, Lyme disease, and legionellosis. Alternatives to the microscopic agglutination test exist (e.g., indirect hemagglutination assay, ELISA) and represent more rapid means of diagnosis, although they are generally less sensitive.

Direct detection is done by observing a smear under dark-field microscopy, with modified silver stains, or by detection of leptospiral antigens in infected tissue specimens by immunohistochemical techniques.

PCR can detect leptospiral DNA in tissue specimens, including urine, serum, aqueous humor, and CSF. It is more sensitive than culture or serology and is most useful during the first 7–10 days before development of humoral immunity and subsequent clearance of leptospiremia. PCR of urine may be positive for several weeks, and that of aqueous humor may remain positive for several months after diagnosis.

Treatment

Difficulty in assessing the efficacy of antibiotics results from the late presentation of many patients with severe disease, after localization of the organism in tissues. Several placebo-controlled trials have shown the efficacy of IV PCN in severe and late disease and PO amoxicillin (Amoxil), ampicillin, tetracycline, and doxycycline for mild to moderate disease (Table 22-1). Mild infection may be treated supportively without antibiotics. Severe disease requires hospitalization; icteric leptospirosis requires ICU management, including cardiac monitoring.

Chemoprophylaxis offers an alternative prevention strategy for persons with exposure to high-risk areas of endemic disease. Doxycycline was shown to be 95% effective in preventing disease.

Prevention

Approved vaccines are available for cattle, dogs, and swine, but vaccination may not protect from a carrier state. The most effective strategy is reducing both direct contact with infected animals and indirect contact with animal urine–contaminated fresh water, soil, and mud, as well as maintaining hygiene practices in farms and abattoirs.

TABLE 22-1. AGENTS RECOMMENDED FOR PROPHYLAXIS AND TREATMENT OF LEPTOSPIROSIS

Indication	Drug	Dosage
Chemoprophylaxis	Doxycycline	200 mg once/wk
Mild disease	Doxycycline	100 mg PO q12h × 7 d
	Ampicillin	500–750 mg PO q6h × 7 d
	Amoxicillin	500 mg PO q6h × 7 d
Moderate to severe disease	PCN G	1.5 million U IV q6h × 5–7 d
	Ampicillin	0.5–1 g IV q6h × 5–7 d

Adapted from Farr RW. Leptospirosis. *Clin Infect Dis* 1995;21:1–8.

RAT-BITE FEVER

Two organisms cause rat-bite fever: *Streptobacillus moniliformis* and *Spirillum minus*. *S. minus* is a gram-negative spirochete that is common in Asia. It is found in the oropharyngeal flora of rodents. Exposure occurs after rodent bites (especially when patients are asleep) or after accidental exposure in lab workers. Rat-bite fever was described in India >2000 yrs ago and first recorded in the United States in 1839. *S. moniliformis* is the organism causing disease in the United States, and the two organisms cause different types of rat-bite fever (Table 22-2).

Clinical Manifestations

At the time of inoculation of *S. minus*, the wound initially heals but 1–4 wks later becomes painful and swollen, associated with regional lymphadenopathy. This is followed by spirochetemia characterized by fever, chills, headache, and malaise; in contrast to streptobacillary fever, myalgias and arthralgias are very rare. The bite wound may progress to chancre-like ulceration and eschar formation. Rash may occur during febrile episodes, which last 3–4 days but may recur every 3–9 days if untreated. Endocarditis is the most serious complication of untreated spirillary fever in patients with valvular abnormalities.

Diagnosis

S. minus cannot be cultured on artificial media. There is no serologic test available for diagnosis. The diagnostic method of choice is direct visualization on blood smears, exudates, or lymph node tissue using Giemsa or Wright's stains or dark-field microscopy. Differential diagnosis includes relapsing fever, malaria, and lymphoma.

Treatment

The usual treatment is PCN G, 1–2 million U IV q4–6h for 10–14 days. Therapy for mild disease can be oral [e.g., amoxicillin plus clavulanate potassium (Augmen-

TABLE 22-2. COMPARISON OF TWO DIFFERENT TYPES OF RAT-BITE FEVER

	Streptobacillus moniliformis	*Spirillum minus*
Organism	Gram-negative bacillus	Gram-negative coiled rod
Geographic distribution	North America, Europe	Asia
Mode of transmission	Rat bite, ingestion	Rat bite
Clinical syndrome		
Ulceration of initial bite wound	No	Yes
Arthritis	Yes	No
Regional lymphadenopathy	No	Yes
Rash	Yes	Yes
Relapsing fever	Yes	Yes
Diagnosis	Culture, serologic tests	Direct visualization, xenodiagnosis
Therapy	PCN G	PCN G

From Washburn RG. *Streptobacillus moniliformis* (rat-bite fever). In: Mandell GL, Bennett JE, Dolin R, eds. *Principles and practice of infectious diseases*, 5th ed. Philadelphia: Churchill Livingstone, 2000:2422–2423, with permission.

tin), 875/125 mg PO bid]. More severe disease should be treated with IV therapy for 5–7 days and then changed to oral therapy if the patient has clinically responded. Oral tetracycline, 500 mg q6h, can be used in PCN-allergic patients. Streptomycin, 7.5 mg/kg IM q12h, can be used as a third-line agent; less experience exists with erythromycin (E-Mycin), chloramphenicol, clindamycin, and ceftriaxone.

The Jarisch-Herxheimer reaction can occur after initiation of therapy. It should be managed conservatively, as in other spirochetal diseases. Endocarditis is rare enough that optimal therapy is unclear, but 4 wks of IV PCN with or without streptomycin is recommended. After a rodent bite, a 3-day course of oral PCN, 2 g/day, is reasonable, although efficiency of prophylaxis in this setting is unknown.

RELAPSING FEVER

The causative agent of relapsing fever is a spirochetal pathogen, the genus of which (*Borrelia*) belongs to the same family that contains *Leptospira* and *Treponema*. It causes relapsing fever in two distinct but similar syndromes. Louse-borne relapsing fever is caused by *Borrelia recurrentis*, which is carried by the human body louse (*Pediculus humanus*), and is currently reported from small endemic foci in the world (Ethiopia, Sudan, Eritrea, Somalia, the Peruvian Andes, and the Himalayas). Tick-borne relapsing fever is caused by many different *Borrelia* species and has a more worldwide distribution, especially in undisturbed rural settings. In the United States, it is mostly localized in the remote western mountainous areas.

Pathophysiology and Clinical Manifestations

The spirochetes of relapsing fever can enter intact skin and mucosae after deposition from the louse or tick. After a 7- to 8-day incubation period, an initial spirochetemia occurs, characterized by abrupt onset of symptoms (e.g., fever, rigors, headache, photophobia, myalgias, arthralgias, abdominal pain, cough, and even neurologic symptoms) without any prodrome. Neurologic symptoms manifest in 30% of patients with coma, cranial nerve palsies, hemiplegia, meningitis, and seizures. Other systemic findings include jaundice, hepatosplenomegaly, mucosal hemorrhages, iridocyclitis, and pneumonia. A truncal skin rash of 1–2 days' duration is common at the end of the primary febrile episode. This episode characteristically terminates abruptly in 3–6 days, although it may be associated with fatal hypotension. The pathophysiology of relapse is due to a cyclic antigenic variation, which prevents the host's defense mechanisms from controlling spirochetemia after an initial episode of infection. This has been suggested to be due to mini-chromosome rearrangements and subsequent production of new proteins. Subsequent periods of relapse are less severe and shorter than the first febrile attack, with each relapse being less severe than the previous one. During febrile periods, *Borrelia* organisms are sequestered in internal organs. The ultimate termination of clinical disease has been attributed primarily to the development of specific anti-*Borrelia* antibody rather than to activity of phagocytic cells.

Louse-Borne Relapsing Fever

Humans are the only known hosts. Disease usually occurs during catastrophic events, such as war or famine, as occurred during World War II in North Africa and Europe with an estimated 50,000 deaths. The body louse ingests *B. recurrentis* from an infected person and carries these organisms in its hemolymph. Dissemination within the louse does not occur, which explains the lack of transovarian transmission to its progeny and the lack of human transmission by its saliva. Infection occurs after crushing the louse, which releases the organism that can then penetrate intact skin. Generally, *B. recurrentis* has a longer incubation period, longer febrile periods, and longer afebrile intervals than does tick-borne disease.

Tick-Borne Relapsing Fever

Tick-borne relapsing fever is usually carried by soft ticks of the genus *Ornithodoros*, which feed on wild rodents and small animals (e.g., chipmunks, squirrels, rabbits, rats, mice, owls, and lizards) and can remain alive and infectious for up to 12 yrs without feeding. These ticks prefer warm and humid environments and altitudes of 1500–6000 ft. Relatively recent outbreaks have been reported in the western United States. Transmission occurs after rodents carry those ticks passively into human dwellings or after the casual intrusion of humans into rodents' environments. Unlike the louse-borne disease, tick-borne *Borrelia* organisms multiply and invade all tissues of the tick, which explains transovarian transmission as well as transmission via tick saliva or excreta while feeding on a human host. (See Chap. 21, Tick-Borne Illnesses.)

Diagnosis

- **Blood smear:** Rapid and definite diagnosis is established by direct observation of spirochetes in the peripheral blood of febrile patients. This is positive in 70% of cases on a Wright's- or Giemsa-stained smear. Sensitivity can be enhanced by staining fixed smears with acridine orange and by dark-field or phase-contrast microscopy of wet-mount preparations.
- **PCR** may be helpful in diagnosis.
- **Serology** is available but not standardized. This may be helpful when paired sera are tested especially in the setting of false-positive VDRL, which can occur in 5–10% of patients, or false-positive Lyme serology.

Diagnosis has to be suspected especially during epidemics or in the right environmental context, as well as on occurrence of relapses. However, the differential diagnosis during the initial febrile episode is broad and includes malaria, typhoid fever, hepatitis, leptospirosis, rat-bite fever, Colorado tick fever, and dengue.

The relative infrequency of relapsing fever makes it more likely to be underrecognized and underreported, and it may be falsely identified as Lyme disease due to false-positive Lyme serology.

Treatment

Tetracycline (500 mg PO qid) is the drug of choice based on clinical experience, although chloramphenicol, PCN, doxycycline, and erythromycin have all been successfully used; the latter is preferred for pregnant women and children <8 yrs old.

For cases of tick-borne relapsing fever (other *Borrelia* species), therapy with tetracycline or erythromycin should last for 5–10 days because of the higher rate of failure for shorter duration.

For cases of *B. recurrentis*, administer a single dose of tetracycline, 500 mg PO, or erythromycin, 500 mg PO.

CNS involvement should be treated by IV therapy with PCN G (24 million U IV qd), cefotaxime (2 g IV qd), or ceftriaxone for ≥14 days.

Treatment is associated with severe Jarisch-Herxheimer reaction in one-third of patients, which typically starts 1–3 hrs after administration of the first dose of therapy on clearing of spirochetemia. It can be described as an exaggeration of the crisis observed in untreated patients, with fever, rigors, hypotension, and leukopenia. It is believed to be related to cytokine release or endogenous opioids; prior administration of antibodies to tumor necrosis factor-alpha can prevent this reaction. Therapy to this reaction remains supportive.

Prevention

Avoidance of exposure to the arthropod vector is the most effective method of prevention. *Ornithodoros* ticks are widely distributed and cannot be eliminated; exposure can be avoided by applying insect repellents to clothing and insecticides to populated areas in natural habitats of the tick. Prevention of louse-borne disease can be accomplished by good personal hygiene and delousing procedures.

KEY POINTS TO REMEMBER

- Diseases caused by spirochetes often present with nonspecific signs and symptoms or as an FUO. A careful history is important to assess exposure risk.
- A high index of suspicion is necessary to make the diagnosis, as proper testing can be technically difficult.

REFERENCES AND SUGGESTED READINGS

Abdulkader RC. Acute renal failure in leptospirosis. *Renal Fail* 1997;19:191–198.

Barbour AG, Restrepo BI. Antigenic variation in vector-borne pathogens. *Emerg Infect Dis* 2000;6:449–457.

Bradley KK. Leptospirosis. *J Okla State Med Assoc* 1999;92:114–115.

Brown PD, Gravekamp C, Carrington DG, et al. Evaluation of the polymerase chain reaction for the early diagnosis of leptospirosis. *J Med Microbiol* 1995;43:110–114.

Calia KE, Calia FM. Tickborne relapsing fever. In: Cunha, BA, ed. *Tickborne infectious diseases: diagnosis and management.* New York: Marcel Dekker, 2000:169.

Centers for Disease Control and Prevention. Relapsing fever. *MMWR Morb Mortal Wkly Rep* 1973;22:242–246.

Centers for Disease Control and Prevention. Summary of notifiable diseases, United States 1994. *MMWR Morb Mortal Wkly Rep* 1994;43:1–80.

Didier R, Roux V. The body louse as a vector of reemerging human diseases. *Clin Infect Dis* 1999;29:888–911.

Dow GR, Rankin RJ, Saunders BW. Rat-bite fever. *N Z Med J* 1992;105:133.

Dworkin MS, Anderson DE Jr, Schwan TG, et al. Tick-borne relapsing fever in the northwestern United States and southwestern Canada. *Clin Infect Dis* 1998;26: 122–131.

Fekade D, Knox K, Hussein K, et al. Prevention of Jarisch-Herxheimer reaction by treatment with antibodies against tumor necrosis factor alpha. *N Engl J Med* 1996;335: 311–315.

Felsenfeld O. Immunity in relapsing fever. In: Johnson RC, ed. *The biology of parasitic spirochetes.* New York: Academic Press, 1976:351–358.

Levett PN. Leptospirosis. *Clin Micro Rev* 2001;14:296–326.

McClain JBL, Ballou WR, Harrison SM, et al. Doxycycline therapy for leptospirosis. *Ann Intern Med* 1984;100:696–698.

Spach DH, Liles WC, Campbell GL, et al. Tick-borne diseases in the United States. *N Engl J Med* 1993;329:936–947.

Washburn RG. *Streptobacillus moniliformis* (rat-bite fever). In: Mandell GL, Bennett JE, Dolin R, eds. *Principles and practice of infectious diseases,* 5th ed. Philadelphia: Churchill Livingstone, 2000:2422–2423.

Washburn RG. *Spirillum minus* (rat-bite fever). In: Mandell GL, Bennett JE, Dolin R, eds. *Principles and practice of infectious diseases,* 5th ed. Philadelphia: Churchill Livingstone, 2000:2518.

Watt G, Padre LP, Tuazon M, et al. Skeletal and cardiac muscle involvement in severe, late leptospirosis. *J Infect Dis* 1990;162:266–269.

World Health Organization. Leptospirosis worldwide, 1999. *Wkly Epidemiol Rec* 1999; 74:237–242.

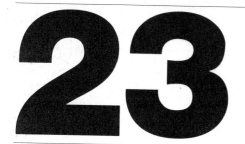

Brucellosis

Michele C. L. Cabellon

INTRODUCTION

Human brucellosis is caused by a group of small, aerobic, nonmotile, non–spore-forming, gram-negative coccobacilli belonging to the genus *Brucella*. The organisms are transmitted to humans through exposure to animals who are infected with the disease for life.

There are four species that cause illness in humans. *Brucella abortus* is present almost worldwide in cattle and also in some populations of buffalo, camel, and yak. *Brucella suis* is found in swine and mainly is seen in the midwestern United States, South America, and southeast Asia. *Brucella melitensis*, found in sheep and goats, is located in the Mediterranean region, the Middle East, Latin America, and the Indian subcontinent. *Brucella canis* can be found in some kennel-raised dogs, mainly in North and South America, Japan, and central Europe. *B. melitensis* and *B. suis* are the most virulent of the four. *B. canis* is rarely seen.

Most cases of brucellosis in the United States have been documented in Texas, California, Virginia, and Florida. The majority presents in the spring and summer months. Brucellosis is a zoonosis, and virtually all cases are **transmitted from animal to human** only. There have been rare reports of human-to-human sexual transmission recorded, with *Brucella* organisms found in human sperm.

PATHOPHYSIOLOGY

The method of human infection is most often through **occupational exposure** or by **consuming contaminated dairy products,** in which high amounts of organisms are shed by the animal. Slaughterhouse workers, farmers, dairy workers, veterinarians, and lab workers are at the greatest risk, usually by contracting particles through an abrasion on the skin or through the conjunctiva. Travelers to endemic areas can also be affected, especially if exposed to unpasteurized milk, goat cheese, butter, or other dairy items. Aerosolization is rare but can be another method of infection.

The organisms penetrate the epithelial cells of the skin, conjunctiva, pharynx, or lungs where they are engulfed by neutrophils. They are then taken to the lymph node system where the *Brucella* can multiply and result in bacteremia, usually approximately 1.5–3 wks after the initial infection. Once in the bloodstream, the organisms can seed any organ, with spleen, liver, and bone marrow being the most common. Granulomas form around the bacteria, and these may also suppurate and lead to continued bacteremia.

DIFFERENTIAL DIAGNOSIS

The differential diagnosis is broad due to the widespread symptoms that may occur. Endocarditis must be a consideration. Other infectious agents, such as rickettsial diseases (Lyme disease, ehrlichiosis) and *Bartonella*, are possibilities. Other categories that often fit into the FUO workup (e.g., rheumatologic diseases and malignancies) may present with the exact same symptoms.

CLINICAL MANIFESTATIONS

The most important pieces of information to obtain are questions regarding **occupation, exposure, food intake, and travel.** These are often the only clues to lead to the diagnosis of brucellosis, because the presentation is otherwise nonspecific. Patients may initially have any one of a spectrum of illnesses, from subclinical disease (which is asymptomatic) to acute or subacute disease (presenting anywhere from 2–3 mos to 1 yr postinfection) to chronic illness (which has been ongoing for >1 yr). The symptoms are very nonspecific. >90% of patients report malaise, fever [often >39.4°C (102.9°F)], chills, sweats, fatigue, weakness, arthralgias, and myalgias. These may present abruptly or insidiously. Because the organisms can affect any organ system, a number of other symptoms might coincide. A hallmark is that depression symptoms may be severe and may override all other physical problems.

DIAGNOSIS

On **physical exam,** splenomegaly and lymphadenopathy (usually axillary, cervical, and supraclavicular) may be present but not in all patients. Osteoarticular complaints are common, and sacroiliitis or arthritis of large weight-bearing joints may occur. Orchitis is present in up to 20% of men infected. Rashes are usually nonspecific. Lung findings may be useful to help localize disease.

Common lab tests may be abnormal but are usually also nonspecific. Anemia, lymphopenia or leukocytosis, and thrombocytopenia may be present. Liver function tests may be slightly elevated but usually always recover. Abnormalities may present with a broad array of different organs involved, and further testing should be tailored to those findings.

Blood cultures are positive in approximately 10–30%, and duration of infection correlates with decreased positivity of cultures. When obtained, the lab should be alerted to the suspected diagnosis and to keep the cultures for ≥4 wks. Bone marrow cultures are often of higher yield in isolating the organism when it appears through other lab tests to be infected (e.g., anemia). Cultures can be taken from biopsies of other areas as well, such as lymph nodes and skin lesions. When CNS involvement is suspected (<5%), CSF has a positive culture in 45%, and the ELISA test can be used to detect *Brucella* antibodies.

Standard tube agglutination is used to detect both IgM and IgG antibodies to three of the four *Brucella* species (not *B. canis*). **Titers** can be considered positive if >1:160 or if there is a fourfold rise in titer level over 1–4 wks. False-positives can occur with *Vibrio cholerae, Francisella tularensis,* or *Yersinia enterocolitica* infection; cholera vaccination; or *Brucella* skin testing. A rapid screening test called the *Rose Bengal test* is available, but all positive tests must be confirmed with standard tube agglutination. A nonagglutinating antibody test called the *anti-*Brucella *Coombs' test* can be used in the acute phase of the disease, with a titer ≥1:320 considered positive. ELISA is also available for further confirmation of *Brucella* antibodies. PCR is still being studied as a method for diagnosis.

TREATMENT

Antibiotics with good intracellular penetration are needed to treat brucellosis. There are no good randomized, controlled studies to definitively support one regimen, but doxycycline, 100 mg PO bid for 6 wks, plus streptomycin, 1 g IM qd (or gentamicin) for the first 3 wks, is the recommended therapy for adults. An alternative to the aminoglycoside is rifampin, 900 mg PO qd for 6 wks, although there is some evidence this is slightly less effective than streptomycin. TMP-SMX (Bactrim) plus an aminoglycoside is the preferred treatment for children <8 yrs old. Pregnant women have been treated with rifampin, 900 mg PO qd, as monotherapy. Triple-therapy combinations with agents such as doxycycline, rifampin, aminoglycosides, and even third-generation cephalosporins (for better CNS penetration) have been used for a minimum of 3 mos for cases of CNS and cardiac involvement. Endocarditis almost always requires surgical valve replacement.

The acute form of brucellosis can be very debilitating, with fatigue and inability to work lasting for months despite treatment. Approximately 10% of cases will **relapse** anywhere from months to years after the initial infection, and this is usually due to organisms that have been hiding intracellularly and become reactivated. The antibiotic regimen used initially can be used again, as resistance rarely develops. Chronic disease for >1 yr usually is due to inadequate treatment or a focus of infection in the bone, spleen, or other organ. This should be distinguished from what is known as a **delayed convalescence,** in which some patients experience extreme fatigue and continued depression without fever or other signs of toxicity. These patients have low or nonexistent antibody titers when tested.

PREVENTION

Efforts to control disease have involved vaccinating domestic animals and isolating those infected. Patients should be advised to avoid unpasteurized dairy products and raw meat. The mainstay for high-risk populations includes protective clothing and eyewear and proper wound coverage. If exposure to a vaccine has occurred, those patients should be treated with a full 6-wk course of antibiotics.

KEY POINTS TO REMEMBER

• Consider brucellosis in patients with appropriate occupational exposure, exposure to contaminated dairy products, and sacroiliitis.
• Serologic testing or tissue cultures may be necessary to make the diagnosis.

REFERENCES AND SUGGESTED READINGS

Salata RA. Brucellosis. In: Goldman LJ, Bennett C, eds. *Cecil textbook of medicine, 21st ed.* Philadelphia: WB Saunders, 2000.

Vidal RP, Pujol XP. Brucellosis. In: Rakel RE, ed. *Conn's current therapy 2001, 53rd ed.* Philadelphia: WB Saunders, 2001.

Young EJ. *Brucella* species. In: Mandell GL, Bennett JE, Dolin R, eds. *Principles and practice of infectious diseases,* 5th ed. Philadelphia: Churchill Livingstone, 2000: 2386–2391.

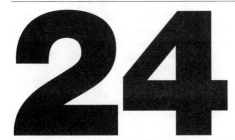

Systemic Mycoses

Anucha Apisarnthanarak

INTRODUCTION

Systemic fungal pathogens are inherently virulent and cause disease in healthy individuals. There are five fungi included in this group: *Histoplasma capsulatum*, *Blastomyces dermatitidis*, *Coccidioides immitis*, *Paracoccidioides brasiliensis*, and *Cryptococcus neoformans*. With the exception of *C. neoformans*, these pathogens are dimorphic and tend to be restricted to particular geographic regions. They grow as filamentous molds in nature and in culture at 25°C (77°F); however, they transform to a unicellular morphology in animal and human hosts and in culture at 37°C (98.6°F). Tissue infections caused by *C. neoformans*, *H. capsulatum*, *B. dermatitidis*, and *P. brasiliensis* are characterized by the presence of budding yeast cells, whereas *C. immitis* infection is characterized by spherules.

PATHOPHYSIOLOGY

Infection with all of the preceding mycoses involves inhalation of the fungal spores into the lung. The primary pneumonic infection may be symptomatic or asymptomatic. The pneumonic process may resolve completely, persist and possibly progress locally, or disseminate. Whether the initial infection resolves or progresses depends on both the virulence of the pathogen and the immunocompetency of the host. Most of these organisms evade the immune system by multiplying intracellularly (*Histoplasma* species, *Blastomyces* species, *Coccidioides* species, and *Paracoccidioides* species), whereas *Cryptococcus* species are surrounded by a capsule that reduces susceptibility to phagocytosis. Some hosts appear to have an innate increased susceptibility to disseminated infection by certain mycoses. For example, African-Americans, Filipinos, Asians, and men appear more likely to develop disseminated coccidioidomycosis.

DIFFERENTIAL DIAGNOSIS

In normal hosts, consider a systemic mycosis infection whenever there are persistent pulmonary infiltrates, nodules, or cavities of undetermined etiology. Systemic mycoses should also be included in the differential diagnosis of the patients with chronic meningitis, lytic bone lesions, chronic skin lesions, culture-negative endocarditis, FUO, and cytopenia (in the elderly).

In an immunocompromised host, systemic mycosis should be considered whenever there are new pulmonary signs or symptoms; symptoms involving the nose, sinus, or orbit; new cutaneous or funduscopic lesions; or persistent fever.

DIAGNOSIS

Frequently, epidemiologic clues help to suggest the diagnosis of endemic mycoses. It is important, therefore, to obtain a travel history and vocational history. Residents of areas in which mycoses are endemic are less subject to infection than are newcomers. Predisposing factors are also helpful in defining host defense. In particular, cell-mediated immunity impairment appears to be of paramount importance in the development of most deep mycoses. Because the treatment strategies for these infections are different in HIV-positive and non–HIV-positive individuals, it is also essential to obtain the patient's history of HIV risk factors. Because systemic mycosis can potentially involve many organ systems, a careful exam should be made of the nares, sinuses, orbit, fundi, lungs, heart, CNS, musculoskeletal system, and skin.

TREATMENT

Table 24-1 lists the treatments for systemic mycoses.

HISTOPLASMOSIS

H. capsulatum grows in soil, especially in areas contaminated with excreta of bats and birds. It occurs worldwide and is particularly common in the midwestern United States, especially the Ohio and Mississippi river valleys and parts of Central and South America.

Clinical Manifestations

In immunocompetent hosts, macrophages acquire fungicidal activity, thereby containing the infection. Transient fungemia, occurring before the development of immunity, accounts for the distribution of calcified granulomas in the liver and spleen. Approximately 5% of infections result in symptomatic disease. However, *H. capsulatum* can also cause progressive and potentially fatal disease when host defenses are impaired. Clinically, histoplasmosis infection ranges from acute and life-threatening disease to chronic, mild, and disseminated histoplasmosis. Fever, night sweats, weight loss, and mucosal lesions are common presentations of this illness.

Diagnosis

The diagnosis of histoplasmosis is based on serologic findings, direct histopathologic exam, and confirmatory culture. Serologic tests are supportive data to the diagnosis of histoplasmosis. Serum complement fixation titers of 1:16 or a fourfold rise in acute to convalescent titer suggest histoplasmosis infection; however, false-positive reactions can occur due to other fungal infections and tuberculosis. The immunodiffusion test detects antibodies to the H and M antigens of *H. capsulatum* and is more specific but less sensitive than the complement fixation test. Intracellular yeast can be seen by direct histopathologic exam of infected tissue, especially bone marrow, blood, and lung. In disseminated histoplasmosis, *H. capsulatum* can be cultured from bone marrow or blood in >75% of cases. However, *H. capsulatum* usually takes 1–2 wks to grow in culture. A urine histoplasma antigen test is also available.

Treatment

Therapy is not indicated for acute presentation of mild pneumonia, histoplasmoma, pericarditis, broncholithiasis, rheumatologic syndromes, or mediastinal fibrosis. Surgery may be beneficial in certain presentations of mediastinal fibrosis. Treatment is indicated for acute pulmonary histoplasmosis with hypoxemia, acute pulmonary histoplasmosis for >1 mo's duration, chronic pulmonary histoplasmosis, esophageal compression or ulceration, granulomatous mediastinitis with obstruction or invasion of tissue, and disseminated histoplasmosis (Table 24-1). All patients with disseminated histoplasmosis should be tested for adrenal insufficiency. Patients with chronic forms of histoplasmosis who are otherwise not immunocompromised may be treated with itraconazole (Sporanox), 200 mg/day PO; ketoconazole (Nizoral), 400 mg/day PO; or amphotericin B (Amphocin, Fungizone), 0.3–0.6 mg/kg/day IV to a total dose of 2–2.5 g. The lung damage associated with chronic pulmonary histoplasmosis is not

TABLE 24-1. TREATMENT FOR SYSTEMIC MYCOSES

Pathogen	Primary treatment	Suppressive therapy
Histoplasma capsulatum		
Acute dissemination; severe disease; AIDS	Amphotericin B, 0.7–1 mg/kg/day IV to a total dose of 1–2 g	Itraconazole, 200 mg/day PO[a]
Chronic forms; immunocompetent moderate disease	Itraconazole, 200–400 mg/day PO for ≥6 mos	Not required
Blastomyces dermatitidis		
Meningeal disease; life-threatening disease; immunocompromised	Amphotericin B, 0.7–1 mg/kg/day IV to a total dose of 1.5–2.5 g	Azoles[a]
Nonmeningeal disease; mild to moderate disease	Itraconazole, 200–400 mg/day PO for 6 mos	Not required
Coccidioides immitis		
Meningeal disease	Amphotericin B, 0.7–1 mg/kg/day IV to a total dose of 2–3 g	Azoles, PO[a]
Nonmeningeal disease	Fluconazole, itraconazole, or ketoconazole for 3–6 mos PO	Azoles, PO[a,b]
Paracoccidioides brasiliensis		
Advanced disease	Amphotericin B, 0.4–0.5 mg/kg/day IV to a total dose of 1.5–2.5 g	Not required
Mild disease	Itraconazole, 200 mg/day PO for 6 mos, or ketoconazole, 400 mg/day for 6–18 mos	Not required
Cryptococcosis neoformans (with meningitis)		
HIV-positive individual	Amphotericin B, 0.7–1 mg/kg/day IV, with or without flucytosine, 100 mg/kg/day[c] for 2 wks; followed by fluconazole, 400 mg/day PO for 8 wks	Fluconazole, 200 mg/day PO[a]
Non–HIV-positive individual	Amphotericin B, 0.3 mg/kg, with flucytosine, 150 mg/kg IV for 6 wks	Not required
C. neoformans (without meningitis)		
HIV-positive individual	Fluconazole, 200–400 mg/day PO or IV[d]	Fluconazole, 200 mg/day PO[e]
Non–HIV-positive individual	Fluconazole, 400 mg/day PO or IV for 8 wks to 6 mos	Not required

[a]Duration of therapy depends on host immune status.
[b]Suppressive therapy is indicated for disseminated disease.
[c]Dose is divided q6h.
[d]Indefinite duration, unless immune reconstitution is achieved.
[e]Need for maintenance therapy with nonmeningeal cryptococcosis is not established.

reversed by medical therapy. Patients with AIDS and acute dissemination are much less likely to be cured and require suppressive therapy. These patients can be treated with amphotericin B, 0.7–1 mg/kg/day IV to a total dose of 1–2 g, followed by switch to itraconazole, 200 mg/day PO, for prolonged periods.

BLASTOMYCOSIS

Blastomycosis is endemic in the Ohio and Mississippi River valleys and, to a lesser extent, the Missouri and Arkansas River basins. Geographically, blastomycosis is limited to the North American continent and parts of Africa. The natural reservoir for the etiologic agent of blastomycosis is unknown. The organism is believed to be present in the soil but flourishes only in a narrow ecologic niche.

Clinical Manifestations

Inhalation of *B. dermatitidis* conidia produces a primary pulmonary infection in the host. The initial infection may be symptomatic or asymptomatic. Primary pulmonary disease results in one of three outcomes: resolution without involvement of other organs, progressive pulmonary disease, or apparent resolution of the pulmonary infection associated with systemic spread of infection with systemic symptoms. Yeast cells proliferate in tissues and are phagocytized by macrophages, allowing dissemination to other organs (e.g., skin). It is important to note that manifestations of symptomatic blastomycosis are most often indicative of systemic spread.

Diagnosis

The role of serologic and immunologic testing for blastomycosis remains underdeveloped. Skin testing and serologic studies are difficult to interpret and tend to be highly cross-reactive with etiologic agents of other systemic mycosis infections, especially *H. capsulatum* and *C. immitis*. The diagnosis of blastomycosis requires identification of the organism in infected tissue or isolation in culture. The characteristic broad-based, budding yeast cells seen in purulent material or biopsies help to distinguish this fungal pathogen from other invasive fungi. The organism grows readily in culture. It is identified by its conversion from the mycelia phase to the yeast phase or by the exoantigen test.

Treatment

Therapy for meningeal or advanced blastomycosis is with IV amphotericin B to a total dose of approximately 2 g (Table 24-1). Less severe blastomycosis may be treated with itraconazole, 200 mg/day PO, or ketoconazole, 400 mg/day PO, for 6 mos to 1 yr. Itraconazole is better tolerated than ketoconazole and is associated with a lower relapse rate. Although disseminated blastomycosis in patients with AIDS is uncommon, when it does occur, the patient should receive chronic suppressive therapy.

COCCIDIOIDOMYCOSIS

The areas of highest endemicity for coccidioidomycosis are semiarid in climate and include the San Joaquin Valley in California, Maricopa and Pima Counties in Arizona, and several western and southern counties in Texas. The organism can be isolated from soil in endemic areas. Although geographically restricted, the organism has, on occasion, spread extensively as a result of dust storms.

Clinical Manifestations

Exposure to *C. immitis* causes a greater percentage of individuals to undergo a mild febrile to moderately severe pulmonary disease. The most common symptoms of primary disease are cough, fever, and chest pain. Night sweats and joint pain are not unusual. Approximately 60% of these infections are asymptomatic and usually self-limited; however, in a small proportion of patients, this organism can cause progressive pulmonary disease or disseminate to produce extrapulmonary disease that mainly involves the meninges or skin.

Diagnosis

The tube precipitin and complement fixation tests are the serologic procedures used to diagnose coccidioidomycosis. Precipitins appear early, approximately 2–4 wks after symptom onset, followed by the appearance of complement-fixing antibodies. Skin test reactivity to coccidioidin develops 2–4 wks after symptoms. New tests that are more sensitive in detecting specific antibodies are agar immunodiffusion and latex particle agglutination. These tests largely replace the tube precipitin and complement fixation tests as routine screening methods. Once the diagnosis has been established, complement fixation titers can yield important prognostic information. Titers >1:16 usually correlate with disseminated disease. The organism can be cultured on conventional media, but it should be handled with caution. The definitive identification is based on conversion to spherules or a specific exoantigen test.

Treatment

Amphotericin B has been the mainstay of treatment for any patient who is critically ill due to coccidioidomycosis. Approximately 60% of patients with extrameningeal disease had a clinical remission when treated with a total dose of amphotericin B, 2–3 g IV. However, amphotericin B penetration into the CSF is poor, and intrathecal administration has been used for meningeal disease. Recently, it has been shown that the clinical response rate of meningeal and nonmeningeal disease to oral or IV fluconazole is approximately equivalent to the response rate with amphotericin B but with less toxicity. Therefore, fluconazole, 400–600 mg/day PO for 6–12 mos, is now used by most providers for primary therapy of coccidioidomycosis (Table 24-1). Recent data indicate that many patients will relapse with active disease if the fluconazole is stopped. Therefore, it is wise to maintain suppressive therapy with fluconazole, 200 mg/day PO, for life. Itraconazole and ketoconazole also have activity in those patients who do not have meningeal involvement.

PARACOCCIDIOIDOMYCOSIS

Epidemiology and Ecology

Paracoccidioidomycosis is restricted to Central and South America, with a high incidence in Brazil, Venezuela, and Colombia. The fungi reside in environments that have high humidity and average temperatures of approximately 23°C (73.4°F). The organism has been isolated from soil on rare occasion.

Clinical Manifestations

Female patients are as susceptible to infections as male patients, but the incidence of clinical disease is approximately ninefold higher in male patients. Primary infection occurs in the lungs as a result of inhaling conidia and is frequently asymptomatic. However, it can develop into severe pulmonary disease or disseminated disease with ulcerative lesions of the buccal, nasal, and GI mucosa.

Diagnosis

Diagnosis of paracoccidioidomycosis is based on detection of specific antibodies, visualization of the organism in histopathologic material, or isolation of the organism in culture. Specific antibodies are measured by complement fixation and immunodiffusion. The presence of multiple, small, budding cells arranged around a large, mature cell in potassium hydroxide or silver-stained tissue is diagnostic of *P. brasiliensis*. Clinical specimens cultured on medium at 25°C (77°F) yield a slow-growing, white mold after 14 days of incubation. Transfer of the culture to incubation at 37°C (98.6°F) yields a yeastlike growth with characteristic multipolar budding cells.

Treatment

Relatively mild cases of paracoccidioidomycosis may be cured by 1 yr of treatment with PO ketoconazole or itraconazole, 200–400 mg/day (Table 24-1). More advanced cases are treated with IV amphotericin B followed by itraconazole.

CRYPTOCOCCOSIS

Epidemiology and Ecology

C. neoformans serotypes A and D are recovered in large numbers from the excreta and debris of pigeons. The organism appears to survive well in a desiccated, alkaline, nitrogen-rich, hypertonic environment. Cryptococcosis occurs throughout the world, but the true prevalence is unknown. Symptomatic cryptococcal disease is frequently seen in individuals who are debilitated, immunosuppressed, or otherwise compromised.

Clinical Manifestations

In contrast to other systemic mycotic agents, dimorphism does not play a role in the pathogenesis of *C. neoformans*. The presentation of primary pulmonary cryptococcosis can range from asymptomatic nodular disease to severe acute respiratory failure, depending on the extent of disease and the underlying status of host immunity. It is important that patients with pulmonary cryptococcal infection have a lumbar puncture performed to rule out concomitant CNS infection. Cryptococcal meningitis is the most frequently diagnosed form of cryptococcosis; CNS involvement occurs in 5–10% of patients with AIDS. Symptoms usually include headache, mental status changes, and fever lasting several days to weeks. Other common manifestations of disseminated cryptococcosis include skin lesions and osteolytic bone lesions.

Diagnosis

The diagnosis of cryptococcosis is based on the detection of antigens. The latex agglutination test for the detection of cryptococcal polysaccharide antigens in CSF and serum is routinely used in clinical labs. A rapid diagnosis of cryptococcal meningitis can also be made by exam of an India ink preparation of CSF. *C. neoformans* appears as a single-cell or budding yeast surrounded by a clear halo because of the exclusion of the ink particles by the polysaccharide capsule. However, the results are positive in only approximately 50% of cryptococcal meningitis cases. Culture remains the definitive method for documenting infection. The organism grows well on standard, nonselective mycologic media.

Treatment

The goal of cryptococcal therapy in **non-HIV individuals** is eradication of infection, which is achievable in many patients. Historically, eradication of cryptococcal infection in patients with advanced HIV disease was often not possible because of persistent immunodeficiency. Therefore, treatment of disseminated cryptococcosis in **HIV and AIDS patients** includes improvement in the host immune function by potent antiretroviral treatment and control of cryptococcal infection by suppressive therapy until immune function is restored. The desired outcome in both groups is the resolution of clinical features that cause morbidity or mortality (e.g., fever, headache, altered mental status, blindness, and elevated ICP).

Pulmonary cryptococcosis is frequently a self-limited infection that can be treated with fluconazole or by careful observation in immunocompetent patients. However, immunocompromised patients with pulmonary cryptococcosis should be assumed to have extrapulmonary disease and treated in the same fashion as patients with CNS disease. For **acute cryptococcal meningitis,** the combination of IV amphotericin B and oral flucytosine for 2 wks, followed by fluconazole (400 mg/day PO) for 8 wks and then suppressive therapy with fluconazole (200 mg/day PO)—the duration of which depends on the host's immunologic status—is the recommended treatment (Table 24-1). During therapy, a **lumbar puncture** should be performed at the second week to assess the requirement for prolonged induction therapy. All patients should be monitored closely for evidence of elevated ICP and managed accordingly. There is no correlation of titers between CSF and serum cryptococcal antigen for management of cryptococcal meningitis. In addition, there is no correlation between changes in serum cryptococcal antigen in patients receiving suppressive therapy who have relapsed. Therefore, management decisions should be made on an individual clinical assessment and should not rely on cryptococcal antigen titers.

KEY POINTS TO REMEMBER

- Always check CSF opening pressure when managing cryptococcal meningitis. Elevated ICP that is not controlled is associated with higher mortality.
- If itraconazole is used, check a drug level during therapy, especially if a PO formulation is used.
- Infections with systemic mycoses are often complex and difficult to treat. ID consultation is advised.

REFERENCES AND SUGGESTED READINGS

Bennett JE. Introduction to mycoses. In: Mandell GL, Bennett JE, Dolin R, eds. *Principles and practice of infectious diseases*, 5th ed. Philadelphia: Churchill Livingstone, 2000:2655–2656.

Chapman SW, Bradsher RW, Campbell GD, et al. Practice guidelines for the management of patients with blastomycosis. *Clin Infect Dis* 2000;30:679–683.

Galgiani JN, Ampel NM, Catanzaro A, et al. Practice guidelines for the treatment of coccidioidomycosis. *Clin Infect Dis* 2000;30:658–661.

Kwong-Chung KJ, Bennet JE. *Medical mycology*. Philadelphia: Lea & Febiger, 1992.

Murray PR, Rosenthal KS, Kobayashi GS, Pfaller MA. *Systemic mycoses*. St. Louis: Mosby, 1998:577–588.

Sagg MS, Graybill RJ, Larsen R, et al. Practice guidelines for the management of cryptococcal disease. *Clin Infect Dis* 2000;30:710–717.

Sobel JD. Practice guidelines for the treatment of fungal infection. *Clin Infect Dis* 2000;30:652.

Sugar SM. *A practical guide to medically important fungi and the diseases they cause*. Philadelphia: Lippincott–Raven, 1997.

Wheat J, Sarosi G, McKinsey D, et al. Practice guidelines for the management of patients with histoplasmosis. *Clin Infect Dis* 2000;30:688–695.

Protozoa

Erik Dubberke

INTRODUCTION

When a patient presents in such a manner or has a risk factor that is concerning for a protozoal infection, it is important to get a thorough history on potential exposures and time course of the illness. A history of immigration from, residence or work in, or travel to areas where various protozoa are endemic may offer a clue as to the causative organism, even if only briefly. In addition, place of residence and available infrastructure, types of activities, and purpose of travel may provide clues. The time to onset and duration of illness may provide clues, as some organisms cause illness in weeks and others in months to years. All ingestions should be sought as well: meats (and how well cooked), eating establishments visited, water sources, and uncooked fruits and vegetables.

PLASMODIUM INFECTIONS

Malaria is caused by four plasmodia (Table 25-1): *Plasmodium vivax* and *Plasmodium falciparum* are more common; *Plasmodium ovale* and *Plasmodium malariae* are less common. The vector and definitive host is the female *Anopheles* mosquito. There are two life cycles: The sexual life cycle (sporogony) occurs in the mosquito, and the asexual life cycle (schizogony) takes place in the mammal host. Malaria is the most common lethal infection worldwide, causing 200 million infections and 1 million deaths/yr. It occurs primarily in tropical and subtropical climates, especially in Asia, Africa, and Central and South America. See Chap. 17, Travel Medicine, for a discussion of malaria chemoprophylaxis.

Pathophysiology

Sporozoites are injected into the human host and are taken up by the liver within 30 mins. They multiply and form merozoites (*P. vivax* and *P. ovale* can also produce hypnozoites that remain latent in the liver). Merozoites are released from the liver and infect erythrocytes. The organisms then differentiate into ringed trophozoites. The trophozoites then develop into merozoites, rupture the host erythrocyte, and infect other erythrocytes. The cycle in the erythrocyte repeats at regular intervals typical for each species [*P. malariae* causes quartan malaria (fever every 72 hrs), and the other species cause tertian malaria (fever every 48 hrs)]. *P. falciparum* causes more severe disease (malignant malaria, cerebral malaria, and blackwater fever) because it infects erythrocytes in all stages of development. *P. vivax* infects only reticulocytes, and *P. malariae* infects only mature red cells.

Differential Diagnosis

The differential diagnosis is nonspecific viral illness, dengue fever, leptospirosis, typhus, meningococcal sepsis, and enteric fever.

Clinical Manifestations

Malaria presents with abrupt onset of fever and chills—accompanied by headache, nausea, vomiting, abdominal pain, myalgias, and arthralgias—approximately 2 wks

TABLE 25-1. FEATURES OF COMMON, MEDICALLY IMPORTANT PROTOZOA

Organism	Disease	Mode of transmission	Occurrence in United States	Diagnosis	Treatment
Plasmodium species	Malaria	*Anopheles* mosquito	Rare	Blood smear	Chloroquine, mefloquine, quinine, primaquine
Leishmania donovani	*Kala-azar*	Sandfly	No	Bone marrow, spleen, lymph node	Stibogluconate
Leishmania tropica, Leishmania mexicana, Leishmania braziliensis	Cutaneous/mucocutaneous leishmaniasis	Sandfly	No	Fluid from lesion	Stibogluconate
Trypanosoma cruzi	Chagas' disease	Reduvid bug	Rare	Blood smear, bone marrow, xenodiagnosis	Nifurtimox
Trypanosoma gambiense, Trypanosoma rhodesiense	African sleeping sickness	Tsetse fly	No	Blood smear	Suramin
Toxoplasma gondii	Toxoplasmosis	Ingestion of cysts in raw meat, contact with soil contaminated with cat feces	Yes	Serology, microscopic exam of tissue	TMP-SMX, pentamidine, atovaquone
Entamoeba	Amebiasis	Ingestion of cysts in food/water	Yes	Trophozoites or cysts in stool, serology	Metronidazole plus iodoquinol
Giardia	Giardiasis	Ingestion of cysts in food/water	Yes	Trophozoites or cysts in stool	Metronidazole
Cryptosporidium	Cryptosporidiosis	Ingestion of cysts in food/water	Yes	Cysts on acid-fast stain	None

Adapted from Levinson WE, Jawetz E, eds. *Medical microbiology and immunology*, 4th ed. New York: McGraw-Hill, 1996.

after the mosquito bite. *P. falciparum* infection can be associated with mental status changes (cerebral malaria) because the high number of infected erythrocytes can aggregate and occlude capillaries. *P. falciparum* infection can also be associated with dark urine secondary to hemoglobinuria from hemolysis (blackwater fever). *P. vivax* and *P. ovale* can cause symptomatic infection years after the mosquito bite because they can form latent hypnozoites that reside in the liver.

In acute, uncomplicated malaria, there are often few clinical findings: fever, tachycardia, malaise, mild anemia, splenomegaly, and possibly hepatomegaly. Mild jaundice may be present as well. In severe *falciparum* malaria, patients may have altered sensorium or impaired consciousness, convulsions, hypoglycemia, respiratory distress, acidosis, hypotension, severe anemia, DIC, and hemoglobinuria.

Diagnosis

Patients typically have a normochromic, normocytic anemia; normal to elevated leukocyte count; low platelets; elevated ESR; and an elevated indirect bilirubin. In severe forms, there may be hemoglobinuria, elevated creatinine, anion gap acidosis, elevated PT or aPTT, elevated ALT or AST, and hypoglycemia. The diagnosis is made on visualization of the parasites on a blood smear. If thick and thin smears are negative and a high index of suspicion remains, smears should be repeated every 12 hrs for 2 days.

Treatment

For benign malaria, chloroquine [Aralen; 1.0 g (or 600 mg base) PO, 0.5 g in 6 hrs, then 0.5 g daily for 2 days] remains the treatment of choice, as well as for *falciparum* malaria in areas where resistance is not a problem. Choices for treating chloroquine-resistant *P. falciparum* include include sulfadoxine and pyrimethamine [Fansidar; 3 tablets (each tablet 25/500 mg) for 1 dose on last day of quinine], quinine (650 mg PO q8h for 3–7 days), tetracycline (250 mg PO qid for 7 days), clindamycin (900 mg PO tid for 3 days), or mefloquine (Lariam PO; 1250 mg for 1 dose). For severe malaria, IV quinine or quinidine is the drug of choice. Primaquine is used to eradicate the hypnozoites of *P. vivax* and *P. ovale* infection. Supportive measures should be provided, and one should be acquainted with the many side effects and adverse reactions of the antimalarial medications. For assistance with antimalarials, the CDC Malaria Hotline can be reached at (770) 488-7788 [on weekends or after hours: (404) 639-2888]. Information is also available at http://www.cdc.gov/travel/diseases.htm#malaria.

BABESIA INFECTIONS

Of the approximately 100 species of *Babesia*, most cases of babesiosis are caused by *Babesia microti* or *Babesia divergens*. Babesiosis is a zoonosis endemic primarily in the coastal areas and islands off the northeastern coast of the United States. Cases have also been reported in Missouri, Wisconsin, Minnesota, Virginia, Georgia, and Mexico. There also have been reports in Russia, Yugoslavia, England, and Ireland. The organism infects rodents and is transmitted by the *Ixodes scapularis* tick.

Pathophysiology

Ticks ingest the organism when feeding, and it multiplies in the tick's GI tract wall. The parasite then travels to the salivary glands. The organism is then injected into the vertebrate host, where it infects erythrocytes. Asexual reproduction occurs within the erythrocyte.

Differential Diagnosis

The differential diagnosis is nonspecific viral illness, Lyme disease, and ehrlichiosis.

Clinical Manifestations

Patients may or may not remember having a tick bite. Influenza-like symptoms begin gradually and may last for months. Patients typically experience fever, chills, malaise, myalgias, and fatigue. Immunocompromised, elderly, and asplenic patients tend to have more severe disease. Patients with *B. divergens* also have more severe illness, with sudden onset of fevers, chills, nausea, vomiting, and hemolytic anemia.

Diagnosis

A definitive diagnosis is made by visualizing the organism on thin or thick smears. An indirect immunofluorescence antibody is useful, but it does not replace the blood smears. Serum antibody titers rise at 2–4 wks and then wane at 6–12 mos; cross-reactions can occur with *Plasmodium*. The exam tends to be nonspecific with hepatosplenomegaly and possibly jaundice. See Chap. 21, Tick-Borne Illnesses, for additional information.

Treatment

B. microti infections in patients with spleens tend to be self-limiting, but patients can have symptoms for months if left untreated. Treatment with quinine (650 mg PO tid for 7 days) and clindamycin (600 mg PO tid for 7 days) for 7–10 days is usually effective, although atovaquone (750 mg PO bid for 7–10 days) and azithromycin (500 mg PO for 1 day then 250 mg PO qd for 6 days) can be used for treatment-resistant cases. Severe cases in asplenic patients can be treated with quinine and clindamycin plus exchange transfusions. See Chap. 21, Tick-Borne Illnesses, for additional information.

LEISHMANIASIS: VISCERAL

Visceral leishmaniasis (*kala-azar*) is caused by *Leishmania donovani* (Table 25-1). The life cycle involves the sandfly as the vector and a variety of mammals as reservoirs. *Kala-azar* occurs in three distinct epidemiologic patterns. In the Mediterranean basin, the Middle East, southern Russia, and parts of China, the reservoir hosts are primarily dogs and foxes. In sub-Saharan Africa, rats and small carnivores are the main reservoirs. In India and neighboring countries, humans appear to be the only reservoir.

Pathophysiology

When the female sandfly takes a blood meal from an infected host, macrophages containing amastigotes are ingested. These turn into promastigotes in the GI tract; they then migrate to the pharynx and multiply, where they can be transmitted with the next bite. Promastigotes are engulfed by macrophages; they transform into amastigotes and divide. The host cell dies, and the amastigotes are taken up by surrounding macrophages, thus continuing the cycle. In *kala-azar*, the organs of the reticuloendothelial system (liver, spleen, and bone marrow) are the most severely affected with subsequent pancytopenia and hepatosplenomegaly. Untreated disease is nearly always fatal as a result of secondary infection.

Differential Diagnosis

The differential diagnosis includes tropical infections that cause fever or organomegaly (e.g., typhoid fever, miliary TB, brucellosis, malaria, schistosomiasis, and tropical splenomegaly syndrome). The differential diagnosis for post–*kala-azar* dermal leishmaniasis includes yaws, syphilis, and leprosy.

Clinical Manifestations

Patients may report fever, malaise, fatigue, increased pigmentation of the skin, and bleeding. The disease may present in an acute, subacute, or chronic fashion, weeks to years after the causative bite. Patients with severe disease usually also experience protein malnutrition.

Patients may have hepatomegaly, although the splenomegaly is usually more impressive and can be massive. Peripheral lymphadenopathy may occur in some settings (e.g., Sudan). Patients may also have a grayish pigmentation to the skin (*kala-azar* is Hindi for "black fever"). Abnormal lab values that can be seen include pancytopenia, hypergammaglobulinemia, and hypoalbuminemia. Causes of anemia may be bone marrow infiltration, autoimmune hemolysis, bleeding, or hypersplenism. Some patients develop post–*kala-azar* dermal leishmaniasis. This is characterized by skin lesions (macules, papules, nodules, or patches) that are most prominent on the face. It can occur during treatment or several years after treatment. These patients can serve as reservoirs.

Diagnosis

The diagnosis is usually made by detecting amastigotes in a bone marrow, spleen, or lymph node biopsy. Patients develop high titers on antibodies. Skin tests are available, although they are negative during active infection and become positive after recovery.

Treatment

Treatment outside of India consists of a pentavalent antimonial compound. If antimonial resistance is high, then amphotericin B can be used. Patients feel better during the first few weeks of therapy. Abnormal lab values and splenomegaly can take months to resolve. The best predictor of cure is no evidence of clinical relapse 6 mos after therapy.

LEISHMANIASIS: CUTANEOUS AND MUCOCUTANEOUS

Leishmania tropica and *Leishmania mexicana* cause cutaneous leishmaniasis, and *Leishmania braziliensis* causes mucocutaneous leishmaniasis (Table 25-1). The vectors are sandflies, and the main reservoirs are forest rodents. Old World cutaneous leishmaniasis (oriental sore, Delhi boil) is caused by *L. tropica* and is endemic in the Middle East, Africa, and India. New World cutaneous leishmaniasis (chicle ulcer, bay sore) is caused by *L. mexicana* and is found in Central and South America. *L. braziliensis* is found mostly in Brazil and Central America. It typically occurs in forestry and construction workers.

Pathophysiology

The lesions of cutaneous leishmaniasis occur only on the skin; the lesions of mucocutaneous leishmaniasis can occur on the mucous membranes, cartilage, and skin. A granulomatous response occurs, and a necrotic ulcer forms at the bite site. The lesions can become superinfected with bacteria.

Clinical Manifestations

Patients will notice a papule that appears weeks to months after the bite that eventually ulcerates. Satellite lesions and lymphadenopathy may occur as well.

The ulcers can be several centimeters in diameter, with an indurated, raised border. Mucocutaneous disease involving cartilage can be disfiguring. Some patients exhibiting anergy may present with diffuse cutaneous leishmaniasis.

Diagnosis

Definitive diagnosis is made by visualizing organisms in a scraping from a lesion. Serology is insensitive, but skin testing is usually positive during active disease.

Differential Diagnosis

The differential diagnosis is traumatic ulcers, venous stasis ulcers, foreign body reactions, superinfected insect bites, myiasis, impetigo, sporotrichosis, mycobacterial disease, sarcoid, neoplastic disease, leprosy, and lupus vulgaris.

Treatment

Treatment may not be needed depending on the location and size of the lesion in an immunocompetent patient. If treatment is needed, pentavalent antimonials are recommended.

CHAGAS' DISEASE

Trypanosoma cruzi is the causative agent of Chagas' disease (Table 25-1). The reduviid bug (kissing bug) is the vector, and both humans and animals (e.g., armadillo, raccoon, rat, and domesticated cats and dogs) act as the reservoirs. Chagas' disease occurs primarily in rural Central and South America and rarely in the southern United States. The reduviid bug lives in the walls of rural huts and feeds at night, preferentially around the mouth and eyes.

Pathophysiology

The reduviid bug ingests trypomastigotes from the blood of an infected host. In the insect's GI tract, they multiply and differentiate to epimastigotes and back to trypomastigotes. When the insect bites again, the site becomes contaminated with feces of the infected bug, and the trypomastigotes enter the bloodstream of the new host and form amastigotes. Any cell can be affected, but myocytes, glial cells, and reticuloendothelial cells are the most frequent sites. The amastigotes can kill cells and cause inflammation. Cardiac myocytes are the most severely affected, and death is typically due to heart failure or arrhythmias. Neuronal damage can lead to loss of tone in the colon (megacolon) or the esophagus (megaesophagus).

Clinical Manifestations

During the acute phase, patients may report facial swelling and erythema, followed by malaise, fever, and anorexia. In chronic infection, patients most commonly present with symptoms of heart failure or heart block. They may also experience (a) dysphagia, odynophagia, or aspiration if the esophagus is involved; or (b) constipation, abdominal pain, and abdominal distention if the colon is involved.

During the acute phase, patients may have a chagoma—an area of induration, erythema, and edema accompanied by local lymphadenopathy where the organism entered the skin. The classic findings of **acute disease** (Romaña's sign) consist of unilateral painless edema of the palpebrae and periocular tissues. This occurs when the conjunctiva is the portal of entry. Patients may also have generalized lymphadenopathy or hepatosplenomegaly. Patients with **chronic disease** present years to decades after the acute infection. Heart failure, often with arrhythmias, due to severely dilated cardiomyopathy is most common. Patients may also present with megacolon or megaesophagus.

Diagnosis

The diagnosis of acute Chagas' disease is made when the organisms are visualized. Parasites may be seen on thick or thin smears of the blood, or microscopic exam of the buffy coat may reveal motile organisms. When attempts to visualize the organism are unsuccessful, mouse inoculation, blood culture in specialized media, or xenodiagnosis (allow uninfected, lab-raised reduviid bugs to feed on the patient; examine the intestinal contents of the insect several weeks later) can be attempted. Serologic testing is of limited usefulness in acute disease. In chronic disease, the diagnosis is usually made by serologic testing. Because of high rates of false-positivity, positives should be confirmed with two other tests.

Treatment

Nifurtimox, 8–10 mg/kg/day PO in 4 divided doses per day (after meals) for 120 days, is the only drug available in the United States that is active against *T. cruzi*, and it results in only a 70% rate of parasitologic cure in acute infection. Nifurtimox should be initiated as soon as possible when acute infection is suspected. The second-line agent is benznidazole, and it has similar efficacy to nifurtimox. Although the utility of treatment for chronic infection is debated, treatment is recommended for chronic infection.

Prevention

Successful vector and blood-bank control programs in endemic countries have decreased the rate of infection in recent years. Vector control involves use of insecticides, improved housing, and education. Travelers to endemic areas should avoid living in dilapidated housing in rural areas. Mosquito nets and insect repellants are useful as well.

SLEEPING SICKNESS

Trypanosoma gambiense and *Trypanosoma rhodesiense* are the causative agents of African sleeping sickness (Table 25-1). The vector is the tsetse fly. Humans are the host for *T. gambiense*, and animals (domestic and wild) are the hosts for *T. rhodesiense*. The disease is endemic in sub-Saharan Africa. *T. gambiense* causes disease along water courses in West Africa; *T. rhodesiense* causes disease in arid East Africa. Both species cause disease in Central Africa.

Pathophysiology

The tsetse fly ingests trypomastigotes from an infected host. The organism multiplies in the GI tract, travels to the salivary gland, transforms into epimastigotes and divides further, and then transforms into metacyclic trypomastigotes. These are then transmitted by the tsetse fly bite. The trypomastigotes travel from the skin to the blood and then to the brain. Patients typically develop somnolence that progresses to coma as a result of a demyelinating encephalitis. The trypanosomes exhibit remarkable antigenic variation and evade the immune system by changing its antigenic type approximately every 10 days.

Clinical Manifestations

A painful chancre appears at the site on inoculation. This is followed by stage I disease, with cyclical high fevers lasting several days followed by afebrile periods, associated with the antigenic variation. Patients may report swollen lymph nodes, pruritus, rash, headache, myalgias, and edema. Stage II disease is associated with CNS invasion. Patients and family members note daytime somnolence and a listless gaze; at night, the patients are often restless and suffer from insomnia.

During stage I, patients may exhibit lymphadenopathy (more prominent in disease caused by *T. gambiense*). The nodes are discrete, mobile, rubbery, and nontender. Cervical nodes are often visible, and enlargement of the nodes of the posterior cervical triangle (Winterbottom's sign) is a classic finding. During stage II, patients may have a listless gaze and loss of spontaneity, and speech may become halting and indistinct. Extrapyramidal signs may develop as well, and patients may appear to have Parkinson's disease. *T. gambiense* disease tends to run a chronic course over years; *T. rhodesiense* disease is acute, often fatal in weeks to months.

Diagnosis

Visualizing the parasite is essential for diagnosis. The organisms may be seen on fluid expressed from a chancre or aspirated from a lymph node. Thick and thin blood smears may be helpful. The organisms can also be recovered from a bone marrow aspirate or the CSF in patients with stage II disease. If the parasites are not seen, quantitative buffy coat analysis tubes are available. The organisms can also be cultured on special media, or *T. rhodesiense* can be inoculated into mice. All patients require a lumbar puncture. An elevation in the cell count is the first abnormality, followed by a rise in the total protein and IgM. Trypanosomes may be seen in the sediment of centrifuged CSF.

Differential Diagnosis

The differential diagnosis includes syphilis, yaws, cutaneous leishmaniasis, and encephalopathy.

Treatment

The drugs used to treat African trypanosomiasis include suramin, pentamidine, organic arsenicals, and eflornithine. Therapy must be individualized on the basis of infecting organism, CNS involvement, adverse drug reactions, and drug resistance.

TOXOPLASMA INFECTIONS

Toxoplasma gondii is the causative agent of toxoplasmosis (Table 25-1). The definitive host is the domestic cat, and humans and other animals are intermediate hosts. Toxoplasmosis occurs worldwide. Approximately 1% of domestic cats in the United States shed *Toxoplasma* cysts.

Pathophysiology

Human infection results when cysts are ingested from undercooked meat or after handling cat feces. The cysts rupture and invade the GI tract wall, where they are ingested by macrophages. Inside the macrophages, they transform into tachyzoites and rapidly divide. Cell-mediated immunity is necessary to contain the infection. The parasites can enter host cells (brain, muscle, and other tissue), where they develop into bradyzoites that can remain dormant for years.

Clinical Manifestations

Most acute infections in immunocompetent hosts are asymptomatic, although toxoplasmosis is a cause of heterophile-negative mononucleosis. Congenital infection can occur during acute infection of the mother. This can result in abortion, stillbirth, or neonatal disease with encephalitis, chorioretinitis, and hepatosplenomegaly. Latent disease can reactivate in patients with depressed cell-mediated immunity. This typically presents as an intracranial mass lesion.

Diagnosis

A positive immunofluorescence for IgM antibodies confirms an acute infection or congenital infection. Isolation of *T. gondii* from body fluids reflects acute infection. Demonstration of cysts in biopsied tissue does not indicate that an acute infection is occurring. A rise in IgG antibodies in an immunocompromised patient with radiographic features consistent with toxoplasmosis is a ground for a presumptive diagnosis; frequently, a biopsy will need to be performed.

Treatment

Immunocompetent adults and children with acute infection do not need treatment unless symptoms are severe or persistent. Sulfadiazine (Microsulfon) with pyrimethamine is the treatment of choice. It is given in conjunction with leucovorin (Wellcovorin) to prevent the bone marrow toxicity associated with pyrimethamine. This regimen is active only against the tachyzoite stage, and immunocompromised patients will require lifelong suppressive therapy. Alternative therapies are available. Dapsone (Dapsone USP, DDS) or clindamycin can be used in place of sulfadiazine. Macrolides in combination therapy can be used as well. Atovaquone is another option.

Prevention

Primary infection can be avoided by not eating undercooked meats and by not handling cat feces.

AMEBIASIS

Entamoeba histolytica is the cause of amebic dysentery and liver abscess (Table 25-1). *E. histolytica* infects only humans and is found worldwide. It is most common in tropical countries in areas with poor sanitation, and it is the third most common cause of death from parasitic infections (behind malaria and schistosomiasis). The prevalence in the United States is 1–2%. The main groups at risk for developing infection are travelers, recent immigrants, homosexual men, and inmates of institutions.

Pathophysiology

E. histolytica is spread by the fecal-oral route. Cysts are ingested. In the small intestine, motile trophozoites are released that then most often become commensals of the colon, releasing cysts in the stool. The cysts can remain infectious for weeks in the proper environment, and they are resistant to killing by chlorination. They are readily killed by boiling and iodination. In patients with active dysentery, trophozoites are present in the stool, although these tend not to be infectious. When trophozoites invade the bowel mucosa, they release enzymes that cause necrosis. Often, there is little inflammation. Submucosal lesions enlarge and form "teardrop" ulcers. Progression can lead to entry into the portal circulation and systemic disease. The most frequent site of systemic disease is the liver, where abscesses form (which resemble anchovy paste).

Differential Diagnosis

Other causes of dysentery include *Shigella*, *Escherichia coli*, *Salmonella*, *Campylobacter*, and some *Vibrio* species. Amebic liver abscess must be differentiated from pyogenic liver abscess, gallbladder disease, pulmonary disease, and echinococcal disease.

Clinical Manifestations

Approximately 90% of patients become asymptomatic carriers. Patients with acute intestinal amebiasis report crampy, lower abdominal discomfort; flatulence; tenesmus; and bloody, mucus-containing diarrhea 2–6 wks after ingestion of cysts. Some patients may develop an ameboma—a submucosal mass of granulation tissue—in response to the infection. Occasionally, amebiasis can be chronic and present with episodic diarrhea, weight loss, and fatigue. Amebic abscess of the liver is characterized by right upper quadrant pain, weight loss, fever, and a tender, enlarged liver.

Diagnosis

Intestinal amebiasis can be diagnosed by visualizing trophozoites in diarrheal stool or cysts in formed stool. Stool samples must be rapidly processed because the trophozoites are killed by water or drying. Trophozoites characteristically contain erythrocytes. Charcot-Leyden crystals may be seen in the stool. There should not be many neutrophils in the stool. Serology may be positive in patients with active disease but is typically negative in individuals who are passing cysts. Hepatic abscesses can be detected with either U/S or CT. An aspiration needs to be performed to differentiate an amebic abscess from a pyogenic abscess.

Treatment

Asymptomatic carriers can be treated with iodoquinol or paromomycin. Patients with active colitis or amebic abscess should be treated with one of the above plus metronidazole.

Prevention

Prevention requires adequate sanitation and elimination of asymptomatic carriers. In high-risk areas, eating unpeeled or uncooked fruits and vegetables should be avoided, and bottled water should be consumed.

FREE-LIVING AMEBAS

Free-living amebas of the genera *Acanthamoeba*, *Balamuthia*, and *Naegleria* are found throughout the world. They reside in a variety of fresh and brackish bodies of water, including lakes, taps, hot springs, swimming pools, and air-conditioning units, as well as in the nasal passages of healthy children. *Naegleria* may be the host for *Legionella pneumophila* in water supplies.

Acanthamoeba

Acanthamoeba causes granulomatous amebic encephalitis in immunocompromised patients. Risk factors include lymphoproliferative disease, chemotherapy, corticosteroids, SLE, and AIDS. It can also cause infections in contact lens wearers. Diagnosis is made by an ophthalmologist, and the treatment is propamidine 1% plus neomycin/gramicidin/polymyxin eyedrops (q waking hour for 1 wk, then slow taper). Infection reaches the CNS hematogenously from a primary focus in the sinuses, skin, or lungs. Onset is insidious. Patients present with altered mental status, headache, and stiff neck. Focal findings may be present, such as cranial nerve palsies, ataxia, and hemiparesis. AIDS patients with CNS disease may have cutaneous ulcers or nodules containing the amebas. Demonstration of trophozoites and cysts on wet mounts or biopsy specimens establishes the diagnosis. CT findings may reveal cortical and subcortical lesions of decreased attenuation that can be confused with embolic infarcts. Some patients develop multiple ring-enhancing lesions that may be confused with toxoplasmosis. Prognosis in encephalitis is poor; there is no proven treatment for encephalitis. Keratitis has been treated successfully with topical therapy or a combination of oral and topical therapy.

Balamuthia

Balamuthia causes amebic meningoencephalitis in immunocompetent hosts. The onset is subacute, with focal neurologic signs, fever, seizures, and headache leading to death several weeks to months after onset. CSF studies reveal a mononuclear pleocytosis with an elevated protein level and low glucose concentration. CT may show multiple hypodense lesions. Diagnosis is usually made postmortem.

Naegleria

Naegleria invades the olfactory epithelium after aspiration of trophozoites in water or cysts in dust and causes meningoencephalitis. After an incubation period of 2–15 days, patients develop severe headache, fever, nausea, vomiting, and meningismus. Photophobia and ocular palsies are common. Rapid progression to seizures and coma follows, and most patients die within 1 wk. Infection typically occurs in otherwise healthy children and young adults with a history of recently swimming in a lake or a pool. CSF findings mimic those of acute bacterial meningitis. The diagnosis should be considered in patients with purulent meningitis and negative Gram's stain and culture. Diagnosis is made by visualizing motile trophozoites on wet preparation of the CSF. The only four known survivors were treated with high-dose amphotericin B and rifampin (Rifadin, Rimactane).

GIARDIA INFECTIONS

Giardia lamblia is the cause of giardiasis (Table 25-1). It occurs worldwide and infects both humans and other mammals. The cysts can live for months in cold water. Chlorination does not kill the cysts, but they can be removed by filtration. It is spread by the fecal-oral route, and the incidence is high among children in day care centers and patients in mental hospitals.

Pathophysiology

Cysts ingested from fecally contaminated food or water exist in the duodenum. The trophozoite then attaches to the GI tract wall but does not invade. Inflammation of the duodenal mucosa occurs, which leads to malabsorption of protein and fat. The immune response to *Giardia* is poorly understood, but humoral mechanisms are believed to be important because patients with hypogammaglobulinemia develop prolonged, severe infections that respond poorly to therapy.

Clinical Manifestations

Disease manifestation varies greatly from asymptomatic to fulminant diarrhea. Symptoms, if they develop, occur after an incubation period of 1–3 wks. Early symptoms include bloating, abdominal pain, nausea, belching, flatus, vomiting, and diarrhea. Symptoms typically last >1 wk. Symptoms may be continuous or episodic for years. Some patients may develop weight loss as a result of malabsorption.

Diagnosis

Giardia is diagnosed by detecting antigen, cysts, or trophozoites in the stool or trophozoites in the duodenum.

Treatment

Metronidazole is the treatment of choice. Other agents include quinacrine, furazolidone, and albendazole.

CRYPTOSPORIDIUM INFECTIONS

Cryptosporidium causes cryptosporidiosis (Table 25-1). It can cause a diarrheal illness in immunocompetent patients and is especially common among patients with AIDS. *Cryptosporidium* can be found in many animals. Oocysts are resistant to chlorination.

Pathophysiology

Oocysts are ingested and exist to liberate sporozoites that enter and invade the intestinal epithelium. Although the parasite resides in a vacuole within the epithelium, the mechanism by which a secretory diarrhea is caused is unknown. In patients with AIDS, it can invade the biliary tree and cause papillary stenosis, sclerosing cholangitis, and cholecystitis.

Clinical Manifestations

Asymptomatic infections can occur in immunocompromised and immunocompetent patients. Immunocompetent patients who develop symptoms have watery diarrhea, abdominal pain, nausea, anorexia, and fever approximately 1 wk after ingestion of the oocyst. This typically subsides in 1–2 wks. In immunocompromised patients, particularly AIDS patients, the diarrhea can be chronic and profuse, causing significant electrolyte fluid and abnormalities. Weight loss and wasting can be severe.

Diagnosis

Stool should be examined for oocysts. They are smaller (4–5 μm) than most other parasites. They are positive with a modified acid-fast stain. Direct immunofluorescent and enzyme immunoassays are available. Multiple stool specimens are often needed to detect the oocysts.

Treatment

There are no effective chemotherapeutic agents available, although paromomycin may be partially effective for patients with HIV. Treatment is otherwise supportive.

ISOSPORA INFECTIONS

Isospora belli is the causative parasite of isosporiasis. After consumption of the oocyst, the parasite invades the intestinal epithelium. The oocysts are not immediately infective after release in the stool but require further maturation. Animals and humans can be infected, and it is more common in tropical and subtropical climates. Similar to *Cryptosporidium* infection, it causes a secretory diarrhea that can be profound in immunocompromised patients. Diagnosis is made by visualizing the large oocysts (25 μm) in stool with a modified acid-fast stain. Often, multiple stool samples need to be obtained to make the diagnosis. If stool samples are repeatedly negative, it may be necessary to get samples of duodenal contents. Therapy involves TMP-SMX or pyrimethamine for those intolerant of sulfonamides.

CYCLOSPORA INFECTIONS

Cyclospora cayetanensis is a parasite found worldwide that can cause a diarrheal illness. The epidemiology is not fully defined, although water-borne transmission and transmission from imported raspberries have been documented. Some patients are asymptomatic, although many develop diarrhea, flu-like symptoms, and flatulence. The disease can be self-limited, wax and wane, or be chronic. The parasite is detectable in epithelial cells of small bowel biopsies. Absence of inflammation is not uncommon. The oocysts can be detected in stool, although routine ova and parasites exam is not sufficient. Special fecal exams must be requested to detect the oocysts, which are variably acid-fast and are fluorescent when viewed under ultraviolet light. Cyclosporiasis can be effectively treated with TMP-SMX.

MICROSPORIDIOSIS

Seven genera of microsporidia are known to cause disease in humans. They are obligate intracellular parasites that can infect animals and humans. Little is known about how microsporidiosis is acquired. Microsporidia are extremely uncommon in immunocompetent patients, but they can cause chronic diarrhea and wasting in AIDS patients, accounting for 10–40% of cases of chronic diarrhea in this population. They have also been known to cause disease of the biliary tract, sinuses, respiratory tract, myositis, and disseminated infection. Microsporidia are small gram-positive organisms. Specialized staining of stool specimens may detect the spores. The organisms may be seen under light microscopy of biopsy samples. Definitive therapies remain to be established. Albendazole may be helpful with some genera.

BALANTIDIASIS

Balantidium coli is the only ciliated protozoan that causes human disease. It is found infrequently in the United States, pigs are the main reservoir, and infection occurs when cysts are ingested. The trophozoites live in the large intestine and cause disease similar to amebiasis, although extraintestinal lesions do not occur.

The diagnosis is made by visualizing trophozoites or cysts in stool. The treatment of choice is tetracycline.

KEY POINTS TO REMEMBER

- Malaria must be considered in the differential diagnosis of travelers with fever returning from malarial regions.
- *Acanthamoeba* can also cause infections in contact lens wearers.
- A thorough history and time course of illness are essential in considering the possibility of a protozoal infection.
- Visceral leishmaniasis and toxoplasmosis can be presenting opportunistic infections with AIDS. Consider obtaining an HIV test in these patients.

REFERENCES AND SUGGESTED READINGS

Bartlett JG. *Pocket book of infectious disease therapy*. Philadelphia: Lippincott Williams & Wilkins, 2000:188–197.

Braunwald E, Fauci AS, Kasper DL, et al., eds. *Harrison's principles of internal medicine*, 15th ed. New York: McGraw-Hill, 2001:1199–1230.

Gilbert DN, Moellering RC, Sande MA. *The Sanford guide to antimicrobial therapy 2003*, 33rd ed. Hyde Park, VT: Antimicrobial Therapy, Inc., 2003:91.

Levinson WE, Jawetz E, eds. *Medical microbiology and immunology*, 4th ed. New York: McGraw-Hill, 1996.

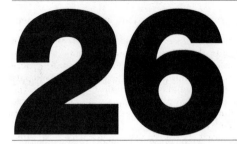

Ectoparasitic Infections

Rebecca E. Chandler

ECTOPARASITES

Ectoparasites are arthropods or helminths that infect the skin or hair of mammals. These organisms attach to their hosts and subsequently burrow beneath the skin. They feed on the blood and tissue of their hosts; in so doing, they may inject toxins into the host that may cause either tissue necrosis or hypersensitivity reactions. The most common organisms causing ectoparasitic infections are scabies (mites) and lice.

SCABIES AND PEDICULOSIS

Scabies is caused by the human itch mite, *Sarcoptes scabiei*; it is approximately 400 μm in diameter and is pearly white with brownish legs and mouth. Transmission of scabies results from close person-to-person contact; surprisingly, transmission by sharing of contaminated clothing or bedding is unlikely because the mite does not survive >24 hrs without its host. Although scabies is more common in those persons living in crowded conditions and poverty, it is not limited to this population; outbreaks occur in households, hospitals, nursing homes, and day care centers. Scabies is known to infest between 300 and 500 million people annually.

Pediculosis is the term given to infestation by lice. There are two genera of these organisms that are known to infect humans: *Pediculus* and *Pthirus*. There are three species in these two genera that are specifically important: *Pediculus humanus corporis* (the body louse), *Pediculus humanus capitis* (the head louse), and *Pthirus pubis* (the crab louse). Lice are wingless insects with three pairs of legs, each terminating with a curved claw. Lice range in size from 0.8 to 4.0 mm and are grayish-white to mahogany in color. Transmission of lice also results from close person-to-person contact; certain populations are more affected by each of these organisms (e.g., body lice in those with poor hygiene, head lice in school children, and pubic lice in sexually active individuals).

Pathophysiology

In scabies, gravid female mites bury beneath the stratum corneum of their host, making burrows into which they deposit their eggs and excreta. Hypersensitivity results to the mite excreta and eggs, causing itching and rash.

In pediculosis, lice grasp the clothes or hairs of their hosts with their curved claws and then proceed to bite their human host to feed on blood. Although the bite of the louse is painless, the saliva of the insect causes an allergic reaction in sensitized individuals.

Patients become sensitized to the ectoparasites approximately 1 mo after the initial infestation occurs; thus, patients without a prior exposure to the organisms do not reveal symptoms or signs until approximately 4 wks after obtaining the parasite. On repeated exposure to the organism, symptoms and signs may appear more rapidly and may be more severe in nature.

Clinical Manifestations

The major symptom of both scabies and pediculosis is an intensely pruritic rash. In scabies, the lesions are typically located in the finger webs, wrists, elbows, and scrotum and along skin folds. Although lesions above the neck are usually rare, these areas may not be spared in patients living in warmer climates. Patients may report that the pruritus is worse at night or after a hot shower or bath. In pediculosis, the pruritus is usually localized to specific lesions that may not be as widespread as those of scabies. Associated symptoms of irritability and sleeplessness may result; it is from this condition that the phrase "feeling lousy" was coined.

The lesions of scabies may be quite varied. The initial rash appears as 1- to 2-mm erythematous papules. These lesions may show signs of excoriation; with chronic infestations, the lesions may become lichenified, hyperpigmented, and scaly. The minute burrows of the gravid females may occasionally be noted, particularly in the webs of the fingers of the patient. Hypersensitized patients may even develop bullae or nodular lesions.

The lesions of pediculosis are also varied, as they occur on different areas of the body. Head lice result in crusted, oozing lesions on the scalp surrounded by matted hair. Body lice result in discrete areas of an erythematous maculopapular rash. Pubic lice also result in localized areas of a bluish maculopapular rash; blepharitis, or infestation of the eyelashes, may also occur.

Diagnosis

The diagnosis of scabies is made by finding the organisms themselves or by finding their eggs or fecal pellets (scybala). This may be accomplished by placing a drop of mineral oil on a suspected lesion, scraping it with a scalpel, and then examining the specimen under a microscope. The burrow ink test may also be performed; blue or black ink, such as in a felt-tip pen, may be applied to a suspected burrow. The burrow is then cleansed with an alcohol pad; if a burrow is present, the ink is partially retained within it.

The diagnosis of pediculosis is made by identifying the eggs, or "nits," at the sites of the lesions. The use of a magnifying glass may be helpful in differentiating the nits from other artifacts, such as dandruff, dried hair spray, or casts of sebum from the hair follicle.

Differential Diagnosis

Scabies and pediculosis must be differentiated from the many other dermatologic entities that cause pruritic, maculopapular rashes. Examples include contact dermatitis, eczema, psoriasis, and even urticaria. Additionally important is the recognition of possible superinfection of the lesions by *Staphylococcus*.

Treatment

The treatment of choice for scabies is 5% permethrin cream. It should be evenly spread onto the body from the chin to the toes; it should then be removed after 8 hrs with soap and water. This process should be repeated within 1 wk. This treatment is safe for all ages >2 mos and for pregnant women. An alternative treatment is a single dose of ivermectin, 200 μg/kg PO.

The treatment of choice for pediculosis is 1% permethrin cream to affected areas. Alternative therapies include 0.5% malathion and 1% lindane; however, these agents are less effective and more toxic. Combs and brushes should be sterilized with hot water (65°C; 149°F) for 5–15 mins. Clothing and bedding should also be sterilized with hot water and drying (54°C; 129.2°F) for 30–45 mins. No specific follow-up is necessary for either scabies or pediculosis.

KEY POINTS TO REMEMBER

- The lesions caused by ectoparasitic infections must be distinguished from the multiple other dermatologic conditions causing pruritic, maculopapular rashes.
- The diagnosis of scabies rests on finding "burrows"; diagnosis of pediculosis depends on finding "nits" at the sites of lesions.

REFERENCES AND SUGGESTED READINGS

Taplin D, Meinking TL. Scabies, lice, and fungal infections. *Primary Care* 1989; 16:551–568.

Wilson WR, Steckelberg JM. Ectoparasitic infestations and arthropod stings and bites. In: Wilson WR, Sande MA, eds. *Current diagnosis and treatment in infectious diseases*. New York: McGraw-Hill, 2001;899–905.

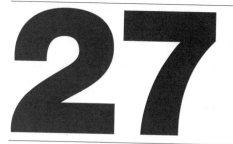

Antimicrobial Agents

David J. Ritchie and
Nathan P. Wiederhold

INTRODUCTION

This chapter provides key microbiologic, pharmacologic, dosing, and safety information for antibacterials, antimycobacterials, antifungals, and antivirals. Throughout this book, readers are referred to this chapter, which is intended to serve as a quick reference to assist prescribers in the clinical use and monitoring of the agents discussed.

The content of this chapter is derived from a multitude of primary, secondary, and tertiary sources. Additional information on products mentioned in this chapter may be obtained from the American Hospital Formulary Service, the *Physicians' Desk Reference*, LexiDrugs PDA reference, *The Pharmacological Basis of Therapeutics* text, product package inserts, and a variety of Web- (e.g., http://www.hopkins-abxguide.org) and print-based sources.

DEFINITIONS

AUC: area under the curve
CrCl: creatinine clearance
CVVHD: continuous venovenous hemodialysis
HD: hemodialysis
PD: peritoneal dialysis
Vd: volume of distribution

ANTIBACTERIAL AGENTS

Beta-Lactams

Beta-lactam antibiotics (PCNs, cephalosporins, carbapenems, monobactams, and carbacephems) **irreversibly bind PCN-binding proteins,** components of the bacterial cell wall, causing osmotic rupture and death. Acquired resistance to beta-lactams occurs in many bacterial species typically through alterations in PCN-binding proteins or the cell wall or through expression of hydrolytic enzymes (beta-lactamases).

The main **side effects** are GI disturbances, hypersensitivity reactions, and phlebitis. Hematologic disturbances, seizures, electrolyte abnormalities, liver function test (LFT) abnormalities, and interstitial nephritis may also rarely occur. Patients receiving high doses of beta-lactams should have their neurologic status **monitored** continuously for the presence of seizure activity. Serum creatinine should be periodically monitored to assess dosing appropriateness and for interstitial nephritis. CBCs should also be monitored for evidence of bone marrow suppression, as should the appearance of the skin for evidence of rash. Serum electrolytes should also be periodically monitored, as electrolyte disturbances may occur.

Penicillins

AMOXICILLIN

Amoxicillin is an oral amino-PCN.

Microbiology: Key Spectrum Aspects
Amoxicillin is similar in spectrum to ampicillin but is more active than ampicillin against *Salmonella* and less active against *Shigella*.

Pharmacokinetics
- **Absorption:** Amoxicillin is 74–92% absorbed into the bloodstream and achieves peak serum concentrations at least twice as high as equivalent doses of PO ampicillin. Food does not significantly decrease the rate and extent of oral absorption of amoxicillin.
- **Distribution:** The Vd is approximately 0.21 L/kg, and the drug is 18% plasma protein bound. Amoxicillin effectively penetrates middle ear fluid.
- **Elimination:** Amoxicillin and its metabolites are primarily excreted in the urine by tubular secretion and glomerular filtration. Approximately 19–33% of amoxicillin is metabolized by hydrolysis to penicilloic acids, which are microbiologically inactive metabolites. Small amounts of the drug are excreted in bile and feces. The elimination half-life is 1.7 hrs in patients with normal renal function but is extended to 5–20 hrs in patients with end-stage renal disease.

Dosing and Administration
The usual dosage range is 250–500 mg q8h or 500–875 mg q12h.
Dosing adjustments:
- **Renal failure:** Patients with CrCl of 10–30 mL/min and <10 mL/min should receive amoxicillin, 250–500 mg q12h and 250–500 mg q24h, respectively.
- **HD:** A dose of 250–500 mg q24 is recommended, with the daily dose administered after each dialysis procedure to account for dialytic elimination.
- **PD:** A dose of 250 mg q12h is recommended.
- **CVVHD:** Amoxicillin is 15–28% eliminated by continuous HD procedures. If the combined dialysate and ultrafiltrate flow rates are ≥1.5 L/hr, the daily dose for HD recommended above should be increased by a factor of 1.4 to compensate for extracorporeal elimination.
- **Hepatic:** No specific dosage adjustments have been recommended.

Safety
- **Drug interactions:** Probenecid increases the peak serum level and half-life by 30–60% and the AUC by 60% due to competitive inhibition of tubular secretion. Administration of amoxicillin with estrogen-containing oral contraceptives may result in decreased contraceptive efficacy.
- **Other key safety issues:** Amoxicillin crosses the placenta and is distributed into breast milk.

AMOXICILLIN/CLAVULANIC ACID

Amoxicillin/clavulanic acid is an oral antibiotic that combines amoxicillin with the beta-lactamase inhibitor clavulanate.

Microbiology: Key Spectrum Aspects
The addition of clavulanic acid to amoxicillin extends or restores the spectrum of amoxicillin to include beta-lactamase–producing strains of oxacillin-sensitive *Staphylococcus aureus* (OSSA), enterococci, anaerobes, *H. influenzae*, *M. catarrhalis*, and some gram-negative bacilli.

Pharmacokinetics
- **Absorption:** Both amoxicillin and clavulanic acid are well absorbed orally into the bloodstream. Food does not significantly affect the rate or extent of oral absorption of amoxicillin or clavulanic acid.
- **Distribution:** The Vd of amoxicillin is approximately 0.21 L/kg, and the drug is 18% plasma protein bound. Clavulanic acid is 22–30% plasma protein bound. Amoxicillin and clavulanic acid both effectively penetrate middle ear fluid.
- **Elimination:** Amoxicillin and its metabolites are primarily excreted in the urine by tubular secretion and glomerular filtration. Approximately 19–33% of amoxicillin is metabolized by hydrolysis to penicilloic acids, which are microbiologically inactive metabolites. Clavulanic acid is extensively metabolized and excreted in the urine by

glomerular filtration. Small amounts of the drug are excreted in bile and feces. The elimination half-lives of amoxicillin and clavulanic acid are 1–1.7 hrs and 0.8–1.2 hrs, respectively, in patients with normal renal function but are extended to up to 7–21 hrs and ≥4–5 hrs, respectively, in patients with severely compromised renal function.

Dosing and Administration
The usual dosage range is (a) 250–500 mg q8h or 500–875 mg q12h of the PO tablets; (b) 90 mg/kg/day divided q12h of the suspension; or (c) 2000 mg PO q12h of the Augmentin XR tablet formulation.

Dosing adjustments:
- **Renal failure:** Patients with CrCl of 15–30 mL/min, 5–15 mL/min, and <5 mL/min should receive amoxicillin/clavulanic acid q12–18h, q24–36h, and q48h, respectively.
- **HD:** A dose of 250–500 mg q24–48h is recommended, with the daily dose on dialysis days administered after the dialysis procedure to account for dialytic elimination.
- **PD:** A dose of 250 mg q12h is recommended.
- **CVVHD:** Consideration could be given to dosing amoxicillin/clavulanic acid like amoxicillin in this setting (see the section Amoxicillin: Dosing and Administration), although no specific guidelines are available.
- **Hepatic:** No specific dosage adjustments have been recommended.

Safety
- **Drug interactions:** Probenecid increases the amoxicillin peak serum level and half-life by 30–60% and the AUC by 60% due to competitive inhibition of tubular secretion. The pharmacokinetics of clavulanic acid are not affected by probenecid. Administration of amoxicillin with estrogen-containing oral contraceptives may result in decreased contraceptive efficacy.
- **Other key safety issues:** Amoxicillin and clavulanic acid both cross the placenta and are distributed into breast milk. The chewable tablets and oral suspension formulations contain aspartame and should thus be used carefully in patients with phenylketonuria.

AMPICILLIN

Ampicillin is an amino-PCN available in parenteral and oral dosage forms.

Microbiology: Key Spectrum Aspects
Ampicillin is considered the drug of choice for treatment of infections caused by susceptible strains of enterococci and *Listeria monocytogenes*.

Pharmacokinetics
- **Absorption:** Oral ampicillin is 30–55% absorbed into the bloodstream. Peak (occurring 2 hrs after an oral dose) and 6-hr trough concentrations of ampicillin, 500 mg PO, are 3–6 and <1 μg/mL, respectively. Food decreases the rate and extent of oral absorption of ampicillin by 50%.
- **Distribution:** The Vd of ampicillin is approximately 0.28 L/kg, and the drug is 18% plasma protein bound. Ampicillin penetrates the CSF poorly; however, when given at high doses in patients with inflamed meninges, it achieves therapeutic concentrations in the CSF.
- **Elimination:** Ampicillin and its metabolites are primarily excreted in the urine by tubular secretion and glomerular filtration. Approximately 7–12% is metabolized by hydrolysis to penicilloic acids, which are microbiologically inactive metabolites. Small amounts of the drug are excreted in bile and feces. The elimination half-life is 1–1.5 hrs in patients with normal renal function but is extended to up to 7–21 hrs in patients with severe renal dysfunction.

Dosing and Administration
The usual dosage range for IV ampicillin is 8–14 g/day administered in divided doses q3–6h or as a continuous infusion. The dose of PO ampicillin is 250–500 mg PO q6h.

Dosing adjustments:
- **Renal failure:** Patients with CrCl of 30–50 mL/min, 10–30 mL/min, and <10 mL/min should receive the usual dose q6–8h, q8–12h, and q12h, respectively.

- **HD:** Patients should receive 25–50% of the normal daily dose (e.g., 2 g IV q12–24h), with one of the daily doses administered after each dialysis procedure to account for dialytic elimination.
- **PD:** Patients should receive a dose of 250 mg–2 g q12h.
- **CVVHD:** Ampicillin is 20–37% eliminated by continuous HD procedures. If the combined dialysate and ultrafiltrate flow rates are ≥1.5 L/hr, the daily dose for HD recommended above should be increased by a factor of 1.6 to compensate for extracorporeal elimination. A suggested dose is 250 mg to 2 g q6–12h.
- **Hepatic:** No specific dosage adjustments have been recommended.

Equivalent oral: ampicillin PO or amoxicillin

Safety
- **Drug interactions:** Probenecid increases the peak serum level and half-life of ampicillin due to competitive inhibition of tubular secretion. Administration of ampicillin with estrogen-containing oral contraceptives may result in decreased contraceptive efficacy.
- **Other key safety issues:** Ampicillin crosses the placenta and is distributed into breast milk.

AMPICILLIN/SULBACTAM

Ampicillin/sulbactam is a parenteral antibiotic that combines ampicillin with the beta-lactamase inhibitor sulbactam.

Microbiology: Key Spectrum Aspects
The addition of sulbactam to ampicillin extends or restores the spectrum of ampicillin to include beta-lactamase–producing strains of methicillin-sensitive *Staphylococcus aureus* (MSSA), enterococci, anaerobes, *Haemophilus influenzae, Moraxella catarrhalis*, and some gram-negative bacilli.

Pharmacokinetics
- **Absorption:** Peak serum concentrations of ampicillin and sulbactam after a 1.5-g dose of ampicillin/sulbactam are 40–71 and 21–40 µg/mL, respectively. Peak serum concentrations of ampicillin and sulbactam after a 3-g dose of ampicillin/sulbactam are 109–150 and 48–88 µg/mL, respectively.
- **Distribution:** The Vd of ampicillin and sulbactam are 0.28 and 0.24–0.4 L/kg, respectively. Ampicillin and sulbactam are 15–28% and 38% plasma protein bound, respectively. Ampicillin and sulbactam penetrate the CSF poorly; however, when given at high doses in patients with inflamed meninges, CSF concentrations are approximately doubled.
- **Elimination:** Ampicillin and sulbactam are primarily (75–92%) excreted in the urine by glomerular filtration and tubular secretion. Approximately 7–12% of ampicillin is metabolized by hydrolysis to penicilloic acids, which are microbiologically inactive metabolites. Small amounts of the drug are excreted in bile and feces. The elimination half-lives of ampicillin and sulbactam are 1–1.5 hrs and 1–1.4 hrs, respectively, in patients with normal renal function. The half-lives of ampicillin and sulbactam are extended to 7–20 hrs and 10–13 hrs, respectively, in patients with end-stage renal disease.

Dosing and Administration
The usual dosage is 1.5–3 g IV q6h.
Dosing adjustments:
- **Renal failure:** Patients with CrCl of 15–30 mL/min and 5–14 mL/min should receive 1.5–3 g IV q12h and q24h, respectively.
- **HD:** A dose of 1.5–3 g IV q24h is recommended, with the daily dose on dialysis days administered after the dialysis procedure to account for dialytic elimination.
- **PD:** A dose of 1.5–3 g IV q24h is recommended.
- **CVVHD:** A dose of 2.25 g IV q12h has been recommended.
- **Hepatic:** No specific dosage adjustments have been recommended.

Equivalent oral: amoxicillin/clavulanic acid (Augmentin)

Safety
- **Drug interactions:** Probenecid increases the peak serum levels and half-lives of ampicillin and sulbactam due to competitive inhibition of tubular secretion. Administration of ampicillin/sulbactam with estrogen-containing oral contraceptives may result in decreased contraceptive efficacy.
- **Other key safety issues:** Ampicillin and sulbactam both cross the placenta and are distributed into breast milk.

DICLOXACILLIN

Dicloxacillin is an orally administered penicillinase-resistant synthetic PCN.

Microbiology: Key Spectrum Aspects
Dicloxacillin is a drug of choice for treating mild MSSA infections, but the agent has minimal activity against enterococci and gram-negative bacteria.

Pharmacokinetics
- **Absorption:** Dicloxacillin is 35–76% absorbed into the bloodstream. Food decreases the rate and extent of oral absorption of dicloxacillin.
- **Distribution:** The Vd is 0.09 L/kg, and the drug is 95–99% plasma protein bound.
- **Elimination:** Approximately 10% of dicloxacillin is metabolized by hydrolysis to penicilloic acids, which are microbiologically inactive metabolites, and by hydroxylation to an active metabolite. Dicloxacillin and its metabolites are primarily excreted in the urine by tubular secretion and glomerular filtration. The drug is also partially excreted in bile and feces. The elimination half-life of dicloxacillin is 0.7 hr in patients with normal renal function but can be extended to 1–2.2 hrs in patients with severely compromised renal function.

Dosing and Administration
The usual dosage range is 125–500 mg q6h.
Dosing adjustments:
- **Renal failure:** No dosage adjustment is required.
- **HD:** No dosage adjustment is required.
- **PD:** No dosage adjustment is required.
- **CVVHD:** No dosage adjustment is required.
- **Hepatic:** Dose reduction is likely unnecessary in patients with hepatic impairment.

Safety
- **Drug interactions:** Probenecid increases the peak serum level and half-life of dicloxacillin due to competitive inhibition of tubular secretion. Administration of dicloxacillin with estrogen-containing oral contraceptives may result in decreased contraceptive efficacy.
- **Other key safety issues:** Dicloxacillin crosses the placenta and is distributed into breast milk.

NAFCILLIN

Nafcillin is a penicillinase-resistant synthetic PCN.

Microbiology: Key Spectrum Aspects
Nafcillin is a drug of choice for treating MSSA infections, but the agent has minimal activity against enterococci and gram-negative bacteria.

Pharmacokinetics
- **Absorption:** Oral nafcillin is poorly absorbed. Food further decreases the rate and extent of oral absorption.
- **Distribution:** The Vd is 0.35 L/kg, and the drug is 89% plasma protein bound.
- **Elimination:** Approximately 60% of nafcillin is metabolized to microbiologically inactive metabolites. Nafcillin and its metabolites are primarily excreted in the bile and urine. The elimination half-life of nafcillin is 1 hr in patients with normal renal function but can be extended to 1.8–2.8 hrs in patients with severely compromised renal function.

Dosing and Administration
The usual dosage range is 4–12 g/day. The usual dose of nafcillin PO is 250–1000 mg q4–6h.

Dosing adjustments:
- **Renal failure:** Nafcillin does not require dosage adjustment in patients with renal failure.
- **HD:** No dosage adjustment is required.
- **PD:** No dosage adjustment is required.
- **CVVHD:** No dosage adjustment is required.
- **Hepatic:** Dose reduction should be considered in patients with significant hepatic impairment, particularly in the setting of combined hepatic and renal insufficiency (consider up to 50% dosage reduction).

Equivalent oral: dicloxacillin or nafcillin

Safety
- **Drug interactions:** Probenecid increases the peak serum level and half-life of nafcillin due to competitive inhibition of tubular secretion. Administration of nafcillin with estrogen-containing oral contraceptives may result in decreased contraceptive efficacy.
- **Other key safety issues:** Neutropenia and interstitial nephritis may occur. Nafcillin crosses the placenta and is distributed into breast milk.
- **Monitoring:** Serum creatinine should be periodically monitored, particularly in patients receiving long courses of nafcillin to monitor for interstitial nephritis. CBCs should be monitored for evidence of bone marrow suppression, particularly neutropenia.

OXACILLIN

Oxacillin is a penicillinase-resistant synthetic PCN.

Microbiology: Key Spectrum Aspects
Oxacillin is a drug of choice for treating MSSA infections, but the agent has minimal activity against enterococci and gram-negative bacteria.

Pharmacokinetics
- **Absorption:** Oral oxacillin is 30–35% absorbed into the bloodstream. Food decreases the rate and extent of oral absorption of oxacillin.
- **Distribution:** The Vd of oxacillin is 0.39–0.43 L/kg, and the drug is 89–94% plasma protein bound.
- **Elimination:** Approximately 49% of oxacillin is metabolized by hydrolysis to penicilloic acids, which are microbiologically inactive metabolites. The drug is also partially metabolized by hydroxylation. Oxacillin and its metabolites are primarily excreted in the urine by tubular secretion and glomerular filtration. Significant amounts of the drug are excreted in bile and feces. The elimination half-life of oxacillin is 0.4–0.7 hrs in patients with normal renal function but can be extended to 0.5–2 hrs in patients with severe renal dysfunction.

Dosing and Administration
The usual dosage range for IV oxacillin is 4–12 g/day. The usual dose of oxacillin PO is 250–500 mg q4–6h.

Dosing adjustments:
- **Renal failure:** Oxacillin does not require dosage adjustment in patients with renal failure.
- **HD:** No dosage adjustment is required.
- **PD:** No dosage adjustment is required.
- **CVVHD:** No dosage adjustment is required.
- **Hepatic:** Dose reduction should be considered in patients with significant hepatic impairment, particularly in the setting of combined hepatic and renal insufficiency (consider up to 50% dosage reduction).

Equivalent oral: dicloxacillin or oxacillin

Safety
- **Drug interactions:** Probenecid increases the peak serum level and half-life of oxacillin due to competitive inhibition of tubular secretion. Administration of oxacillin with estrogen-containing oral contraceptives may result in decreased contraceptive efficacy.
- **Other key safety issues:** Hepatitis may occur, particularly when given at doses ≥12 g/day. Neutropenia has also been associated with oxacillin. Oxacillin crosses the placenta and is distributed into breast milk.
- **Monitoring:** Serum creatinine should be periodically monitored, particularly in patients receiving long courses of oxacillin to monitor for interstitial nephritis. LFTs should be obtained periodically to monitor for hepatotoxicity, especially in patients receiving ≥12 g/day.

PENICILLIN G

Aqueous PCN G is the primary IV preparation of PCN and is available as potassium and sodium salts. PCN VK potassium is the primary oral PCN in use today.

Microbiology: Key Spectrum Aspects
PCN G remains among the drugs of choice for syphilis, *Pasteurella multocida*, *Actinomyces*, and some anaerobic infections. PCN is the drug of choice for group A streptococcal pharyngitis and for prophylaxis of rheumatic fever and poststreptococcal glomerular nephritis.

Pharmacokinetics
- **Absorption:** 1 U each of PCN G sodium and potassium is equivalent to 0.6 and 0.625 μg, respectively. IV doses of PCN G, 2 million U q2h or 3 million U q3h, produce mean serum concentrations of approximately 20 μg/mL.
- **Distribution:** The Vd is 0.53–0.67 L/kg, and the drug is 45–68% plasma protein bound. PCN G penetrates the CSF poorly; however, when given at high doses in patients with inflamed meninges, it achieves therapeutic concentrations in the CSF. Procaine PCN G is an IM form of PCN G rarely used today that maintains measurable serum concentrations of PCN G for 24 hrs after a dose. Benzathine PCN is a long-acting repository form of PCN G commonly used for treating syphilis that provides low and sustained serum levels of PCN for up to 2–3 wks.
- **Elimination:** PCN G and its metabolites are primarily excreted in the urine by tubular secretion, although there is also a small amount of biliary excretion. A total of 16–30% of PCN is metabolized to penicilloic acid, a microbiologically inactive metabolite. Small amounts of PCN are also hydroxylated. The elimination half-life is 0.4–0.9 hrs in patients with normal renal function but is extended to up to 20 hrs in patients with severe renal dysfunction.

Dosing and Administration
The usual dosage range for IV PCN G is 12–30 million U/day administered in divided doses q2–4h or as a continuous infusion. The dose of oral PCN VK is 250–500 mg q6h. The usual dose of procaine PCN is 0.6–1.2 million U/day. The usual dose of benzathine PCN is 1.2–2.4 million U administered intermittently.
Dosing adjustments:
- **HD:** A daily dose equivalent to 20–50% of the normal daily dose (e.g., 2–3 million U/day) is recommended, with one of the daily doses administered after each dialysis procedure to account for dialytic elimination.
- **PD:** 20–50% of the normal daily dose is recommended.
- **CVVHD:** Patients should receive 20–50% of the normal daily dose, as only 12–24% is eliminated by continuous dialysis procedures.
- **Hepatic:** No specific dosage adjustments have been recommended.

Equivalent oral: PCN VK

Safety
- **Drug interactions:** Probenecid increases the peak serum level and half-life of PCN by 24–75% and the AUC by 60–124% due to competitive inhibition of tubular secre-

tion. Administration of PCN VK with estrogen-containing oral contraceptives may result in decreased contraceptive efficacy.
- **Other key safety issues:** Hyperkalemia (particularly with PCN G potassium) and hypokalemia (with PCN G sodium) may occur. Although the potassium salt is the more commonly used PCN G preparation, the sodium salt is available and should be given in the setting of hyperkalemia or azotemia. PCN G crosses the placenta and is distributed into breast milk.

PIPERACILLIN

Piperacillin is an extended-spectrum parenteral PCN.

Microbiology: Key Spectrum Aspects
The extended-spectrum PCNs, including piperacillin, have improved gram-negative activity over other PCN derivatives, including antipseudomonal activity (typically when combined with an aminoglycoside). Piperacillin also has significant activity against enterococci and anaerobes.

Pharmacokinetics
- **Absorption:** The mean peak serum concentration range after a 4-g IV dose is 155–298 μg/mL.
- **Distribution:** The Vd is 0.18 L/kg, and the drug is 16–22% plasma protein bound. Piperacillin penetrates the CSF poorly, but CSF concentrations are increased in the presence of inflamed meninges.
- **Elimination:** Piperacillin is extensively excreted in the urine by glomerular filtration and tubular secretion. A total of 10–20% of the drug is excreted in bile and feces. The elimination half-life of piperacillin is 0.9 hrs in patients with normal renal function but is extended to up to 6 hrs in patients with CrCl <10 mL/min.

Dosing and Administration
The usual dosage range for piperacillin is 2–4 g IV q4–6h.
Dosing adjustments:
- **Renal failure:** Patients with CrCl of 20–40 mL/min and <20 mL/min should receive 3–4 g q8h and 3–4 g q12h, respectively.
- **HD:** Patients on HD should receive 2 g q8h, with one of the daily doses on dialysis days administered after the dialysis procedure to account for dialytic elimination.
- **PD:** A dose of 2 g q8h is recommended.
- **CVVHD:** A dose of 2–4 g q6–8h is recommended, as 17–32% of the drug is removed.
- **Hepatic:** No specific dosage adjustments have been recommended.

Equivalent oral: ciprofloxacin, levofloxacin, or gatifloxacin (for UTI) or ciprofloxacin + either clindamycin or metronidazole (for other systemic infections)

Safety
- **Drug interactions:** Probenecid increases the peak serum level, half-life, and AUC of piperacillin due to competitive inhibition of tubular secretion.
- **Other key safety issues:** Piperacillin crosses the placenta and is distributed into breast milk.

PIPERACILLIN/TAZOBACTAM

Piperacillin is a parenteral combination product containing an extended-spectrum PCN (piperacillin) and a beta-lactamase inhibitor (tazobactam).

Microbiology: Key Spectrum Aspects
The addition of tazobactam to piperacillin enhances the spectrum of piperacillin to include beta-lactamase–producing strains of anaerobes, gram-negative bacilli, staphylococci, and enterococci.

Pharmacokinetics
- **Absorption:** The mean peak serum concentrations of piperacillin and tazobactam after a 3.375-g IV dose (3 g piperacillin, 375 mg tazobactam) are 242 and 24 μg/mL,

respectively. Mean peak serum concentrations after a 4.5-g IV dose (4 g piperacillin, 500 mg tazobactam) are 298 and 34 μg/mL, respectively.

- **Distribution:** The Vd of piperacillin is 0.18 L/kg, and the drug is 16–22% plasma protein bound. Tazobactam is also widely distributed in the body and is 30% plasma protein bound. Piperacillin/tazobactam penetrates the CSF poorly, but CSF concentrations are increased in the presence of inflamed meninges.
- **Elimination:** Piperacillin and tazobactam are extensively excreted in the urine by glomerular filtration and tubular secretion. A total of 10–20% of the drugs are excreted in bile and feces. The elimination half-lives of piperacillin and tazobactam are 0.7–1.2 hrs in patients with normal renal function but are extended 2–4 times in patients with CrCl <20 mL/min.

Dosing and Administration
The usual dosage is 3.375–4.5 g IV q6h.

Dosing adjustments:

- **Renal failure:** Patients with CrCl of 20–40 mL/min and <20 mL/min should receive 2.25 g IV q6h and 2.25 g IV q8h, respectively.
- **HD:** Patients on HD should receive 2.25 g q8h, with one of the daily doses on dialysis days administered after the dialysis procedure to account for dialytic elimination.
- **PD:** A dose of 2.25 g q8h is recommended.
- **CVVHD:** A dose of 2.25 g q6–8h is recommended, as 17–32% of piperacillin is removed.
- **Hepatic:** No specific dosage adjustments have been recommended.

Equivalent oral: PO fluoroquinolone + either clindamycin or metronidazole (for systemic mixed infections)

Safety

- **Drug interactions:** Probenecid increases the half-lives of piperacillin and tazobactam by 21% and 71%, respectively, due to competitive inhibition of tubular secretion.
- **Other key safety issues:** Piperacillin crosses the placenta and is distributed into breast milk. The extent to which tazobactam crosses the placenta and is distributed into breast milk is unknown, although the combination is rated pregnancy category B.

TICARCILLIN/CLAVULANATE

Ticarcillin/clavulanate is a parenteral combination product containing an extended-spectrum PCN (ticarcillin) and a beta-lactamase inhibitor (clavulanate).

Microbiology: Key Spectrum Aspects
The addition of clavulanate to ticarcillin enhances the spectrum of ticarcillin to include beta-lactamase–producing strains of anaerobes, gram-negative bacilli, and staphylococci.

Pharmacokinetics

- **Absorption:** The mean peak serum concentrations of ticarcillin and clavulanate after a 3.1-g IV dose (3 g ticarcillin, 100 mg clavulanic acid) are 324 and 8 μg/mL, respectively.
- **Distribution:** The Vd of ticarcillin is 0.21 L/kg, and the drug is 65% plasma protein bound. Clavulanate has a Vd of 0.31–0.34 L/kg and is 9–30% plasma protein bound. Ticarcillin/clavulanate penetrates the CSF poorly, but CSF concentrations are increased in the presence of inflamed meninges.
- **Elimination:** Ticarcillin/clavulanate is extensively excreted in the urine by glomerular filtration and tubular secretion. The drug is partially excreted in bile and feces. The elimination half-lives of ticarcillin and clavulanate are 1.1–1.2 hrs and 1.1–1.5 hrs, respectively, in patients with normal renal function but are extended to 8.5 hrs and 2.9 hrs, respectively, in patients with CrCl <8 mL/min.

Dosing and Administration
The usual dosage is 3.1 g IV q4–6h.

Dosing adjustments:

- **Renal failure:** Patients with CrCl of 30–60 mL/min, 10–30 mL/min, and <10 mL/min should receive 2 g q4h, 2 g q8h, and 2 g q12h, respectively.

- **HD:** Patients on HD should receive 2 g q12h, with an additional 3.1-g supplemental dose administered after each dialysis session.
- **PD:** A dose of 3.1 g q12h is recommended.
- **CVVHD:** A dose of 2 g q8h is recommended.
- **Hepatic:** Patients with hepatic dysfunction and CrCl <10 mL/min should receive 2 g q24h.

Equivalent oral: PO fluoroquinolone + either clindamycin or metronidazole (for systemic mixed infections)

Safety
- **Drug interactions:** Probenecid increases the peak serum level, half-life, and AUC of ticarcillin due to competitive inhibition of tubular secretion. Serum levels of clavulanate are not affected by probenecid.
- **Other key safety issues:** Fluid overload may occur as a result of the substantial sodium load in the product. Ticarcillin and clavulanate cross the placenta and are distributed into breast milk.

Carbapenems

ERTAPENEM

Microbiology: Key Spectrum Aspects
Ertapenem possesses a broad spectrum of activity that encompasses most strains of anaerobes, gram-negative bacilli, and gram-positive cocci, including strains of these organisms that produce a variety of beta-lactamases. However, ertapenem does not provide reliable coverage against *Pseudomonas aeruginosa, Acinetobacter*, enterococci, methicillin-resistant Staphylococcus aureus (MRSA), and *Stenotrophomonas maltophilia* and is thus not suitable for empiric therapy of nosocomial infections.

Pharmacokinetics
- **Absorption:** The mean peak serum concentration of ertapenem after a 1-g IV dose is 155 μg/mL, with a 24-hr trough level of 1 μg/mL.
- **Distribution:** The Vd is 8.2 L, and the drug is 85–95% plasma protein bound.
- **Elimination:** Ertapenem is eliminated primarily in the urine as both unchanged drug and a metabolite. The half-life is approximately 4 hrs in patients with normal renal function but is significantly extended in patients with CrCl ≤30 mL/min.

Dosing and Administration
The usual dosage is 1 g IV q24h.
Dosing adjustments:
- **Renal failure:** Patients with CrCl ≤30 mL/min should receive 500 mg q24h.
- **HD:** Patients on HD should receive 500 mg q24h, with the daily dose on dialysis days administered after the dialysis procedure to account for dialytic elimination. Alternatively, if ertapenem is given within 6 hrs before any HD session, a 150-mg postdialysis supplemental dose may be given.
- **PD:** No specific dosage adjustments have been recommended.
- **CVVHD:** No specific dosage adjustments have been recommended.
- **Hepatic:** No specific dosage adjustments have been recommended.

Equivalent oral: PO fluoroquinolone + either clindamycin or metronidazole (for systemic mixed infections)

Safety
- **Drug interactions:** Concomitant administration of ertapenem with probenecid results in a slight increase in the ertapenem half-life.
- **Other key safety issues: Seizures may occur,** particularly in patients with renal failure and prior CNS disorders. Patients allergic to PCN may exhibit cross-hypersensitivity reactions with ertapenem. Ertapenem is rated pregnancy category B but should be used in pregnant women with caution due to the minimal experience in this setting. The drug is distributed into breast milk.

- **Monitoring:** Patients receiving ertapenem should have their neurologic status monitored continuously for the presence of seizure activity. Serum creatinine should be periodically monitored to assess dosing appropriateness in an effort to decrease seizure risk.

IMIPENEM/CILASTATIN

Imipenem/cilastatin is a combination product containing a carbapenem (imipenem) and a renal dehydropeptidase inhibitor (cilastatin).

Microbiology: Key Spectrum Aspects
Imipenem possesses an extremely broad spectrum of activity that encompasses most strains of anaerobes, gram-negative bacilli, and gram-positive cocci, including strains of these organisms that produce a variety of beta-lactamases. However, imipenem does not provide reliable coverage against MRSA, *Enterococcus faecium*, and *Stenotrophomonas maltophilia*. Cilastatin is microbiologically inactive but is added to imipenem to prevent renal metabolism by dehydropeptidase I, thus increasing urinary levels of imipenem.

Pharmacokinetics
- **Absorption:** The mean peak serum concentration of imipenem after a 500-mg IV dose is 21–58 μg/mL.
- **Distribution:** The Vd of imipenem is 0.23–0.35 L/kg, and the drug is 13–21% plasma protein bound. Low concentrations (1–10% serum levels) of imipenem reach the CSF.
- **Elimination:** Imipenem is extensively excreted in the urine by glomerular filtration and tubular secretion. <1% of the drug is excreted in bile and feces. The elimination half-life of imipenem is 0.8–1.1 hrs in patients with normal renal function but is extended to 2.7–3.7 hrs in patients with CrCl <10 mL/min.

Dosing and Administration
The usual dosage is 500 mg IV q6h.
Dosing adjustments:
- **Renal failure:**

Body weight (kg)	CrCl (mL/min)			
	≥71	41–70	21–40	6–20
≥70	500 mg q6h	500 mg q8h	250 mg q6h	250 mg q12h
60	500 mg q8h	250 mg q6h	250 mg q8h	250 mg q12h
50	250 mg q6h	250 mg q6h	250 mg q8h	250 mg q12h
40	250 mg q6h	250 mg q8h	250 mg q12h	250 mg q12h
30	250 mg q8h	125 mg q6h	125 mg q8h	125 mg q12h

- **HD:** Patients on HD should receive the dosage recommended in the table above for CrCl 6–20 mL/min adjusted for body weight, with one of the daily doses on dialysis days administered after the dialysis procedure to account for dialytic elimination.
- **PD:** A dosage reduction to 25% of the usual dose is recommended.
- **CVVHD:** Patients should receive the dosage recommended in the 6–20 mL/min CrCl column above, as only 7–15% of imipenem is removed.
- **Hepatic:** No specific dosage adjustments have been recommended.

Equivalent oral: PO fluoroquinolone + either clindamycin or metronidazole (for systemic mixed infections)

Safety
- **Drug interactions:** Concomitant administration of imipenem and ganciclovir may result in an increased risk for seizures.

- **Other key safety issues: Seizures may occur,** particularly in patients with renal failure and prior CNS disorders. Patients allergic to PCN may exhibit cross-hypersensitivity reactions with imipenem. Imipenem crosses the placenta and is distributed into breast milk.
- **Monitoring:** Patients receiving imipenem should have their neurologic status monitored continuously for the presence of seizure activity. Serum creatinine should be periodically monitored to assess dosing appropriateness in an effort to decrease seizure risk.

MEROPENEM

Meropenem is a synthetic carbapenem antibiotic that readily penetrates the cell wall of most gram-positive and gram-negative bacteria to reach PCN-binding protein targets.

Microbiology: Key Spectrum Aspects
Meropenem has a broad spectrum of activity against many gram-positive species, gram-negative aerobes, and anaerobic species. Compared to imipenem, meropenem has slightly more activity against gram-negative organisms and slightly less activity against gram-positive organisms. Meropenem lacks activity against *Stenotrophomonas maltophilia*, *Enterococcus faecium*, and MRSA.

Pharmacokinetics
- **Absorption:** Peak plasma concentrations of meropenem after a 1-g IV dose average 49 μg/mL.
- **Distribution:** The drug distributes widely, including into the CSF. After doses of 2 g three times daily, peak and trough CSF concentrations have been reported as 16 and 0.5 μg/mL, respectively. The Vd of meropenem is 12–20 L with low protein binding (approximately 2%).
- **Elimination:** 62–83% of meropenem is excreted unchanged in the urine. The elimination half-life in patients with normal renal function is approximately 1 hr but increases to ≥6 hrs in patients with CrCl <50 mL/min.

Dosing and Administration
Meropenem may be administered as an IV bolus or infusion over 30 mins. The usual dose is 1 g q8h for systemic infections and 2 g q8h for meningitis.
Dosing adjustments:
- **Renal failure:**

CrCl (mL/min)	Dosing interval
>50 mL/min	1 g q8h
26–50 mL/min	1 g q12h
10–25 mL/min	500 mg q12h
<10 mL/min	500 mg q24h

- **HD:** Dose for CrCl <10 mL/min, with the daily dose given after dialysis.
- **PD:** Dose for CrCl <10 mL/min.
- **CVVHD:** 500 mg q12h.

Equivalent oral: PO fluoroquinolone + either clindamycin or metronidazole (for systemic mixed infections)

Safety
- **Drug interactions:** Probenecid competes with meropenem for active tubular secretion, thus inhibiting the renal excretion of meropenem. This interaction increases the elimination half-life of meropenem and the extent of systemic exposure.
- **Other key safety issues: Seizures may occur,** particularly in patients with renal failure and prior CNS disorders. Patients allergic to PCN may exhibit cross-hypersensitivity reactions with meropenem. The extent of excretion in breast milk is not

known, and meropenem should be used during pregnancy and lactation only if clearly indicated.

- **Monitoring:** Patients receiving meropenem should have their neurologic status monitored continuously for the presence of seizure activity. Serum creatinine should be periodically monitored to assess dosing appropriateness in an effort to decrease seizure risk.

Monobactam

AZTREONAM

Aztreonam is the sole monobactam antibiotic available for clinical use.

Microbiology: Key Spectrum Aspects
Aztreonam possesses a clinically relevant spectrum of activity that encompasses only gram-negative bacteria, including many strains of *P. aeruginosa* and other organisms that produce a variety of beta-lactamases. Aztreonam does not provide reliable coverage against gram-positive or anaerobic bacteria and is also not stable to (a) type I chromosomal cephalosporinases produced by *Enterobacter, Citrobacter freundii, Serratia,* or *Morganella*; or (b) extended-spectrum plasmid-mediated beta-lactamases produced by *Klebsiella, Escherichia coli,* and other gram-negative bacilli.

Pharmacokinetics
- **Absorption:** The mean peak serum concentration of aztreonam after a 1-g IV dose is 90–164 μg/mL.
- **Distribution:** The Vd is 0.11–0.22 L/kg, and the drug is 46–60% plasma protein bound. Aztreonam penetrates the CSF at concentrations 2–30% of serum concentrations in patients with uninflamed meninges; however, CSF concentrations are increased to 3–52% of serum concentration in the presence of inflamed meninges.
- **Elimination:** Aztreonam is extensively excreted in the urine by glomerular filtration and tubular secretion. Up to 11% of the drug is excreted in bile and feces. The elimination half-life of aztreonam is 1.3–2.2 hrs in patients with normal renal function but is extended to approximately 9 hrs in anuric patients.

Dosing and Administration
The usual dosage is 1–2 g IV q8h.
Dosing adjustments:
- **Renal failure:** Patients with CrCl of 10–30 mL/min and <10 mL/min should receive 50% and 25% of the normal dose, respectively.
- **HD:** Patients on HD should receive 1 g IV q24h, with the daily dose on dialysis days administered after the dialysis procedure to account for dialytic elimination.
- **PD:** A dose of 125–500 mg IV q8h is recommended.
- **CVVHD:** A dosage reduction to 50–75% the usual dosage is recommended.
- **Hepatic:** No specific dosage adjustments in patients with hepatic dysfunction have been recommended.

Equivalent oral: PO fluoroquinolone

Safety
- **Drug interactions:** Aztreonam does not appear to have clinically significant drug interactions.
- **Other key safety issues:** Aztreonam crosses the placenta and is distributed into breast milk in low concentrations. In contrast to cephalosporins and carbapenems, aztreonam is considered safe to use in patients with a history of beta-lactam allergy.

Cephalosporins
Cephalosporins kill bacteria by **interfering with cell wall synthesis** by the same mechanism as PCNs. These agents are well tolerated and have a broad spectrum of activity. **First-generation cephalosporins** have activity against staphylococci; streptococci; and many community-acquired *E. coli, Klebsiella* species, and *Proteus* species. These agents have limited activity against other enteric gram-negative rods and anaerobes. Cefazolin is

the most commonly used parenteral first-generation cephalosporin. Cefadroxil, cephalexin, and cephradine are oral preparations of the parenteral first-generation cephalosporins.

Second-generation cephalosporins have expanded coverage against enteric gram-negative rods and are divided into "above the diaphragm" and "below the diaphragm" agents. Cefuroxime is considered an "above the diaphragm" agent and has reasonable staphylococcal and streptococcal activity in addition to an extended spectrum against gram-negative aerobes. This agent does not cover *Bacteroides fragilis*. Cefoxitin and cefotetan are the cephamycins and are considered "below the diaphragm" agents. These agents do not have dependable staphylococcal or streptococcal activity but have an extended spectrum against gram-negative aerobes and anaerobes, including *B. fragilis*. These antibiotics are typically used for intraabdominal or gynecologic surgical prophylaxis and infections, including diverticulitis and PID. Cefuroxime axetil, cefprozil, cefdinir, and cefaclor are oral second-generation cephalosporins typically used for bronchitis, sinusitis, otitis media, UTIs, local soft tissue infections, and step-down therapy for pneumonia or cellulitis responsive to parenteral second-generation cephalosporins. Loracarbef is a carbacephem, rather than a cephalosporin, and is used for generally the same indications as the oral second-generation cephalosporins, with the additional indication for uncomplicated pyelonephritis.

Third-generation cephalosporins have broad coverage against enteric aerobic gram-negative rods, and most retain good activity against streptococci. They have moderate gram-positive anaerobic activity but do not cover *B. fragilis*. Ceftazidime is the only third-generation cephalosporin useful for treating serious *P. aeruginosa* infections. Several of these agents have good CNS penetration and are useful in treating meningitis. Third-generation cephalosporins are not reliable for treatment of organisms producing type I beta-lactamases regardless of the results of susceptibility testing. These microbes should be treated with cefepime, carbapenems, or fluoroquinolones. Ceftriaxone, cefotaxime, and ceftizoxime are very similar in terms of spectrum. Ceftibuten, cefixime, cefpodoxime proxetil, and cefditoren pivoxil are oral third-generation cephalosporins.

The fourth-generation cephalosporin, cefepime, provides the broadest spectrum of the cephalosporins against aerobic gram-negative bacilli, including *P. aeruginosa* and many gram-negative bacilli resistant to third-generation cephalosporins. Cefepime also has significant activity against staphylococci and streptococci but not against *B. fragilis*. Because of its stability to type I beta-lactamases, it is a suitable agent for treatment of infections involving organisms producing these enzymes.

All cephalosporins have been associated with anaphylaxis, interstitial nephritis, anemia, and leukopenia. All patients should be asked about PCN or cephalosporin **allergies.** Patients allergic to PCNs have approximately a 10% incidence of a cross-hypersensitivity reaction to cephalosporins. These agents should not be used in a patient with a reported allergy without prior skin testing or desensitization. Prolonged therapy (>2 wks) is typically monitored with weekly serum creatinine and CBC. Ceftriaxone (and possibly cefoperazone) can cause biliary sludging and symptomatic gallbladder disease requiring discontinuation of the medication. Cefotetan has an *N*-methylthiotetrazole side chain that interferes with vitamin K–dependent clotting factor metabolism and is associated with disulfiram-like reactions with ethanol intake. Cephalosporins containing the *N*-methylthiotetrazole side chain should be avoided when a prolonged course of therapy is likely, as a coagulopathy may develop.

Patients receiving cephalosporins, particularly at high doses and in the presence of renal failure, should have their neurologic status **monitored** continuously for the presence of seizure activity. Serum creatinine should be periodically monitored to assess dosing appropriateness. CBCs should also be monitored for evidence of bone marrow suppression, as should the appearance of the skin for evidence of rash.

FIRST-GENERATION CEPHALOSPORINS

CEFADROXIL

Pharmacokinetics
- **Absorption:** Cefadroxil is extensively absorbed after oral administration, the extent of which is unaffected by food. The mean peak serum concentration after a 1-g oral dose is 24–35 μg/mL.

- **Distribution:** The Vd is 0.22 L/kg, and the drug is 20% plasma protein bound.
- **Elimination:** Cefadroxil is extensively excreted in the urine by glomerular filtration and tubular secretion. Only a minimal amount of the drug is excreted via nonrenal routes. The elimination half-life is 1.1–2 hrs in patients with normal renal function but is extended to up to 26 hrs in patients with CrCl <20 mL/min.

Dosing and Administration
The usual dosage is 1 g twice daily.
Dosing adjustments:
- **Renal failure:** Patients with CrCl of 10–25 mL/min and ≤10 mL/min should receive 1 g q24h and 1 g q36h, respectively.
- **HD:** Patients receiving HD should receive 1 g q24–48h, with the daily dose on dialysis days administered after the dialysis procedure to account for dialytic elimination.
- **PD:** A dose of 500 mg q24h is recommended.
- **CVVHD:** No data are available.
- **Hepatic:** No specific dosage adjustments have been recommended.

CEFAZOLIN

Microbiology: Key Spectrum Aspects
Cefazolin possesses activity against aerobic gram-positive cocci and a limited number of gram-negative bacilli. Cefazolin does not have activity against methicillin-resistant staphylococci, enterococci, *P. aeruginosa*, and other gram-negative organisms that produce a variety of beta-lactamases.

Pharmacokinetics
- **Absorption:** The mean peak serum concentration after a 1-g IV dose is 188 μg/mL.
- **Distribution:** The Vd is 0.12 L/kg, and the drug is 74–86% plasma protein bound. Only low concentrations of cefazolin penetrate the CSF even in the presence of meningeal inflammation; therefore, the agent should not be used for treatment of meningitis.
- **Elimination:** Cefazolin is extensively excreted in the urine by glomerular filtration and tubular secretion. Only a minimal amount of the drug is excreted via nonrenal routes. The elimination half-life of cefazolin is 1.2–2.2 hrs in patients with normal renal function but is extended to up to 57 hrs in anuric patients.

Dosing and Administration
The usual dosage is 1–2 g IV q8h.
Dosing adjustments:
- **Renal failure:** Patients with CrCl of 11–34 mL/min and ≤10 mL/min should receive 1 g q12h and 1 g q24h, respectively.
- **HD:** Patients receiving HD should receive 1 g q24h, with the daily dose on dialysis days administered after the dialysis procedure to account for dialytic elimination.
- **PD:** A dose of 500 mg IV q12h is recommended.
- **CVVHD:** A dose of 1 g q12h is recommended.
- **Hepatic:** No specific dosage adjustments have been recommended.

Equivalent oral: cephalexin or cefadroxil

CEPHALEXIN

Pharmacokinetics
- **Absorption:** Cephalexin is extensively absorbed after oral administration, the extent of which is unaffected by food. The mean peak serum concentration after a 500-mg oral dose is 15–18 μg/mL.
- **Distribution:** The Vd is 0.26 L/kg, and the drug is 14% plasma protein bound.
- **Elimination:** Cephalexin is extensively excreted in the urine by glomerular filtration and tubular secretion. Only a minimal amount of the drug is excreted via nonrenal routes. The elimination half-life is 0.5–1.2 hrs in patients with normal renal function but is extended to up to 14 hrs in anuric patients.

Dosing and Administration
The usual dosage is 250–500 mg PO q6h.
Dosing adjustments:
- **Renal failure:** Patients with CrCl of 11–40 mL/min and ≤10 mL/min should receive 500 mg q8–12h and 250–500 mg q12–24h, respectively.
- **HD:** Patients receiving HD should receive 250–500 mg q12–24h, with one of the daily doses on dialysis days administered after the dialysis procedure to account for dialytic elimination.
- **PD:** A dose of 500 mg q12h is recommended.
- **CVVHD:** As 32–52% is eliminated, a dose of 500 mg q12h (i.e., twice the anuric dose) seems reasonable.
- **Hepatic:** No specific dosage adjustments have been recommended.

CEPHRADINE

Pharmacokinetics
- **Absorption:** Cephradine is extensively absorbed after oral administration, the extent of which is unaffected by food. The mean peak serum concentration after a 500-mg oral dose is 15–18 μg/mL.
- **Distribution:** The Vd is 0.25 L/kg, and the drug is 14% plasma protein bound.
- **Elimination:** Cephradine is extensively excreted in the urine by glomerular filtration and tubular secretion. Only a minimal amount of the drug is excreted via nonrenal routes. The elimination half-life is 0.7–2 hrs in patients with normal renal function but is extended to up to 60 hrs in patients with CrCl <10 mL/min.

Dosing and Administration
The usual dosage is 250–500 mg q6h.
Dosing adjustments:
- **Renal failure:** Patients with CrCl of 5–20 mL/min and ≤5 mL/min should receive 250 mg q6h and 250 mg q12h, respectively.
- **HD:** Patients receiving HD should receive 500 mg q24h, with the daily dose on dialysis days administered after the dialysis procedure to account for dialytic elimination.
- **PD:** A dose of 500 mg q24h is recommended.
- **CVVHD:** As 23–40% is eliminated, a dose of 500 mg q12–24h (i.e., up to 1.5–2 times the anuric dose) seems reasonable.
- **Hepatic:** No specific dosage adjustments have been recommended.

SECOND-GENERATION CEPHALOSPORINS

CEFACLOR

Pharmacokinetics
- **Absorption:** Cefaclor is well absorbed from the GI tract. The extent of absorption is not affected by food. Mean peak serum concentrations after 250- and 500-mg oral doses are 5–7 μg/mL and 13–15 μg/mL, respectively.
- **Distribution:** The Vd is 0.36 L/kg, and the drug is 25% plasma protein bound.
- **Elimination:** Cefaclor is extensively excreted in the urine. Only a minimal amount of the drug is excreted via nonrenal routes. The elimination half-life is 0.5–1 hr in patients with normal renal function but is extended to up to 2.8 hrs in anuric patients.

Dosing and Administration
The usual dosage is 250–500 mg PO q8h for the standard-release preparation or 375 mg q12h for the extended-release preparation.
Dosing adjustments:
- **Renal failure:** Patients with CrCl of 10–50 mL/min and ≤10 mL/min should receive 50–100% of full dosage and 50% of dosage, respectively.
- **HD:** Patients receiving HD should receive 250 PO q8h, with one of the daily doses on dialysis days administered after the dialysis procedure to account for dialytic elimination.
- **PD:** A dose of 250 mg PO q8–12h is recommended.

- **CVVHD:** As only 6–14% of the drug is removed, a dose of 250 mg PO q8h seems reasonable.
- **Hepatic:** No specific dosage adjustments have been recommended.

Safety
Cefaclor has been associated (0.5%) with serum sickness–like reactions, most commonly in children <6. Symptoms of this reaction include rash, arthritis, arthralgia, and fever usually occurring 2–11 days into therapy. Symptoms typically resolve within a few days after discontinuation.

CEFDINIR

Pharmacokinetics
- **Absorption:** Cefdinir has an oral bioavailability of 16–25% that is decreased by 10% in the presence of food. The mean peak serum concentrations after 300- and 600-mg oral doses are 1.6 and 2.9 μg/mL, respectively.
- **Distribution:** The Vd is 0.35–0.67 L/kg, and the drug is 60–70% plasma protein bound.
- **Elimination:** Cefdinir is excreted primarily in the urine, with no appreciable metabolism. The elimination half-life is 1.7–1.8 hrs in patients with normal renal function but is extended to up to 9 hrs in patients with CrCl <30 mL/min.

Dosing and Administration
The usual dosage is 600 mg PO q24h or 300 mg PO q12h.
Dosing adjustments:
- **Renal failure:** Patients with CrCl <30 mL/min should receive 300 mg q24h.
- **HD:** Patients receiving HD should receive 300 mg q24–48h, with the daily dose on dialysis days administered after the dialysis procedure to account for dialytic elimination.
- **PD:** No specific recommendations are available.
- **CVVHD:** No specific recommendations are available.
- **Hepatic:** No specific dosage adjustments have been recommended.

CEFOTETAN

Pharmacokinetics
- **Absorption:** The mean peak serum concentration after a 1-g IV dose is 126–158 μg/mL.
- **Distribution:** The Vd is 0.13 L/kg, and the drug is 88% plasma protein bound. Cefotetan achieves only low concentrations in the CSF and should not be used to treat meningitis.
- **Elimination:** Cefotetan is extensively excreted in the urine by glomerular filtration and tubular secretion. Approximately 20% of the drug is excreted in bile and feces. The elimination half-life is 2.8–4.6 hrs but is extended to up to 35 hrs in patients with CrCl <15 mL/min.

Dosing and Administration
The usual dosage is 1–2 g IV q12h.
Dosing adjustments:
- **Renal failure:** Patients with CrCl of 10–30 mL/min and <10 mL/min should receive 1 g IV q24h and 1 g IV q48h, respectively.
- **HD:** Patients receiving HD should receive 250–500 mg IV q24h on days between dialysis and 500–1000 mg on dialysis days, with the daily dose on dialysis days administered after the dialysis procedure to account for dialytic elimination.
- **PD:** A dose of 1 g IV q24 is recommended.
- **CVVHD:** A dose of 750 mg IV q12h is recommended.
- **Hepatic:** No specific dosage adjustments have been recommended.

Equivalent oral: amoxicillin/clavulanate or (fluoroquinolone + metronidazole)

Safety
Cefotetan may cause bleeding and the disulfiram reaction (when administered concomitantly with alcohol) due to an *N*-methylthiotetrazole side chain contained on the molecule.

CEFOXITIN

Pharmacokinetics
- **Absorption:** The mean peak serum concentration after a 1-g IV dose is 110–125 μg/mL.
- **Distribution:** The Vd is 0.31 L/kg, and the drug is 73% plasma protein bound. Cefoxitin achieves only low concentrations in the CSF and should not be used to treat meningitis.
- **Elimination:** Cefoxitin is extensively excreted in the urine by glomerular filtration and tubular secretion. Approximately 20% of the drug is excreted in bile and feces. The elimination half-life is 0.7–1.1 hrs but is extended to up to 22 hrs in patients with CrCl approximately 2 mL/min.

Dosing and Administration
The usual dosage is 1–2 g IV q6–8h.
Dosing adjustments:
- **Renal failure:** Patients with CrCl of 30–50 mL/min, 10–29 mL/min, 5–9 mL/min, and <5 mL/min should receive 1–2 g q8–12h, 1–2 g q12–24h, 500 mg to 1 g q12–24h, and 500 mg to 1 g q24–48h, respectively.
- **HD:** Patients receiving HD should receive 500 mg to 1 g q24–48h, with the daily dose on dialysis days administered after the dialysis procedure to account for dialytic elimination.
- **PD:** A dose of 1 g IV q24h is recommended.
- **CVVHD:** As 14–27% is eliminated, a dose of 1–2 g q8–12h is recommended.
- **Hepatic:** No specific dosage adjustments have been recommended.

Equivalent oral: amoxicillin/clavulanate or (fluoroquinolone + metronidazole)

CEFPROZIL

Pharmacokinetics
- **Absorption:** Cefprozil is well absorbed from the GI tract, with a bioavailability of 90–95% that is not affected by food. Mean peak serum concentrations after 250- and 500-mg oral doses are 6.1 and 10.5 μg/mL, respectively.
- **Distribution:** The Vd is 0.23 L/kg, and the drug is 35–45% plasma protein bound.
- **Elimination:** Cefprozil is extensively excreted in the urine by glomerular filtration and tubular secretion. Only a minimal amount of the drug is excreted via nonrenal routes. The elimination half-life is 1–1.4 hrs in patients with normal renal function but is extended to up to 5.9 hrs in patients with renal impairment.

Dosing and Administration
The usual dosage is 250–500 mg PO q12h.
Dosing adjustments:
- **Renal failure:** Patients with CrCl <30 mL/min should receive 250–500 mg PO q24h.
- **HD:** Patients receiving HD should receive 250–500 PO q24h, with the daily dose on dialysis days administered after the dialysis procedure to account for dialytic elimination.
- **PD:** A dose of 250–500 mg PO q24h is recommended.
- **CVVHD:** A dose of 250–500 mg PO q24h is recommended.
- **Hepatic:** No specific dosage adjustments have been recommended.

CEFUROXIME

Pharmacokinetics
- **Absorption:** The mean peak serum concentration after a 750-mg IV dose is 51 μg/mL.
- **Distribution:** The Vd is 0.19 L/kg, and the drug is 33% plasma protein bound. Cefuroxime achieves low concentrations in the CSF, but therapeutic CSF levels may be achieved in the presence of inflamed meninges.
- **Elimination:** Cefuroxime is extensively excreted in the urine by glomerular filtration and tubular secretion. Only a minimal amount of the drug is excreted via nonrenal routes. The elimination half-life of cefuroxime is 1–2 hrs in patients with normal renal function but is extended to up to 15–22 hrs in anuric patients.

Dosing and Administration
The usual dosage is 750 mg to 1.5 g IV q8h.
Dosing adjustments:
- **Renal failure:** Patients with CrCl of 10–20 mL/min and ≤10 mL/min should receive 750 mg IV q12h and 750 mg IV q24h, respectively.
- **HD:** Patients receiving HD should receive 750 mg q24h, with the daily dose on dialysis days administered after the dialysis procedure to account for dialytic elimination.
- **PD:** A dose of 750 mg q24h is recommended.
- **CVVHD:** As 47–67% of the drug is removed, a dose of 1 g IV q12h is recommended.
- **Hepatic:** No specific dosage adjustments have been recommended.

Equivalent oral: cefuroxime axetil

CEFUROXIME AXETIL

Pharmacokinetics
- **Absorption:** Cefuroxime axetil is absorbed from the GI tract and hydrolyzed to cefuroxime by esterases in the intestine. The bioavailability is 37% and 52% in fasting and fed states, respectively. Mean peak serum concentrations of cefuroxime after 250- and 500-mg oral doses are 4.1 and 7 μg/mL, respectively.
- **Distribution:** The Vd is 0.19 L/kg, and the drug is 33% plasma protein bound.
- **Elimination:** Cefuroxime is extensively excreted in the urine by glomerular filtration and tubular secretion. Only a minimal amount of the drug is excreted via nonrenal routes. The elimination half-life is 1–2 hrs in patients with normal renal function but is extended to up to 15–22 hrs in anuric patients.

Dosing and Administration
The usual dosage is 250–500 mg PO q12h.
Dosing adjustments:
- **Renal failure:** Patients with CrCl of 10–50 mL/min and ≤10 mL/min may still receive 250–500 mg PO q12h.
- **HD:** Patients receiving HD should receive 250–500 mg PO q12h, with one of the daily doses on dialysis days administered after the dialysis procedure to account for dialytic elimination.
- **PD:** A dose of 250–500 mg PO q12h is recommended.
- **CVVHD:** As 47–67% of the drug is removed, a dose of 500 mg PO q12h seems reasonable.
- **Hepatic:** No specific dosage adjustments have been recommended.

THIRD-GENERATION CEPHALOSPORINS

CEFDITOREN PIVOXIL

Pharmacokinetics
- **Absorption:** Cefditoren pivoxil is hydrolyzed to cefditoren in the GI tract where it is absorbed. The absolute bioavailability under fasting conditions or with a low-fat meal ranges from 14% to 16%. Administration with a high-fat meal increases AUC and peak concentrations by 70% and 50%, respectively. Concomitant ingestion with magnesium- and aluminum-containing antacids and H_2-blockers decreases absorption of cefditoren. The mean peak serum concentration after a 400-mg oral dose is 4.4 μg/mL.
- **Distribution:** The Vd is 9.3 L, and the drug is 88% plasma protein bound.
- **Elimination:** Cefditoren is excreted primarily in the urine. The elimination half-life is 1.6 hrs in patients with normal renal function but is extended in patients with renal insufficiency.

Dosing and Administration
The usual dosage is 200–400 mg PO q12h with food.
Dosing adjustments:
- **Renal failure:** Patients with CrCl of 30–49 mL/min and <30 mL/min should receive 200 mg PO q12h and 200 mg PO q24h, respectively.

- **HD:** HD removes 30% of cefditoren but does not affect the elimination half-life. No dosage recommendations have been made in this setting.
- **PD:** No recommendations are available.
- **CVVHD:** No recommendations are available.
- **Hepatic:** No specific dosage adjustments have been recommended.

Miscellaneous: Cefditoren decreases serum levels of carnitine, the clinical significance of which is unknown. However, carnitine levels normalize after 7–10 days. The tablets are also formulated with sodium caseinate (milk protein), and patients with a history of milk protein sensitivity should not receive cefditoren tablets.

CEFIXIME

Pharmacokinetics
- **Absorption:** Cefixime is 30–50% absorbed from the GI tract. Food decreases the rate but not the extent of absorption. The mean peak serum concentrations after 200- and 400-mg oral doses are 2 and 3.7 μg/mL, respectively.
- **Distribution:** The Vd is 0.1 L/kg, and the drug is 65–70% plasma protein bound.
- **Elimination:** Cefixime is excreted in the urine by glomerular filtration and tubular secretion. A significant amount of the drug (up to 60%) is eliminated by nonrenal routes, including biliary excretion. The elimination half-life is 2.4–4 hrs in patients with normal renal function but is extended to up to 11.5 hrs in patients with CrCl of 5–20 mL/min.

Dosing and Administration
The usual dosage is 400 mg PO q24h or 200 mg PO q12h.
Dosing adjustments:
- **Renal failure:** Patients with CrCl of 21–60 mL/min and <20 mL/min should receive 300 mg q24h and 200 mg PO q24h, respectively.
- **HD:** Patients receiving HD should receive 300 mg q24h, with the daily dose on dialysis days administered after the dialysis procedure to account for dialytic elimination.
- **PD:** A dose of 200 mg PO q24h is recommended.
- **CVVHD:** No specific recommendations are available.
- **Hepatic:** No specific dosage adjustments have been recommended.

CEFOTAXIME

Pharmacokinetics
- **Absorption:** The mean peak serum concentration after a 1-g IV dose is 41–46 μg/mL. Serum levels 6 hrs after a 1-g dose average 1.1–1.6 μg/mL.
- **Distribution:** The Vd is 0.23 L/kg, and the drug is 36% plasma protein bound. Cefotaxime penetrates the CSF and achieves concentrations clinically useful for treatment of meningitis.
- **Elimination:** Cefotaxime is partially metabolized in the liver to a microbiologically active metabolite, desacetylcefotaxime. Cefotaxime and desacetylcefotaxime are extensively eliminated in the urine. The elimination half-lives of cefotaxime and desacetylcefotaxime are 1–1.7 hrs and 1.4–1.9 hrs, respectively. The half-lives of cefotaxime and desacetylcefotaxime are extended to up to 1.4–11.5 hrs and 8.2–56.8 hrs, respectively, in patients with CrCl <10 mL/min.

Dosing and Administration
The usual dosage is 1 g q6–8h for most infections and 2 g q4h for treatment of meningitis.
Dosing adjustments:
- **Renal failure:** The dose should be reduced to 1 g q8–12h and 1 g q24h in patients with CrCl of 10–50 mL/min and <10 mL/min, respectively.
- **HD:** Patients receiving HD should receive 1 g q24h, with the daily dose on dialysis days administered after the dialysis procedure.
- **PD:** A dose of 1 g q24h is recommended.
- **CVVHD:** A dose of 1 g q12–24h is recommended, as only 7–14% of the drug is removed.
- **Hepatic:** No specific dosage adjustments in patients have been recommended.

Equivalent oral: cefpodoxime, cefixime, ceftibuten, moxifloxacin, gatifloxacin, levofloxacin

CEFPODOXIME PROXETIL

Pharmacokinetics
- **Absorption:** Cefpodoxime is 50% absorbed from the GI tract, and bioavailability is increased 21–33% in the presence of food. Cefpodoxime is a prodrug that must be hydrolyzed to active cefpodoxime by esterases in the GI tract. The mean peak serum concentrations after 100-, 200-, and 400-mg oral doses are 1.4, 2.3, and 3.9 μg/mL, respectively.
- **Distribution:** The Vd is 0.7–1.2 L/kg, and the drug is 21–29% plasma protein bound.
- **Elimination:** Cefpodoxime is excreted in the urine (53%) and feces (43%). The elimination half-life is 2.1–2.9 hrs in patients with normal renal function but is extended to up to 9.8 hrs in patients with CrCl of 5–29 mL/min.

Dosing and Administration
The usual dosage is 100–400 mg PO q12h.
Dosing adjustments:
- **Renal failure:** Patients with CrCl <30 mL/min should receive 100–400 mg q24h.
- **HD:** Patients receiving HD should receive 100–400 mg q24–48h, with the daily dose on dialysis days administered after the dialysis procedure to account for dialytic elimination.
- **PD:** A dose of 100–400 mg PO q24–48h is recommended.
- **CVVHD:** No specific recommendations are available.
- **Hepatic:** No specific dosage adjustments have been recommended.

CEFTAZIDIME

Pharmacokinetics
- **Absorption:** The mean peak serum concentration after a 1-g IV dose is 69 μg/mL. Serum levels 8 hrs after a 1-g dose average 1.9–3.2 μg/mL.
- **Distribution:** The Vd is 0.23 L/kg, and the drug is 21% plasma protein bound. Ceftazidime penetrates the CSF and achieves concentrations clinically useful for treatment of gram-negative meningitis.
- **Elimination:** Ceftazidime is excreted extensively in the urine by glomerular filtration. The elimination half-life is approximately 1.6 hrs in patients with normal renal function but is extended to up to 12–35 hrs in patients with CrCl <10 mL/min.

Dosing and Administration
The usual dosage is 1–2 g q8h for most infections and 2 g q8h for treatment of gram-negative meningitis.
Dosing adjustments:
- **Renal failure:** Patients with CrCl of 10–50 mL/min and <10 mL/min should receive 1 g q12–24h and 1 g q24–48h, respectively.
- **HD:** A dose of 1 g q24–48h is recommended, with the daily dose on dialysis days administered after the dialysis procedure.
- **PD:** A dose of 500 mg q24h is recommended.
- **CVVHD:** A dose of 1 g q24h seems reasonable, as 38–58% of the drug is removed.
- **Hepatic:** No specific dosage adjustments have been recommended.

Equivalent oral: ciprofloxacin

CEFTIBUTEN

Pharmacokinetics
- **Absorption:** Ceftibuten is extensively absorbed from the GI tract, with a bioavailability of 75–90% that is decreased 8–17% in the presence of food. The mean peak serum concentration after a 400-mg oral dose is 15–17.6 μg/mL.
- **Distribution:** The Vd is 0.21–0.5 L/kg, and the drug is 65% plasma protein bound.
- **Elimination:** Ceftibuten is excreted in the urine (57–70%) and feces (39%). The elimination half-life is 2–2.6 hrs in patients with normal renal function but is extended to up to 22.3 hrs in patients with CrCl <5 mL/min.

Dosing and Administration
The usual dosage is 400 mg PO q24h.
Dosing adjustments:
- **Renal failure:** Patients with CrCl of 30–49 mL/min and 5–29 mL/min should receive 200 mg PO q24h and 100 mg PO q24h, respectively.
- **HD:** Patients receiving HD should receive 400 mg q24–48h, with the daily dose on dialysis days administered after the dialysis procedure to account for dialytic elimination.
- **PD:** A dose of 100 mg PO q24h (i.e., 25% usual dose) is recommended.
- **CVVHD:** A dose of 200 mg PO q24h is recommended.
- **Hepatic:** No specific dosage adjustments have been recommended.

CEFTIZOXIME

Pharmacokinetics
- **Absorption:** The mean peak serum concentration after a 1-g IV dose is 84.4 μg/mL. Serum levels 8 hrs after a 1-g dose average 1.4 μg/mL.
- **Distribution:** The Vd is 0.36 L/kg, and the drug is 28% plasma protein bound. Ceftizoxime penetrates the CSF in the presence of inflamed meninges, but clinical data and experience are lacking in this setting relative to cefotaxime and ceftriaxone.
- **Elimination:** Ceftizoxime is primarily eliminated in the urine by glomerular filtration and tubular secretion. The elimination half-life is 1.4–1.9 hrs but is extended to 30 hrs in patients with CrCl of 0–1.2 mL/min.

Dosing and Administration
The usual dosage is 1–2 g q8–12h.
Dosing adjustments:
- **Renal failure:** The dose should be reduced to 1 g q12–24h and 1 g q24h in patients with CrCl of 10–50 mL/min and <10 mL/min, respectively.
- **HD:** Patients receiving HD should receive 1 g q24h, with the daily dose on dialysis days administered after the dialysis procedure.
- **PD:** A dose of 500 mg to 1 g q24h is recommended.
- **CVVHD:** A dose of 1 g q12–24h is recommended.
- **Hepatic:** No specific dosage adjustments have been recommended.

Equivalent oral: cefpodoxime, cefixime, or ceftibuten

CEFTRIAXONE

Pharmacokinetics
- **Absorption:** The mean peak serum concentration after a 1-g IV dose is 123–151 μg/mL. Serum levels 24 hrs after a 1-g dose average 4.6–9.3 μg/mL.
- **Distribution:** The Vd is 0.16 L/kg, and the drug is 90–95% plasma protein bound. Ceftriaxone penetrates the CSF and achieves concentrations clinically useful for treatment of meningitis.
- **Elimination:** Ceftriaxone undergoes both biliary excretion into feces and renal elimination via glomerular filtration. The elimination half-life is approximately 7.3 hrs in patients with normal renal function but is extended to up to 12–18 hrs in patients with CrCl <5 mL/min.

Dosing and Administration
The usual dosage is 1–2 g q24h for most infections and 2 g q12h for treatment of meningitis.
Dosing adjustments:
- **Renal failure:** No dosage adjustments are recommended in patients with impaired renal function.
- **HD:** No dosage adjustments are recommended, as ceftriaxone is not removed by HD.
- **PD:** No dosage adjustments are recommended, as ceftriaxone is not removed by PD.
- **CVVHD:** No dosage adjustments are recommended, as only 12–23% of the drug is removed.
- **Hepatic:** No specific dosage adjustments have been recommended.

Equivalent oral: cefpodoxime, cefixime, ceftibuten, moxifloxacin, gatifloxacin, or levofloxacin

Safety
Ceftriaxone may cause biliary sludging and stones due to its high extent of biliary excretion and resultant precipitation with bile salts.

FOURTH-GENERATION CEPHALOSPORINS

CEFEPIME

Pharmacokinetics
- **Absorption:** The mean peak serum concentration after a 1-g IV dose is 66–82 μg/mL. Serum levels 8 hrs after a 1-g dose average 2.4 μg/mL.
- **Distribution:** The Vd is 13–22 L, and the drug is 20% serum protein bound. Cefepime penetrates the CSF and achieves concentrations clinically useful for treatment of meningitis.
- **Elimination:** Cefepime is primarily eliminated in the urine by glomerular filtration. The elimination half-life is 2–2.3 hrs in patients with normal renal function but is extended to up to 13.5 hrs in patients with CrCl <10 mL/min.

Dosing and Administration
The usual dosage is 1–2 g q8–12h for most infections and 2 g q8h for use in febrile neutropenia.
Dosing adjustments:
- **Renal failure:** The dose should be reduced to 1–2 g q24h, 500 mg to 1 g q24h, and 250–500 mg q24h in patients with CrCl of 30–60 mL/min, 11–29 mL/min, and <11 mL/min, respectively.
- **HD:** Patients receiving HD should receive 250–500 mg q24h, with the daily dose on dialysis days administered after the dialysis procedure.
- **PD:** A dose of 1 g q24–48h is recommended.
- **CVVHD:** A dose of 1 g q12h is recommended.
- **Hepatic:** No specific dosage adjustments have been recommended.

Equivalent oral: ciprofloxacin

CARBACEPHEM

LORACARBEF

Pharmacokinetics
- **Absorption:** Loracarbef is 90% absorbed from the GI tract. Food decreases the peak concentration by approximately 50%, but the AUC remains unaffected by food. The mean peak serum concentrations of cefpodoxime after 200- and 400-mg oral doses are 8 and 14 μg/mL, respectively, for the tablets and 17 μg/mL for a 400-mg dose of the suspension.
- **Distribution:** Loracarbef has a Vd of 0.27–0.39 L/kg, and the drug is 25% plasma protein bound.
- **Elimination:** Loracarbef is extensively eliminated in the urine. The elimination half-life is 1 hr in patients with normal renal function but is extended to up to 32 hrs in patients with CrCl <10 mL/min.

Dosing and Administration
The usual dosage is 200–400 mg PO q12h on an empty stomach.
Dosing adjustments:
- **Renal failure:** Patients with CrCl of 10–50 mL/min and <10 mL/min should receive 200–400 mg q24h and 200–400 mg PO q3–5d, respectively.
- **HD:** Patients receiving HD should receive 200–400 mg q3–5d and after each dialysis session.
- **PD:** A dose of 200–400 mg PO q3–5d is recommended.
- **CVVHD:** A dose of 200–400 mg q24h is recommended.
- **Hepatic:** No specific dosage adjustments have been recommended.

Macrolides and Azalides

Macrolides and azalides block protein synthesis in bacteria by binding the 50S subunit of the bacterial ribosome. These antibiotics are commonly used to treat upper and lower respiratory tract infections. Macrolides and azalides possess activity against many typical and atypical respiratory tract pathogens, including *Streptococcus pneumoniae*, *Mycoplasma pneumoniae*, *Chlamydia pneumoniae*, and *Legionella pneumophila*. In addition, clarithromycin and azithromycin provide coverage against *H. influenzae* as well as *Mycobacterium avium* complex infections.

AZITHROMYCIN

Microbiology: Key Spectrum Aspects
Azithromycin provides reliable coverage against *H. influenzae*; in addition, it is therapeutically useful for treatment of *M. avium* complex infections and some STDs (chlamydia, gonorrhea, PID, chancroid).

Pharmacokinetics
- **Absorption:** The drug has an oral bioavailability of 34–52% that is unaffected by food. The mean peak serum concentration after a 500-mg oral dose is 0.41 μg/mL. The trough concentration 24 hrs after 250 mg oral daily dosing is 0.05 μg/mL. The mean peak and trough concentrations after a 500-mg IV dose are 3.6 and 0.2 μg/mL, respectively.
- **Distribution:** Azithromycin distributes widely into infected tissues and cells, achieving concentrations in these sites significantly exceeding serum concentrations. The drug is 7–51% plasma protein bound and has a Vd of 31 L/kg.
- **Elimination:** Azithromycin is eliminated primarily by biliary excretion and transintestinal elimination. The drug is only minimally excreted in the urine. The elimination half-life is 68 hrs.

Dosing and Administration
The usual dosage is 250–500 mg PO q24h or 500 mg IV q24h.
Dosing adjustments:
- **Renal failure:** Dose reduction is not required in the presence of renal insufficiency.
- **HD:** No dosage adjustment is required.
- **PD:** No dosage adjustment is required.
- **CVVHD:** No dosage adjustment is required.
- **Hepatic:** No specific dosage adjustments have been recommended.

Safety
- **Adverse effects:** Adverse effects include GI disturbances, elevations in LFTs, hepatic dysfunction, IV site reactions, rash, and, rarely, ototoxicity at high sustained doses.
- **Drug interactions:** Unlike erythromycin and clarithromycin, azithromycin does not inhibit cytochrome P450 hepatic enzymes and is not associated with drug interactions involving this mechanism.
- **Other key safety issues:** Azithromycin is pregnancy category B and has been safely used in pregnant women. The drug is also distributed in breast milk.

CLARITHROMYCIN

Microbiology: Key Spectrum Aspects
Clarithromycin provides reliable coverage against *H. influenzae* primarily by virtue of its active 14-hydroxy metabolite (14-hydroxyclarithromycin); in addition, it is therapeutically useful for treatment of *M. avium* complex infections and *Helicobacter pylori*–associated peptic ulcer disease.

Pharmacokinetics
- **Absorption:** The drug has an oral bioavailability of 50–55% that is unaffected by food. The mean peak serum concentration after a 500-mg oral dose of standard-release clarithromycin is 3–4 μg/mL. The mean peak serum concentration after a 1000-mg dose of the extended-release formulation is 2–3 μg/mL.

- **Distribution:** Clarithromycin is 42–72% plasma protein bound and has a Vd of 2.6 L/kg.
- **Elimination:** Clarithromycin is eliminated by both hepatic metabolism and renal excretion (40%). The elimination half-life is 5–7 hrs.

Dosing and Administration

The usual dosage is 250–500 mg PO q12h or 1000 mg PO q24h for the extended-release formulation.

Dosing adjustments:
- **Renal failure:** Patients with CrCl <30 mL/min should receive 50% of the usual dose.
- **HD:** No dosage adjustment is required.
- **PD:** No dosage adjustment is required.
- **CVVHD:** No dosage adjustment is required.
- **Hepatic:** No specific dosage adjustments in patients with hepatic dysfunction have been recommended, but some reduction in dose may be advisable, as 25% higher peak concentrations have been achieved in these patients.

Safety

- **Adverse effects:** Adverse effects include GI disturbances, taste disturbances, elevations in LFTs, hepatic dysfunction, headache, rash, and, rarely, ototoxicity at high doses.
- **Drug interactions:** Clarithromycin is a significant inhibitor of hepatic cytochrome P450 enzymes and can increase serum levels of pimozide, cisapride, carbamazepine, HMG CoA reductase inhibitors, cyclosporine, tacrolimus, theophylline, warfarin, ergotamine, dihydroergotamine, triazolam, and possibly many other drugs.
- **Other key safety issues:** Clarithromycin is pregnancy category C and should be avoided in pregnancy.

ERYTHROMYCIN

Microbiology: Key Spectrum Aspects

Erythromycin does not provide reliable coverage against *H. influenzae*, but it does possess clinically useful activity against *Chlamydia trachomatis* and *Campylobacter*.

Pharmacokinetics

- **Absorption:** The mean peak serum concentrations after 250-mg oral doses of erythromycin base, estolate, and stearate are approximately 0.3–0.4, 1.4, and 0.4 μg/mL, respectively. A 400-mg oral dose of erythromycin ethylsuccinate produces similar peak concentrations. A 200-mg IV dose of erythromycin lactobionate produces a peak serum concentration of 3 μg/mL.
- **Distribution:** The Vd of erythromycin is 0.78 L/kg, and the drug is 84% serum protein bound. Only low concentrations of erythromycin are achievable in the CSF. The drug does cross the placenta and is distributed in breast milk.
- **Elimination:** Erythromycin is primarily eliminated unchanged in the bile. The drug is also partially metabolized in the liver to inactive metabolites and undergoes minimal renal elimination. The elimination half-life is 1.6 hrs.

Dosing and Administration

The usual dosage of erythromycin is 250–500 mg PO q6h (base, estolate, stearate), 333 mg PO q8h (base), or 400 mg PO q6h (ethylsuccinate). The usual IV dose of erythromycin lactobionate is 500 mg to 1 g IV q6h.

Dosing adjustments:
- **Renal failure:** Dose reduction is not required in the presence of renal insufficiency.
- **HD:** No dosage adjustment is required.
- **PD:** No dosage adjustment is required.
- **CVVHD:** No dosage adjustment is required.
- **Hepatic:** No specific dosage adjustments in patients with hepatic dysfunction have been recommended, but some reduction in dose may be advisable, as 25% higher peak concentrations have been achieved in these patients.

Safety

- **Adverse effects:** Adverse effects include GI disturbances, elevations in LFTs, hepatic dysfunction, phlebitis (with IV), rash, and ototoxicity at high doses.

- **Drug interactions:** Erythromycin is a significant inhibitor of hepatic cytochrome P450 enzymes and can increase serum levels of pimozide, cisapride, carbamazepine, hepatic 3-methylglutaryl coenzyme A (HMG CoA) reductase inhibitors, cyclosporine, tacrolimus, theophylline, warfarin, ergotamine, dihydroergotamine, triazolam, and possibly many other drugs.
- **Other key safety issues:** Erythromycins cross the placenta and are distributed in breast milk. Erythromycin may be safely used in pregnant and lactating women.

Aminoglycosides

Aminoglycosides kill bacteria by **binding to the bacterial ribosome** causing misreading during translation of bacterial messenger RNA into proteins. These drugs are commonly used in severe infections caused by gram-negative aerobes as adjunctive agents and may also be used to provide synergistic activity with beta-lactams and vancomycin in the treatment of severe gram-positive infections. These agents have diminished activity in the low-pH/low-oxygen environment of abscesses and do not have activity against anaerobes. Use of these antibiotics is limited by significant nephrotoxicities and ototoxicities. Resistance to one aminoglycoside is not routinely associated with resistance to all members of this class; in cases of serious infections, susceptibility testing with each aminoglycoside is appropriate.

Traditional dosing of aminoglycosides is q8h, with the upper end of the dose range reserved for life-threatening infections. Peak and trough levels should be obtained with the third or fourth dose and then every 3–4 days along with a serum creatinine. Increasing serum creatinine or peaks/troughs out of the acceptable range require immediate attention. Traditional dosing should be used for pregnant patients and in patients with endocarditis, burns covering >20% of the body, cystic fibrosis, anasarca, and CrCl <20 mL/min. For all other indications, extended-interval dosing is more convenient for both the patient and physician.

Extended-interval dosing of aminoglycosides is an alternative method of administration. Extended-interval doses are given below with each drug. A drug level is obtained 6–14 hrs after the first dose, and a nomogram is consulted to determine the dosing interval. Monitoring includes obtaining a drug level at 6–14 hrs after the dosage every week and a serum creatinine thrice weekly. In patients who are not responding to therapy a 12-hr level should be checked; if that level is undetectable, extended-interval dosing should be abandoned in favor of traditional dosing. For obese patients [actual weight >20% above **ideal body weight (IBW)**], an **obese dosing weight (ODW)** must be used for determining doses in either traditional or extended-interval dosing:

$$ODW = IBW + 0.4 \text{ (actual weight } - IBW)$$

Ototoxicity and nephrotoxicity are associated with administration of aminoglycosides. Nephrotoxicity usually occurs after ≥5 days of therapy and is characterized by a reduction in glomerular filtration rate (GFR). Risk factors include hypotension, duration of therapy, associated liver disease, increased serum trough concentrations, advanced age, and coadministration of other nephrotoxic agents. The renal dysfunction noted is generally nonoliguric and is usually reversible with discontinuation of the agent. Ototoxicity associated with aminoglycosides is usually irreversible and may be vestibular or auditory. The hearing loss typically affects high-tone frequencies. Vestibular damage may manifest as nystagmus, vertigo, nausea, or vomiting. Aminoglycosides may also rarely cause neuromuscular blockade. Underlying conditions or the use of other medications that affect the neuromuscular junction enhances this effect. Hypokalemia and hypomagnesemia may also occur.

Patients receiving aminoglycosides should be **monitored** for nephrotoxicity and ototoxicity. Serum creatinine should be monitored closely as well as serum drug levels, with the dose and frequency adjusted accordingly. Patients receiving aminoglycosides for extended periods should have baseline and regularly scheduled audiometric studies to assess for ototoxicity. Patients receiving other nephrotoxic or ototoxic agents should receive aminoglycosides with caution and be monitored closely.

Aminoglycosides can cause fetal harm when given to pregnant women. These agents are able to cross the placenta and may cause otologic damage. These agents should only be used during pregnancy if the potential benefits outweigh the possible risks to the fetus.

AMIKACIN

Microbiology: Key Spectrum Aspects

Amikacin has *in vitro* activity against a wide range of aerobic gram-negative bacilli and methicillin-susceptible *S. aureus*. When organisms are susceptible to gentamicin, amikacin offers no therapeutic advantage. However, amikacin does offer advantages for treating infections caused by organisms resistant to other aminoglycosides. Amikacin is also useful in the treatment of infections caused by *Nocardia asteroides*, *M. avium-intracellulare*, and certain species of rapid-growing mycobacteria (*Mycobacteria chelonae* and *Mycobacteria fortuitum*). As with other aminoglycosides, amikacin lacks activity against anaerobic organisms and *S. maltophilia*.

Pharmacokinetics

- **Absorption:** Amikacin should be administered IV or IM. After IM administration, amikacin is completely absorbed, with maximum serum levels being reached in 30–90 mins.
- **Distribution:** The Vd is 0.2–0.3 L/kg, with approximately 4% bound to proteins. The Vd increases in edematous states, including ascites, in burn patients, and in some severe infections. Amikacin, as with other aminoglycosides, poorly crosses the blood-CSF and blood-brain barriers. Therapeutic concentrations are achieved in the heart, bone, gallbladder, and lung tissue. Amikacin is also well distributed into bile; sputum; bronchial secretions; and interstitial, pleural, and synovial fluids.
- **Elimination:** In adults, 94–98% of a single IM or IV dose is excreted unchanged in the urine by glomerular filtration. The plasma elimination half-life is usually 2–3 hrs in adults with normal renal function but may increase to 30–86 hrs in patients with severe renal impairment.

Dosing and Administration

Amikacin may be given in multiple daily doses. The multiple daily dosing regimen usually consists of doses of 5–7.5 mg/kg q8h. This dose is calculated on IBW, unless the patient is obese (actual body weight >1.2 × IBW) or if actual body weight is <IBW. For obese patients, the ODW is calculated using the following equation:

$$ODW = IBW + 0.4 \text{ (actual weight} - IBW)$$

With the multiple daily dose regimens, serum peaks and troughs should be measured once the patient is at steady state. Serum peak concentrations should be 20–30 μg/mL, with troughs of 5–10 μg/mL.

Amikacin may also be given as a single daily dose. The recommended dose with this regimen is 15 mg/kg, with a random level checked 6–14 hrs after the initial dose. The dosing interval should then be adjusted based on this random level using a nomogram.

Single daily dosing is not recommended for use in patients with enterococcal endocarditis, pregnant patients, children, patients with severe renal insufficiency or renal failure, those with cystic fibrosis, and patients with increased Vds (e.g., anasarca, burn patients).

Dosing adjustments:

- **HD:** 50–100% of a dose may be removed by HD. 50–100% of the full dose may be administered after dialysis on dialysis days only, with close monitoring of serum levels to avoid toxicity.
- **CAPD:** Dose for CrCl <20 mL/min.
- **CVVHD:** 100% of dose q24–48h, with close monitoring of serum levels.

- **Renal failure:** In patients with renal insufficiency receiving multiple daily doses (5–7.5 mg/kg), the interval should be adjusted to maintain a steady-state trough concentration of 5–10 μg/mL. Estimated dosing intervals are as follows:

CrCl (mL/min)	Frequency
>60	q8h
40–60	q12h
20–40	q24h
<20	× 1, monitor levels

Equivalent oral: ciprofloxacin

GENTAMICIN

Microbiology: Key Spectrum Aspects

Gentamicin has *in vitro* activity against a wide range of aerobic gram-negative bacilli as well as methicillin-susceptible *S. aureus*. Gentamicin lacks *in vitro* activity against a number of bacteria, including *S. pneumoniae*, *S. maltophilia*, *Burkholderia cepacia*, and anaerobic organisms. It may be used in combination with a cell wall–active agent for the treatment of viridans group streptococci as well as susceptible *Enterococcus* species.

Pharmacokinetics

- **Absorption:** Gentamicin should be administered IV or IM. After IM administration, gentamicin is completely absorbed, with maximum serum levels being reached in 30–90 mins.
- **Distribution:** The Vd is 0.2–0.3 L/kg, with approximately 10% bound to proteins. The Vd increases in edematous states, including ascites, in burn patients, and in some severe infections. Gentamicin poorly crosses the blood-CSF and blood-brain barriers and is found in small concentrations within bronchial secretions.
- **Elimination:** Gentamicin is almost completely excreted (>90%) as unchanged drug in the urine within the first 24 hrs after a dose. The half-life is 2–3 hrs but increases in patients with renal insufficiency.

Dosing and Administration

Gentamicin may be given in multiple daily doses. The multiple daily dosing regimen usually consists of doses of 1–1.5 mg/kg q8h. This is calculated on IBW, unless the patient is obese (actual body weight >1.2 × IBW) or if actual body weight is <IBW. For obese patients, the ODW is calculated using the following equation:

$$ODW = IBW + 0.4 \text{ (actual weight} - IBW)$$

Loading doses may be used in severely ill patients and range from 2 to 2.5 mg/kg. With the multiple daily dosing regimens, serum peaks and troughs should be measured once the patient is at steady state. For UTIs and gram-positive synergy, the recommended peak concentration (measured 30 mins after the end of the infusion or ≥1 hr after an IM dose) is 3–5 μg/mL, with troughs of <2 μg/mL. For severe systemic infections, higher peaks of 6–10 μg/mL may be needed.

Gentamicin may also be given as a single daily dose. The recommended dose with this regimen is 5 mg/kg, with a random level checked 6–14 hrs after the initial dose. The dosing interval should then be adjusted based on this random level using a nomogram. Estimated dosing intervals are as follows:

CrCl (mL/min)	Dosing interval
≥60	q24h
40–59	q36h
20–39	q48h
<20	Do not use nomogram

Single daily dosing is not recommended for use in patients with enterococcal endocarditis, pregnant patients, children, patients with severe renal insufficiency or failure, those with cystic fibrosis, and patients with increased Vds (e.g., anasarca, burn patients).

Dosing adjustments:

- **Renal failure:** In patients with renal insufficiency receiving multiple daily doses (1–1.5 mg/kg), the interval should be adjusted to maintain a steady-state trough concentration of $<2\,\mu g/mL$.
- **HD:** 50% of a dose may be removed by HD. 50–100% of the full dose may be administered after dialysis on dialysis days only, with close monitoring of serum peak levels to avoid toxicity.
- **PD:** 1 mg/kg may be given q12h after a loading dose of 2 mg/kg, with close monitoring of serum levels.
- **CVVHD:** 30–70% of the usual dose may be given q12h, with close monitoring of serum levels.

Equivalent oral: ciprofloxacin

STREPTOMYCIN

Microbiology: Key Spectrum Aspects

Streptomycin is generally less active than other aminoglycosides against aerobic gram-negative bacilli. Like other aminoglycosides, it does have activity against tularemia and plague. Streptomycin also has some activity against *Mycobacterium tuberculosis*.

Pharmacokinetics

- **Absorption:** Streptomycin should be administered IM. Although not approved for IV administration, streptomycin has been safely administered by this route in situations in which IM administration is impractical. After IM administration, streptomycin is completely absorbed, with maximum serum levels reached in 1–2 hrs and reported between 25 and 50 $\mu g/mL$ after a single 1-g dose.
- **Distribution:** The Vd is 0.25 L/kg, with 48% bound to plasma proteins. The Vd increases in edematous states, including ascites, in burn patients, and in some severe infections. Streptomycin is distributed into most body tissues and fluids with the exception of the CNS. Substantial amounts have been reported in the pleural fluid and within tuberculous cavities.
- **Elimination:** 30–90% of a single IM dose is excreted unchanged in the urine by glomerular filtration. The plasma half-life is usually 2–3 hrs in adults with normal renal function but may increase to up to 110 hrs in patients with severe renal impairment.

Dosing and Administration

Tuberculosis

- Daily therapy: 15 mg/kg/day (maximum, 1 g)
- Twice-weekly therapy: 25–30 mg/kg (maximum, 1.5 g)
- thrice-weekly therapy: 25–30 mg/kg (maximum, 1.5 g)

Tularemia and Synergy for Endocarditis

15 mg/kg (up to 1 g) q12h in combination with cell wall–active agent (e.g., PCN, ampicillin)

Brucellosis

15 mg/kg (up to 1 g) once to twice daily for the first week of therapy, followed by once-daily dosing for ≥1 additional wk

Elderly

In elderly patients, doses of 10 mg/kg/day to a maximum of 750 mg/day have been recommended.

Calculation

The dose is calculated on IBW, unless the patient is obese (actual body weight $>1.2 \times$ IBW) or if actual body weight is <IBW. For obese patients, the ODW is calculated using the following equation:

$$ODW = IBW + 0.4 \text{ (actual weight} - IBW)$$

Monitoring

Serum concentrations should be monitored once steady state is achieved and the frequency or dose modified in response. Peak levels should be 20–30 μg/mL, and serum troughs should be <5 μg/mL.

Dosing adjustments

- **Renal failure:** In patients with renal insufficiency, the interval should be adjusted to maintain a steady-state trough concentration of <5 μg/mL. In persons with mild renal insufficiency (i.e., CrCl of 50–80 mL/min), a loading dose of 1 g may be administered, followed by maintenance doses of 7.5 mg/kg q24h. For patients with a CrCl estimated to be 10–50 mL/min and <10 mL/min, doses should be administered q24–72h and q72–96h, respectively.
- **HD:** Streptomycin is removed by HD. 50–100% of the usual dose should be administered postdialysis days, with close monitoring of serum levels.
- **CVVHD:** Dose q24–72h, with close monitoring of serum levels.

Safety

IM injections of streptomycin are often painful. Hot, tender masses may develop at sites of injection.

TOBRAMYCIN

Microbiology: Key Spectrum Aspects

- Tobramycin's *in vitro* activity is very similar to that of gentamicin, covering a wide range of aerobic gram-negative bacilli and methicillin-susceptible *S. aureus*. Its *in vitro* activity against some strains of *Acinetobacter* species and *P. aeruginosa* may be greater than that of gentamicin. Organisms that are resistant to gentamicin are also usually resistant to tobramycin. Tobramycin lacks *in vitro* activity against a number of bacteria, including *S. pneumoniae*, *S. maltophilia*, *B. cepacia*, and anaerobic organisms. It may be used in combination with a cell wall–active agent for the treatment of viridans group streptococci as well as susceptible *Enterococcus* species.

Pharmacokinetics

- **Absorption:** Tobramycin should be administered IV or IM. After IM administration, tobramycin is completely absorbed, with maximal serum levels achieved in 30–90 mins.
- **Distribution:** The Vd is approximately 0.25 L/kg, with between 0 and 30% protein binding. The Vd increases in edematous states, including ascites, in burn patients, and in some severe infections. After systemic administration, tobramycin does distribute to bronchial secretions.
- **Elimination:** The majority of tobramycin (60–85%) is excreted unchanged in the urine. The half-life is 1.6–3 hrs in patients with normal renal function. This half-life increases to >50 hrs in patients with renal failure.

Dosing and Administration

Tobramycin may be given in multiple daily doses. The multiple daily dosing regimen usually consists of doses of 1–1.5 mg/kg q8h. This is calculated on IBW, unless the patient is obese (actual body weight >1.2 × IBW) or if actual body weight is <IBW. For obese patients, the ODW is calculated using the following equation:

$$ODW = IBW + 0.4 \text{ (actual weight} - IBW)$$

Loading doses may be used in severely ill patients and range from 2 to 2.5 mg/kg. With the multiple daily dose regimens, serum peaks and troughs should be measured once the patient is at steady state. For UTIs and gram-positive synergy, the recommended peak concentration (measured 30 mins after the end of the infusion or ≥1 hr after an IM dose) ranges between 3 and 5 μg/mL, with troughs of <1–2 μg/mL. For severe systemic infections, higher peaks of 6–10 μg/mL may be needed.

Tobramycin may also be given as a single daily dose. The recommended dose with this regimen is 5 mg/kg, with a random level checked 6–14 hrs after the initial dose. The dosing interval should then be adjusted based on this random level using a nomogram. Estimated dosing intervals are as follows:

CrCl (mL/min)	Dosing interval
≥60	q24h
40–59	q36h
20–39	q48h
<20	Do not use nomogram

Single daily dosing is not recommended for use in patients with enterococcal endocarditis, pregnant patients, children, patients with severe renal insufficiency or failure, those with cystic fibrosis, and patients with increased Vds (e.g., anasarca, burn patients).

Dosing adjustments:

- **Renal failure:** In patients with renal insufficiency receiving multiple daily doses (1–1.5 mg/kg), the interval should be adjusted to maintain a steady-state trough concentration of <2 μg/mL.
- **HD:** 50% of a dose may be removed by HD. 50–100% of the full dose may be administered after dialysis on dialysis days only, with close monitoring of serum peak levels to achieve the target level and to avoid toxicity.
- **PD:** 1 mg/kg may be given q12h after a loading dose of 2 mg/kg, with close monitoring of serum levels.
- **CVVHD:** 30–70% of the usual dose may be given q12h, with close monitoring of serum levels.

Equivalent oral: ciprofloxacin

Fluoroquinolones

Fluoroquinolones kill bacteria by **inhibiting bacterial DNA gyrase** and **topoisomerase** critical for DNA replication. In general, these antibiotics are well absorbed orally, with serum levels that approach parenteral therapy. With the addition of new fluoroquinolones, the spectrum of activity in this class of antibiotics rivals that of the cephalosporins. These agents typically have poor activity against enterococci, although they may have some efficacy for UTIs when other agents are inactive or contraindicated. Newer fluoroquinolones have activity against MSSA but should be considered only when oxacillin, nafcillin, and first-generation cephalosporins are contraindicated or inactive. Moxifloxacin and gatifloxacin have reasonable anaerobic activity, possibly expanding their role in mixed aerobic or anaerobic infections. Moxifloxacin, gatifloxacin, and levofloxacin are useful for sinusitis, bronchitis, COPD, and community-acquired pneumonia. These agents are also reasonable therapy for soft tissue infections if PCNs or cephalosporins are inactive or contraindicated. These newer quinolones should not be routinely used to treat diabetic foot infections until there are clinical trials to support their use for this indication. Some of these agents have reasonable activity against mycobacteria and have a potential role in treating drug-resistant TB and atypical mycobacterial infections.

The principal **adverse reactions** with fluoroquinolones include nausea, CNS disturbances (drowsiness, headache, restlessness, and dizziness, especially in the elderly), rashes, and phototoxicity. These agents can cause prolongation of the QT interval and should not be used in patients with known conduction abnormalities on ECG, patients with bradycardia, those with uncorrected hypokalemia, and those receiving class IA or III antiarrhythmic agents. It should also be used with caution in patients receiving agents that may have an additive effect in prolonging the QT interval (e.g., cisapride, erythromycin, antipsychotics, and TCAs) and in patients with ongoing proarrhythmic conditions (e.g., significant bradycardia, acute myocardial ischemia). Patients at risk should be monitored closely with the use of ECGs. In patients with hepatic dysfunction or those receiving other hepatotoxic drugs, LFTs should be monitored.

Fluoroquinolones should not be used routinely in patients <18 yrs or in pregnant or lactating women. They cause an age-related arthropathy and should be discontinued in patients who develop joint pain or tendinitis (Achilles tendon). Aluminum- and magnesium-containing antacids, sucralfate, bismuth, oral iron, oral calcium, and oral zinc preparations can markedly impair absorption of oral quinolones.

Animal studies have shown fluoroquinolones to cause chondrocyte toxicity. As a class, these agents have been associated with arthralgias and tendon disorders with the possibility of tendon rupture. **Fluoroquinolones should only be used during pregnancy if the potential benefits outweigh the possible risks to the fetus.**

During therapy, patients should be **monitored** for possible CNS side effects, such as dizziness, confusion, and lightheadedness. Patients should be counseled to use caution when performing tasks requiring alertness or coordination. They should also be counseled to not take products containing divalent metallic cations at the same time as PO ciprofloxacin but to separate the doses. Excess sunlight should also be avoided.

CIPROFLOXACIN

Microbiology: Key Spectrum Aspects
Ciprofloxacin has *in vitro* activity against a wide range of gram-negative aerobes, including Enterobacteriaceae, *P. aeruginosa*, and other non-Enterobacteriaceae. It does possess *in vitro* activity against some gram-positive aerobes, such as *S. aureus* and *Enterococcus* species. However, ciprofloxacin may not be clinically reliable in the treatment of infections caused by these organisms.

Pharmacokinetics
- **Absorption:** The bioavailability is 60–70% after oral administration. Maximum serum concentrations of 2.4 and 4.6 μg/mL are reached after an oral dose of 500 mg and an IV dose of 400 mg, respectively. Approximately 40% of the drug is bound to plasma proteins.
- **Distribution:** Ciprofloxacin distributes widely, with a Vd of 1.2–2 L/kg. Tissues and fluids to which ciprofloxacin distributes include bile, CSF, gallbladder, vagina, endometrium, myometrium, liver, pleural fluid, prostatic tissue, peritoneal fluid, sputum, and synovial fluid, as well as the tonsils. Tissues and fluids in which concentrations exceed those found in the serum include prostate tissue, bile, and lung tissue.
- **Elimination:** 30–60% of a dose is excreted as unchanged drug in the urine. Ciprofloxacin is metabolized by the liver to at least four metabolites. The half-life is 4–6 hrs.

Dosing and Administration
For most infections, an oral dose of 500 mg q12h may be used. For more severe or complicated infections, up to 750 mg q12h may be used. The normal IV dose is 400 mg q12h. For uncomplicated acute cystitis, doses of 100–250 mg q12h or 500 mg qd of the extended-release formulation for 3 days have been used successfully. Duration of therapy depends on the type and severity of infection. The usual IV dose is 400 mg IV q12h. For more severe respiratory tract infections, doses of 400 mg q8h have also been used.

Dosing adjustments:
- **Renal failure:** The half-life of ciprofloxacin is increased in patients with decreased renal function. The normal doses may be used until estimated CrCl falls <30 mL/min. At this point, ciprofloxacin may be administered q24h.
- **HD:** Doses of 200–400 mg q24h (administered after dialysis on days receiving dialysis) may be used.
- **PD:** A dose of 200–250 mg q8h has been recommended.
- **CVVHD:** A dose of 200–400 mg q12h may be used.

GATIFLOXACIN

Gatifloxacin is an 8-methoxy-fluoroquinolone antibiotic that inhibits topoisomerase II (DNA gyrase) and topoisomerase IV, which are required for bacterial DNA replication, transcription, repair, and recombination. Its structure contains a methoxy group at the C-8 position.

Microbiology: Key Spectrum Aspects

Gatifloxacin has a broad spectrum of activity, including gram-positive and gram-negative bacteria. Its *in vitro* activity against *S. pneumoniae* is greater than that of ciprofloxacin and levofloxacin. However, gatifloxacin's activity against gram-negative bacilli, including *P. aeruginosa*, is inferior to ciprofloxacin. The *in vitro* activity against anaerobes is similar to that of moxifloxacin.

Pharmacokinetics

- **Absorption:** The oral bioavailability is 96% and is unaffected by food. Peak serum concentrations of 3.4–4.3 μg/mL are achieved 1–2 hrs after a 400-mg oral dose and 4.6 μg/mL after a 400-mg IV dose. Approximately 20% of the medication is bound to plasma proteins.
- **Distribution:** Gatifloxacin has a Vd of 1.7–2.0 L/kg and is widely distributed. Concentrations similar to those found in the plasma are achieved in prostatic fluid, saliva, and seminal fluid. Concentrations found in the kidneys and lungs exceed those obtained in the plasma.
- **Elimination:** >70% of a dose is excreted as unchanged drug in the urine, with concentrations reaching 440 μg/mL after a single oral 400-mg dose. The half-life is 7–8 hrs.

Dosing and Administration

The usual recommended dose is 400 mg IV or PO for 7–10 days.

Dosing adjustments:

- **Renal failure, HD, PD:** The elimination of gatifloxacin is affected by renal insufficiency. In patients with an estimated CrCl <40 mL/min or those receiving HD or PD, the manufacturer recommends an initial dose of 400 mg followed by a subsequent dose of 200 mg q24h.

GEMIFLOXACIN

Gemifloxacin is an oral fluoroquinolone antibiotic that inhibits topoisomerase II (DNA gyrase) and topoisomerase IV, which are required for bacterial DNA replication, transcription, repair, and recombination.

Microbiology: Key Spectrum Aspects

Gemifloxacin's spectrum of activity includes both gram-positive and gram-negative bacteria. Its *in vitro* activity against *S. pneumoniae* is greater than that of ciprofloxacin, levofloxacin, gatifloxacin, and moxifloxacin. The drug possesses significant activity against *Haemophilus influenzae*, *Moraxella catarrhalis*, and the atypical respiratory tract pathogens and also provides some activity against many *Enterobacteriaceae* and *Pseudomonas aeruginosa*.

Pharmacokinetics

- **Absorption:** Gemifloxacin has an oral bioavailability of 71% that is unaffected by food. The mean peak serum concentration and AUC are 1.6 μg/mL and 9.9 μg $\times$ hr/mL, respectively.
- **Distribution:** The volume of distribution is 4.2 L/kg, and the drug is 60–70% protein bound. The drug is extensively distributed in respiratory tissues.
- **Elimination:** Gemifloxacin undergoes renal excretion and a limited degree of hepatic metabolism not mediated by cytochrome P450 enzymes. The elimination half-life is 7 hrs.

Dosing and Administration

The usual dosage is 320 mg PO q24h.

Dosing adjustments:

- **Renal failure:** The dose should be decreased to 160 mg q24h for CrCl ≤40 mL/min.

- **HD:** A dose of 160 mg q24h is recommended.
- **PD:** No recommendations are available.
- **CVVHD:** No recommendations are available.
- **Hepatic:** Dosage reduction is unnecessary in patients with mild to moderate hepatic dysfunction.

Safety
- **Other key safety issues:** Skin rash occurs in 2.8% of patients; approximately 10% of these cases are severe. The incidence of skin rash may be >15% in women under age 40 yrs who receive 10 days of therapy. Women, patients under the age of 40 yrs, and postmenopausal women receiving hormone replacement therapy are at increased risk of rash.

LEVOFLOXACIN

Levofloxacin is the active *l*-isomer of racemate ofloxacin. Levofloxacin inhibits topo-isomerase II (DNA gyrase) and topoisomerase IV, which are required for bacterial DNA replication, transcription, repair, and recombination.

Microbiology: Key Spectrum Aspects
Levofloxacin's spectrum of activity includes gram-positive and gram-negative bacteria. Its *in vitro* activity against *S. pneumoniae* is greater than that of ciprofloxacin but less than that of gatifloxacin and moxifloxacin. Levofloxacin's activity against gram-negative bacilli, including *P. aeruginosa*, is inferior to ciprofloxacin.

Pharmacokinetics
- **Absorption:** Levofloxacin has excellent bioavailability, with approximately 99% absorbed after an oral dose. After an oral dose of 500 mg, peak serum concentrations of 5.2–5.7 μg/mL are reached within 1.1–1.3 hrs. After IV administration, a peak concentration of 6.4 μg/mL is obtained.
- **Distribution:** The Vd is 1.1–1.3 L/kg. 24–38% of the drug is bound to plasma proteins. Levofloxacin is widely distributed into many sites, including the CNS, ocular fluid, prostate tissue, maxillary sinus mucosa, tonsils, and salivary glands. Lung tissue concentrations generally exceed those found in the plasma.
- **Elimination:** Levofloxacin is primarily eliminated in the urine, with approximately 60–80% found as unchanged drug in the urine. Minimal hepatic metabolism to inactive metabolites does occur. The half-life of levofloxacin is 6–8 hrs.

Dosing and Administration
The usual recommended dose is 500 mg IV or PO q24h. Doses of 750 mg q24h have been used for complicated skin and skin structure infections and pneumonia.

Dosing adjustments:
- **Renal failure:** Levofloxacin requires adjustment for renal dysfunction as follows:

	CrCl (mL/min)		
Dose	**≥50**	**20–49**	**10–19**
500 mg	500 mg q24h	500 mg × 1, 250 mg q24h	500 mg × 1, 250 mg q48h
750 mg	750 mg q24h	750 mg × 1, 500 mg q24h	750 mg × 1, 500 mg q48h

- **HD, PD:** An initial dose of 500 mg should be given, followed by 250 mg q48h.
- **CVVHD:** An initial dose of 500 mg should be given, followed by 250 mg q24–48h.

MOXIFLOXACIN

Moxifloxacin is an 8-methoxy-fluoroquinolone antibiotic that inhibits topoisomerase II (DNA gyrase) and topoisomerase IV, which are required for bacterial DNA replication, transcription, repair, and recombination. Its structure contains a methoxy group at the C-8 position.

Microbiology: Key Spectrum Aspects

Moxifloxacin has a broad spectrum of activity, including gram-positive and gram-negative bacteria. Its *in vitro* activity against *S. pneumoniae* is greater than that of ciprofloxacin and levofloxacin. However, moxifloxacin's activity against gram-negative bacilli, including *P. aeruginosa*, is inferior to ciprofloxacin. The *in vitro* activity against anaerobes is similar to that of gatifloxacin.

Pharmacokinetics

- **Absorption:** Moxifloxacin is nearly completely absorbed after oral administration, with an oral bioavailability of 86–90%. After multiple oral doses of 400 mg, daily peak plasma concentrations (Cmax) have been reported to be 3.8–4.6 mg/L, with a time to maximum plasma concentration of 1.25–1.5 hrs.
- **Distribution:** The Vd is 2.0–3.5 L/kg, with 40–50% bound to serum proteins.
- **Elimination:** Moxifloxacin is metabolized via glucuronide and sulfate conjugation to inactive metabolites without the involvement of the cytochrome P450 system. The half-life is 12 hrs, and approximately 45% of a PO or IV dose is excreted as unchanged drug (approximately 20% in the urine and approximately 25% in the feces).

Dosing and Administration

The recommended dose is 400 mg IV or PO once daily. The duration of therapy depends on the type of infection but ranges from 5 to 14 days.

Dosing adjustments:
- **Renal failure, HD, PD, CVVHD:** Moxifloxacin's pharmacokinetics are not significantly altered by renal impairment, and no dosage adjustments are necessary. However, the effect of HD, PD, or CVVHD on moxifloxacin has not been studied.

Other Antibacterials

CHLORAMPHENICOL

Microbiology: Key Spectrum Aspects

Chloramphenicol is a bacteriostatic antibiotic that binds to the 50S ribosomal subunit blocking protein synthesis in susceptible bacteria. It has broad activity against aerobic and anaerobic gram-positive and -negative bacteria, including *S. aureus*, enterococci, some Enterobacteriaceae, and *Bacteroides*. It also is active against spirochetes, *Rickettsia*, *Mycoplasma*, and *Chlamydia*. Today, it is used almost exclusively as an alternative treatment for serious VRE infections.

Pharmacokinetics

- **Absorption:** Chloramphenicol is no longer available as a PO preparation in the United States. Peak serum levels after a 1-g IV dose are 4.9–12 μg/mL. Peak serum levels should be monitored to ascertain that concentrations are kept below 25 μg/mL, at which point the risk of hematologic toxicity increases.
- **Distribution:** Chloramphenicol is widely distributed in tissues and fluids, including the CSF where it achieves concentrations that are 21–89% of serum levels. The drug is 60% plasma protein bound and has a Vd of 0.94 L/kg.
- **Elimination:** Chloramphenicol is primarily metabolized in the liver but also is 5–30% excreted unchanged in the urine. The half-life is 1.5–4.1 hrs.

Dosing and Administration

The usual dose is 50–100 mg/kg/day given in divided doses q6h. The dose should be adjusted based on the results of plasma concentration monitoring to achieve concentrations below 25 μg/mL and $\geq$5 μg/mL.

Dosing adjustments:
- **Renal failure:** No dosage adjustment is required.
- **HD:** No dosage adjustment is required.
- **PD:** No dosage adjustment is required.

- **CVVHD:** No dosage adjustment is required.
- **Hepatic:** A 50% initial dosage reduction in patients with severe hepatic dysfunction should be considered. Subsequent dosage should be determined based on plasma concentrations.

Safety
- **Adverse effects:** Idiosyncratic (non–dose-related) aplastic anemia (approximately 1/30,000) and dose-related bone marrow suppression are the principal toxicities. Peak drug levels (1 hr postinfusion) should be checked every 3–4 days (goal peak, <25 μg/mL), and doses should be adjusted accordingly. CBCs and serum iron (which typically increases with developing dose-related hematologic toxicity) should be carefully monitored. Dosage adjustment is necessary in the presence of significant liver disease. Other possible side effects include circulatory collapse (gray syndrome), GI disturbances, hypersensitivity reactions, and optic neuritis.
- **Drug interactions:** Chloramphenicol can increase serum levels of warfarin, phenytoin, and tolbutamide. Phenobarbital may decrease chloramphenicol concentrations.
- **Other key safety issues:** Chloramphenicol crosses the placenta and distributes into breast milk. Therefore, the agent should be avoided or used only with extreme caution in these populations to minimize the possibility of circulatory collapse (gray syndrome) in infants.

CLINDAMYCIN

Microbiology: Key Spectrum Aspects
Clindamycin is a lincosamide with predominantly a gram-positive spectrum similar to that of erythromycin, with inclusion of activity against most anaerobes, including *B. fragilis*. Clindamycin also provides activity against a significant number of MRSA isolates. Clindamycin is commonly used to treat osteomyelitis, anaerobic pulmonary infections, peritonsillar/retropharyngeal abscesses, necrotizing fasciitis, and group A streptococcal infections. Metronidazole is more commonly used for intraabdominal infections due to its superior activity against *B. fragilis* relative to clindamycin. Clindamycin has additional uses, including treatment of babesiosis (in combination with quinine), toxoplasmosis (in combination with pyrimethamine), and *Pneumocystis jiroveci* pneumonia (in combination with primaquine).

Pharmacokinetics
- **Absorption:** The drug has an oral bioavailability of 90% that is unaffected by food. The mean peak serum concentration after a 150-mg oral dose is 1.9–3.9 μg/mL, with a trough concentration of 0.7 μg/mL 6 hrs later. The mean peak concentration after a 600-mg IV dose is 10 μg/mL.
- **Distribution:** Clindamycin distributes widely into tissues and fluids except the CSF. The drug penetrates bone and joints at concentrations of 60–80% of the concomitant serum levels. The drug is 93% plasma protein bound and has a Vd of 1.1 L/kg.
- **Elimination:** Clindamycin is extensively metabolized in the liver to active and inactive metabolites. The drug is only minimally excreted in the urine. The elimination half-life is 2–3 hrs.

Dosing and Administration
The usual dosage is 150–450 mg PO q6h or 300–900 mg IV q8h.
Dosing adjustments:
- **Renal failure:** Dose reduction is not required in the presence of renal insufficiency.
- **HD:** No dosage adjustment is required.
- **PD:** No dosage adjustment is required.
- **CVVHD:** No dosage adjustment is required.
- **Hepatic:** No specific dosage adjustments have been recommended.

Safety
- **Adverse effects:** GI disturbances (including *Clostridium difficile* colitis), elevations in LFTs, IV site reactions (with IV), rash, and neuromuscular blockade may occur.
- **Drug interactions:** Clindamycin may enhance the activity of neuromuscular blockers and should be used cautiously in this setting.

- **Other key safety issues:** Clindamycin is pregnancy category B and distributes in breast milk.

COLISTIN

Microbiology: Key Spectrum Aspects
Colistin is a bactericidal polypeptide antibiotic that acts by disrupting the cell membrane of gram-negative bacteria. This drug has a role in the treatment of multiple drug-resistant gram-negative rods (except *Proteus* and *Serratia*), primarily *P. aeruginosa* in patients with cystic fibrosis or bronchiectasis; however, it should only be given under guidance of an experienced clinician, as parenteral therapy has significant CNS side effects and potential nephrotoxicity. Inhaled colistin is better tolerated with only mild upper airway irritation and has some efficacy as adjunctive therapy for *P. aeruginosa*. The drug is not active against gram-positive bacteria.

Pharmacokinetics
- **Absorption:** The peak serum level is approximately 5–7 μg/mL after a 2.5-mg/kg dose.
- **Distribution:** The drug distributes into many tissues and fluids, except CSF, synovial, pleural, or pericardial fluids likely due to the large molecular size of the drug. Colistin is 50% plasma protein bound.
- **Elimination:** The drug is excreted mainly by the kidneys unchanged and as metabolites. The half-life is 10–20 hrs but may be prolonged to 2–3 days in patients with severe renal failure.

Dosing and Administration
The usual dose of colistin IV is 2.5–5 mg/kg/day divided into two to four doses, with a maximum dose of 5 mg/kg/day. The usual dose of inhaled colistin is 75–150 mg inhaled two to three times daily.

Dosing adjustments:
- **Renal failure:** Colistin accumulates in patients with renal failure. Patients with CrCl of 5–20 mL/min should receive 1.25–2.5 mg/kg/day divided q12h. Patients with CrCl <5 mL/min should receive 0.75–1.5 mg/kg/day divided q12h.
- **HD:** A dose of 2–3 mg/kg after each dialysis session has been recommended.
- **PD:** A dose of 0.75–1.5 mg/kg/day divided q12h seems reasonable, as there is not appreciable PD removal.
- **CVVHD:** No specific recommendations are available.

Safety
- **Adverse effects:** Nephrotoxicity, neurotoxicity (paresthesias, neuromuscular blockade), and hypersensitivity reactions are the most significant adverse effects. Serum creatinine should be monitored daily early in therapy and then at regular intervals for the duration of therapy.
- **Drug interactions:** Ideally, colistin should not be coadministered with aminoglycosides, other known nephrotoxins, or neuromuscular blockers due to possible potentiation of toxicity.

DAPTOMYCIN

Daptomycin is a parenteral, cyclic, lipopeptide antibacterial agent that binds to and depolarizes the bacterial cell membrane. The drug is rapidly bactericidal against gram-positive bacteria.

Microbiology: Key Spectrum Aspects
- Daptomycin is active against MSSA, MRSA, and enterococci, including strains that are vancomycin resistant. The drug is also active against streptococci and *Corynebacteria*.

Pharmacokinetics
- **Absorption:** The mean peak serum concentrations after 4 mg/kg, 6 mg/kg, and 8 mg/kg doses are 57.8, 98.6, and 133 μg/mL, respectively.
- **Distribution:** The volume of distribution is 0.09 L/kg, and the drug is 92% protein bound. The drug has been found to bind to surfactant in the lung, which extensively reduces the activity of daptomycin in this site.

- **Elimination:** Daptomycin is eliminated primarily by renal excretion. The drug is not a substrate or an inhibitor of cytochrome P450 enzymes.

Dosing and Administration
The usual dosage is 4 mg/kg IV q24h. Higher doses have been used but are not currently approved by the FDA.

Dosing adjustments:
- **Renal failure:** Patients with CrCl <30 mL/min should receive 4 mg/kg q48h.
- **HD:** A dose of 4 mg/kg q48h is recommended.
- **PD:** A dose of 4 mg/kg q48h is recommended.
- **CVVHD:** No recommendations are available.
- **Hepatic:** No dosage adjustments are required in patients with mild to moderate hepatic dysfunction.

Safety
- **Adverse effects:** Gastrointestinal disturbances, rash, abnormal liver function tests, hypotension, and dyspnea may occur. Elevations in creatine phosphokinase (CPK) as well as muscle pain and weakness may occur, necessitating baseline and serial monitoring of CPK. The drug should be discontinued in patients with unexplained myopathy and a CPK >1000 U/L and in patients without muscle symptoms who have CPK >2000 U/L.
- **Drug interactions:** Receipt of HMG CoA reductase inhibitors in combination with daptomycin may increase the risk of myopathy and should be avoided.
- **Other key safety issues:** Daptomycin is rated pregnancy category B. It is unknown if daptomycin is excreted in breast milk.

DOXYCYCLINE

Microbiology: Key Spectrum Aspects
Doxycycline, a member of the tetracycline class of antibiotics, is a bacteriostatic antibiotic that binds the 30S ribosomal subunit, which results in protein synthesis inhibition. This drug is the treatment of choice for most rickettsial infections, including Rocky Mountain spotted fever and ehrlichiosis, and can also be used to treat *Chlamydia*, *Mycoplasma*, syphilis, and outpatient community-acquired respiratory tract infection.

Pharmacokinetics
- **Absorption:** Doxycycline is 90–100% absorbed orally and achieves peak serum concentrations of approximately 1.5–3 µg/mL after doses of 100–200 mg. Food or milk decreases oral absorption by up to 20%, but this effect is not believed to be clinically important.
- **Distribution:** The drug is widely distributed into most tissues and fluids. Penetration into the CSF (approximately 26%) is enhanced in the presence of inflamed meninges. The Vd is 0.75 L/kg, and the drug is 88% plasma protein bound.
- **Elimination:** Doxycycline is primarily eliminated by fecal and renal excretion, undergoing minimal to no hepatic metabolism. The elimination half-life is 14–24 hrs.

Dosing and Administration
The usual dose is 100 mg PO/IV q12h.

Dosing adjustments:
- **Renal failure:** No dosage reduction is required.
- **HD:** No dosage reduction is required.
- **PD:** No dosage reduction is required.
- **CVVHD:** No dosage reduction is required.
- **Hepatic:** No dosage adjustments have been recommended.

Safety
- **Adverse effects:** GI disturbances and photosensitivity are common side effects. Esophageal ulceration, hepatic impairment, and pseudotumor cerebri may also occur. Doxycycline should not be given to children because of its ability to discolor tooth enamel.

- **Drug interactions:** Doxycycline absorption may be decreased by concomitant administration with polyvalent metallic ions (e.g., magnesium, aluminum, iron). Barbiturates, phenytoin, and carbamazepine can decrease the half-life of doxycycline.
- **Other key safety issues:** Oral doxycycline should be administered with a full glass of water to decrease the possibility of esophageal ulceration. The drug is pregnancy category D and should be avoided in pregnancy. It is distributed in breast milk and should be avoided in nursing mothers.

FOSFOMYCIN

Microbiology: Key Spectrum Aspects
Fosfomycin is a bactericidal oral (sachet dosing form) antibiotic approved for treatment of uncomplicated UTIs. It kills bacteria by inhibiting an early step in cell wall synthesis and has a spectrum of activity that includes most of the major urinary pathogens and difficult-to-treat organisms, including *P. aeruginosa*, *Enterobacter* species, and enterococci (including VRE). It may be used to treat uncomplicated UTIs in women with susceptible strains of *E. coli* and *E. faecalis* but should not be used to treat pyelonephritis or systemic infections.

Pharmacokinetics
- **Absorption:** The drug has an oral bioavailability of 37% that is only reduced to 30% when taken with food. The peak serum concentration achieved after a single 3-g oral dose is 17.6 μg/mL.
- **Distribution:** The drug is distributed into the kidneys and bladder, with a Vd of 136 L. The drug is not bound to plasma proteins.
- **Elimination:** Fosfomycin is excreted unchanged in both urine and feces. The half-life is 5.7 hrs in patients with normal renal function but can be extended to up to 50 hrs in patients with CrCl <10 mL/min.

Dosing and Administration
The recommended dose is a 3-g sachet dissolved in cold water PO once. The drug should only be administered once, as repeat dosing does not improve clinical outcomes.
Dosing adjustments:
- **Renal failure:** There are no guidelines for its use in significant renal impairment.

Safety
- **Adverse effects:** The main side effects are GI disturbances, headache, and vaginitis.
- **Drug interactions:** Metoclopramide decreases fosfomycin absorption and subsequent renal excretion.
- **Other key safety issues:** The drug is rated pregnancy category C and should be avoided in pregnant women. The drug should also be used cautiously, if at all, in lactating women due to its possible excretion in breast milk.

LINEZOLID

Linezolid is an oxazolidinone antibiotic that inhibits bacterial protein synthesis. Agents of this class bind to the 50S ribosomal subunit near the interface with the 30S subunit. This binding inhibits the formation of the 70S initiation complex, causing early inhibition of translation.

Microbiology: Key Spectrum Aspects
Linezolid is active against both MSSA and MRSA as well as coagulase-negative staphylococci. It also has activity against vancomycin-susceptible enterococci and VRE. Linezolid also has activity against all *Streptococcus* species, including *Streptococcus pyogenes* and *S. pneumoniae*. *In vitro* activity has also been demonstrated against *Bacillus* species, *Corynebacterium* species, and *L. monocytogenes*. *In vitro* studies also suggest it may be active against some gram-negative anaerobes and mycobacteria.

Pharmacokinetics

- **Absorption:** Linezolid is rapidly and extensively absorbed after an oral dose, with a bioavailability of 100%. After oral administration of a single 600-mg tablet, a maximum serum concentration of 12.7 μg/mL is achieved within 1–2 hrs. A serum concentration of 21.2 μg/mL is achieved after multiple doses of 600 mg PO q12h. The IV formulation produces a peak serum concentration of 15.1 μg/mL after repeated doses of 600 mg q12h.
- **Distribution:** The Vd is 0.6 L/kg, with approximately 31% bound to proteins.
- **Elimination:** Linezolid is primarily metabolized by serum and hepatic oxidation to inactive metabolites. Hepatic metabolism does not appear to occur through the cytochrome P450 enzyme system. Approximately 30% of a dose is eliminated as unchanged drug in the urine. The half-life is 4.4–5.4 hrs.

Dosing and Administration

The recommended dose is 600 mg IV or PO q12h.

Dosing adjustments:

- **Renal failure:** Similar plasma concentrations are achieved regardless of renal function. Currently, no adjustments are recommended for patients with renal dysfunction. However, accumulation of two primary metabolites may occur. The clinical significance of this has not been determined.
- **HD:** Both linezolid and its two primary metabolites are eliminated by HD. Approximately 30% of a dose is eliminated during a 3-hr dialysis session. Linezolid should still be administered q12h, with one of the doses given postdialysis.
- **CVVHD:** No dosage adjustment is required.

Safety

- **Adverse effects:** The most commonly reported adverse effects include diarrhea, headache, nausea, and rash. Thrombocytopenia has been reported to occur especially in patients receiving courses of >2 wks. Myelosuppression (anemia, leukopenia, and pancytopenia) has also been reported. These hematologic parameters may return to pretreatment values following discontinuation of the drug. Peripheral and optic neuropathy may also occur.
- **Drug interactions:** Linezolid is a reversible, nonselective MAOI. The consumption of large amounts of tyramine in the diet should be avoided while on linezolid to prevent possible elevations in BP. Linezolid also has the potential for interaction with adrenergic and serotonergic agents, causing a reversible enhancement of the pressor response to agents such as dopamine or epinephrine and a risk of serotonin syndrome in patients receiving concomitant serotonergic agents, such as SSRIs and TCAs.
- **Other key safety issues:** Embryo and fetal toxicities have been seen in animal studies. There are no adequate and well-controlled studies in pregnant women. Linezolid should only be used during pregnancy if the potential benefit justifies the potential risk to the fetus. Linezolid has been seen in the milk of lactating rats. It is unknown if it is excreted in breast milk. Caution should be used when this agent is administered to nursing women.
- **Monitoring:** CBCs should be monitored weekly in patients receiving linezolid. This is especially important in patients receiving this medication for durations >2 wks, those with preexisting myelosuppression, and those receiving concomitant drugs that cause bone marrow suppression. Drug profiles should also be prospectively screened for potential drug interactions.

METRONIDAZOLE

Microbiology: Key Spectrum Aspects

Metronidazole kills anaerobic bacteria and some protozoans by accumulation of toxic metabolites that interfere with multiple biologic processes. Metronidazole is more active against gram-negative versus gram-positive anaerobes, but it does possess activity against *Clostridium perfringens* and *C. difficile*. It is used as monotherapy to treat *C. difficile* colitis and bacterial vaginosis; in combination with other antibiotics, it is used to treat intraabdominal infections and brain abscesses. Protozoan infections routinely treated with metronidazole include *Giardia*, *Entamoeba histolytica*, and *Trichomonas vaginalis*.

Pharmacokinetics

- **Absorption:** Metronidazole is ≥80–99% absorbed orally and achieves peak and 8-hr trough serum concentrations of approximately 11.5–13 and 4–5 μg/mL, respectively, after a 500-mg oral dose. A 750-mg dose of the extended-release oral formulation produces steady-state peak serum concentrations of 12.5–19.4 μg/mL.
- **Distribution:** The drug is widely distributed into most tissues and fluids, including abscess cavities, bone, and the CNS. The Vd is 0.74 L/kg, and the drug is 10–20% plasma protein bound.
- **Elimination:** Metronidazole is extensively metabolized in the liver to active and inactive metabolites, which are excreted in the urine. The drug is also partially excreted in the bile, feces, and urine as unchanged drug. The elimination half-life is 6–8 hrs.

Dosing and Administration

The usual dose is 250–500 mg PO/IV q6–12h. A single 2000-mg dose may be used to treat trichomoniasis.

Dosing adjustments:

- **Renal failure:** Dose reduction is not required in the presence of renal insufficiency.
- **HD:** The usual dose may be given; however, one of the daily doses should be administered after each dialysis session, as the drug is removed by HD.
- **PD:** The drug is not removed by PD and may be administered at the usual dose.
- **CVVHD:** No dosage adjustment is required, as only 10–20% of the drug is removed.
- **Hepatic:** A dose reduction may be warranted for patients with decompensated liver disease.

Safety

- **Adverse effects:** GI disturbances (nausea, vomiting, diarrhea), dysgeusia, disulfiram-like reactions to alcohol, and mild CNS disturbances (headache, restlessness) may occur. Rarely, seizures and peripheral neuropathy may occur.
- **Drug interactions:** Metronidazole can increase the procoagulant effects of warfarin. Concomitant administration of metronidazole with disulfiram may result in psychosis and confusion and should be avoided.
- **Other key safety issues:** Alcohol ingestion should be avoided with metronidazole and for 1–3 days after the last dose of the drug to prevent the disulfiram reaction from occurring. The drug is pregnancy category B but should be avoided during the first trimester of pregnancy. It is distributed in breast milk.

NITROFURANTOIN

Microbiology: Key Spectrum Aspects

Nitrofurantoin is a bactericidal oral antibiotic useful for uncomplicated UTIs. The drug is metabolized by bacteria into toxic intermediates that inhibit multiple bacterial processes. This drug has had a modest resurgence, as it is frequently effective against uncomplicated VRE UTIs. It has minimal activity against *P. aeruginosa*, *Serratia*, or *Proteus*. This drug should not be used for pyelonephritis or any other systemic infections due to its poor systemic availability.

Pharmacokinetics

- **Absorption:** The drug is well absorbed orally, particularly when taken with food. However, therapeutically relevant serum levels are not achieved due to the short half-life of the drug.
- **Distribution:** Therapeutic levels are not attained in most tissues and fluids, except the urine. The drug is 20–60% plasma protein bound, and the Vd is 0.58 L/kg.
- **Elimination:** Nitrofurantoin is eliminated primarily by renal excretion but also undergoes partial hepatic metabolism. The half-life is only 20 mins.

Dosing and Administration

The usual dose is 50–100 mg qid for the macrocrystals and 100 mg q12h as the dual-release formulation.

Dosing adjustments:
- **Renal failure:** The drug should be avoided in patients with CrCl <60 mL/min, as these patients do not achieve adequate urinary levels and are at increased risk for toxicity.
- **HD:** The drug should be avoided.
- **PD:** The drug should be avoided.
- **CVVHD:** The drug should be avoided.
- **Hepatic:** No dosage adjustments have been recommended.

Safety
- **Adverse effects:** GI disturbances and headache are the most common side effects. Peripheral neuropathy, pulmonary reactions, hepatotoxicity, hemolytic anemia, brown urine, and rash may also occur.
- **Drug interactions:** Probenecid and sulfinpyrazone may decrease the efficacy of nitrofurantoin by decreasing its renal elimination. Magnesium trisilicate antacids may decrease the absorption of nitrofurantoin.
- **Other key safety issues:** Although nitrofurantoin has been commonly used for UTI suppression therapy, this should be avoided because prolonged therapy is associated with chronic pulmonary syndromes that can be fatal. Although the drug is rated pregnancy category B, it should be avoided in pregnant women at term or when labor is imminent due to risk of hemolysis. It is also contraindicated in children <1 mo of age also due to hemolysis risk. The drug is distributed in breast milk.

QUINUPRISTIN/DALFOPRISTIN

Quinupristin/dalfopristin is a combination product containing two streptogramin antibiotics that act synergistically with one another primarily against gram-positive bacteria.

Microbiology: Key Spectrum Aspects
Quinupristin/dalfopristin has activity against antibiotic-resistant gram-positive organisms, especially VRE, MRSA, vancomycin-intermediate *S. aureus*, and antibiotic-resistant strains of *S. pneumoniae*. Quinupristin/dalfopristin may be used for serious infections with MRSA and *S. pneumoniae* when other agents cannot be tolerated. Quinupristin/dalfopristin is bacteriostatic for enterococci and can be used to treat systemic VRE infections, but the drug has minimal activity against *Enterococcus faecalis* and should not be used to treat this organism.

Pharmacokinetics
- **Absorption:** Peak steady-state serum concentrations of quinupristin and dalfopristin at a dose of 7.5 mg/kg IV q8h are approximately 3.2 and 8 μg/mL, respectively.
- **Distribution:** The product distributes widely into tissues, with Vds of 0.45 and 0.24 L/kg for quinupristin and dalfopristin, respectively.
- **Elimination:** The product is primarily eliminated by biliary elimination and fecal excretion. Only 15–19% of the drug is eliminated in the urine. The half-lives of quinupristin and dalfopristin are approximately 3 hrs and 1 hr, respectively.

Dosing and Administration
The recommended dose is 7.5 mg/kg IV q8–12h.
Dosing adjustments:
- **Renal failure:** No dosage adjustment is required.
- **HD:** No dosage adjustment is required.
- **PD:** No dosage adjustment is required.
- **CVVHD:** No specific recommendations have been made.
- **Hepatic:** Dosage reduction should be considered in this setting, as the AUCs of quinupristin and dalfopristin and their metabolites are increased 180% and 50%, respectively, in patients with hepatic insufficiency.

Safety
- **Adverse effects:** The main adverse effects are arthralgias and myalgias (which are frequent and can force discontinuation of therapy), IV site pain and thrombophlebitis (common when the drug is administered through the peripheral vein), and elevated LFTs.
- **Drug interactions:** Quinupristin/dalfopristin is a significant inhibitor of CYP 3A4 and can increase serum levels of drugs metabolized by that enzyme, including but not limited to carbamazepine, HMG CoA reductase inhibitors, cyclosporine, tacrolimus, midazolam, triazolam, calcium channel blockers, and possibly many other drugs as well.
- **Other key safety issues:** The product is rated as pregnancy category B, is likely excreted in breast milk, and should be used cautiously in these settings.

RIFAXIMIN

Rifaximin is an oral, nonsystemic antibacterial agent that is a structural analog of rifampin. The drug binds to DNA-dependent RNA polymerase and inhibits RNA synthesis.

Microbiology: Key Spectrum Aspects
Rifaximin is active against enterotoxigenic and enteroaggregative strains of *E. coli*. Rifaximin has not been shown to be effective in the treatment of gastrointestinal infections due to *Campylobacter jejuni*, *Salmonella* species, or *Shigella* species.

Pharmacokinetics
- **Absorption:** Rifaximin is not appreciably absorbed from the gastrointestinal tract and can be administered without regard to food.
- **Distribution:** The drug is at least 80–90% concentrated in the gastrointestinal tract.
- **Elimination:** Rifaximin is 97% eliminated in the feces. Because of its lack of systemic absorption, rifaximin does not appear to interact with any drugs *in vivo*.

Dosing and Administration
The usual dosage is 200 mg PO tid for 3 days.
Dosing adjustments:
- **Renal failure, HD, PD, CVVHD:** Rifaximin has not been studied in renal failure, but it appears that dosage adjustments are unlikely given the lack of systemic absorption.
- **Hepatic:** No dosage adjustments are required given the lack of systemic absorption.

Safety
- **Adverse effects:** Gastrointestinal disturbances and hypersensitivity reactions (rash, urticaria) may occur.
- **Drug interactions:** Rifaximin does not appear to have any *in vivo* drug interactions due to its lack of systemic absorption.
- **Other key safety issues:** Rifaximin is rated pregnancy category C. It is unknown if rifaximin is excreted in breast milk.

TELITHROMYCIN

Microbiology: Key Spectrum Aspects
Telithromycin is an oral antibacterial member of the ketolide class of antibacterials, which is closely related to macrolides. The drug possesses clinically useful activity against multidrug–resistant pneumococci, *Haemophilus influenzae*, *Moraxella catarrhalis*, and the atypical respiratory tract pathogens.

Pharmacokinetics
- **Absorption:** The mean peak serum concentration 1 hr after an 800-mg oral dose is $2\,\mu g/mL$. The absolute oral bioavailability is 57% and is unaffected by food intake.
- **Distribution:** The volume of distribution of telithromycin is 2.9 L/kg, and the drug is 60–70% serum protein bound. Telithromycin is highly distributed into respiratory tissues.

- **Elimination:** Telithromycin is 65–70% metabolized in the liver, 50% of which is mediated by cytochrome P450 enzymes. The remaining drug is eliminated in the urine (20–25%) and feces (10–15%) as unchanged drug. The elimination half-life is 7.2–9.8 hrs.

Dosing and Administration
The usual dosage of telithromycin is 800 mg PO q24h.
Dosing adjustments:
- **Renal failure:** Dose reduction may be required for CrCl <30 mL/min; however, no dosage recommendations are available.
- **HD:** Dosage not established.
- **PD:** Dosage not established.
- **CVVHD:** Dosage not established.
- **Hepatic:** No specific dosage adjustment is recommended in patients with hepatic impairment.

Safety
- **Adverse effects:** Gastrointestinal disturbances, visual disturbances (blurred vision, diplopia, difficulty focusing vision), dizziness, elevations in liver function tests, hepatic dysfunction, and rash may occur. Telithromycin also has been associated with myasthenia gravis exacerbations and has the potential to prolong the QTc interval.
- **Drug interactions:** Telithromycin is a significant inhibitor of hepatic cytochrome P450 enzymes and can increase serum levels of pimozide, cisapride, carbamazepine, HMG CoA reductase inhibitors, cyclosporine, tacrolimus, theophylline, warfarin, ergotamine, dihydroergotamine, triazolam, and possibly many other drugs as well. Telithromycin is specifically contraindicated with pimozide, and HMG CoA inhibitors should be avoided. Telithromycin metabolism is increased by rifampin, and the combination should be avoided. Phenytoin, carbamazepine, and phenobarbital may also decrease telithromycin concentrations.
- **Other key safety issues:** Telithromycin has not been adequately studied in pregnant women and is likely excreted in breast milk. Patients should be cautioned about the possibility of visual disturbances and advised not to operate potentially dangerous machinery should these effects occur.

TRIMETHOPRIM-SULFAMETHOXAZOLE (TMP-SMX)

Microbiology: Key Spectrum Aspects
TMP-SMX is a combination antibiotic (IV or PO) with a 1:5 ratio of TMP to SMX. The drug slowly kills bacteria by inhibiting folic acid metabolism. This combination agent is commonly used for uncomplicated UTIs and is the therapy of choice for treatment of *P. jiroveci* pneumonia, *Nocardia*, and *S. maltophilia* infections. Many strains of MRSA are susceptible to TMP-SMX.

Pharmacokinetics
- **Absorption:** TMP-SMX is 95–100% absorbed orally and achieves peak serum concentrations of approximately 1–2 and 40–60 µg/mL of TMP and SMX, respectively, with a dose of TMP-SMX DS (160 mg TMP, 800 mg SMX).
- **Distribution:** TMP-SMX is widely distributed in tissues and fluids, including the CSF where it achieves concentrations that are 40–50% of serum levels. TMP and SMX are 44% and 70% plasma protein bound, respectively. The Vds of SMX and TMP are 0.26 L/kg and 1.6 L/kg, respectively.
- **Elimination:** TMP-SMX undergoes both hepatic metabolism and renal excretion. The half-lives of TMP and SMX are 8–11 hrs and 10–13 hrs, respectively.

Dosing and Administration
The usual dose is 160 mg TMP/800 mg SMX bid. For *P. jiroveci* pneumonia and other serious systemic infections, the dose is 15 mg/kg/day based on the TMP component.
Dosing adjustments:
- **Renal failure:** The dose should be reduced by 50% in patients with CrCl of 15–30 mL/min. Although the drug is not routinely recommended by its manufacturers in

patients with CrCl <15 mL/min, it has been used at doses of 25–50% of the usual dose in this population. Serum concentrations of the drug may be measured, with a goal peak TMP level of 5–10 μg/mL.

- **HD:** The dose for CrCl <15 mL/min should be given, with one of the usual daily doses on dialysis days administered after the dialysis session.
- **PD:** 25–50% of the usual dose should be given.
- **CVVHD:** 50% of the usual daily dose should be given.
- **Hepatic:** No specific dosage adjustments have been recommended.

Safety
- **Adverse effects:** GI disturbances, hypersensitivity reactions, and hematologic abnormalities are common side effects. Headache, hepatitis, interstitial nephritis, hyperkalemia, and crystalluria may also occur.
- **Drug interactions:** TMP-SMX can increase the hypoprothrombinemic effect of warfarin. TMP-SMX can also potentiate the activity of phenytoin and PO hypoglycemic agents.
- **Other key safety issues:** Oral TMP-SMX should be administered with a full glass of water to decrease the possibility of crystalluria. The drug is pregnancy category C and should be avoided when possible in pregnancy, particularly during the third trimester, to minimize the possibility of kernicterus. It is distributed in breast milk and should be avoided in nursing mothers, particularly of infants <2 mos.

VANCOMYCIN

Microbiology: Key Spectrum Aspects
Vancomycin is a glycopeptide antibiotic that kills gram-positive bacteria by interfering with cell wall synthesis. Vancomycin binds a D-alanyl-D-alanine precursor critical for peptidoglycan cross-linking in most gram-positive (not gram-negative) bacterial cell walls. Vancomycin provides clinically useful activity against important gram-positive pathogens, including enterococci, methicillin-resistant staphylococci, and drug-resistant pneumococci.

Most institutions have reported vancomycin-resistant *E. faecium*, and there are increasing reports of vancomycin-intermediate and now vancomycin-resistant *S. aureus*. Therefore, vancomycin should be **restricted** to use in the following circumstances:

- Treatment of serious infections caused by MRSA
- Treatment of serious infections caused by ampicillin-resistant enterococci
- Treatment of serious infections caused by gram-positive bacteria in patients allergic to all other appropriate therapies
- Oral treatment of *C. difficile* colitis that has not responded to two courses (10 days each) of metronidazole or in patients not responding to metronidazole with a potentially life-threatening colitis
- Surgical prophylaxis for placement of prosthetic devices at institutions with known high rates of MRSA or in patients known to be colonized with MRSA
- Empiric use for meningitis until an organism has been identified and sensitivities known
- Life-threatening sepsis syndrome in a patient with known MRSA colonization or extended hospitalization until pathogen(s) identified

Vancomycin should **not** be routinely used in the following circumstances:

- Routine surgical prophylaxis
- Empiric therapy for nonseptic neutropenic fever
- Treatment of single blood culture isolates of coagulase-negative staphylococci or treatment of coagulase-negative staphylococci blood cultures in cases in which the site of infection is inconsistent with the organism (e.g., community-acquired pneumonia and intraabdominal infection)
- Routine treatment of *C. difficile* colitis
- To complete a course of therapy in the absence of MRSA or ampicillin-resistant enterococci
- To prevent against catheter infection

- Use in topical application or irrigation
- Use in dialysis patients in whom MRSA is unlikely strictly for purposes of dosing conveniences

Pharmacokinetics
- **Absorption:** A 1-g IV dose produces peak serum concentrations averaging 25 μg/mL. Although, in general, the PO form of the drug is not appreciably absorbed from the GI tract, some absorption may occur in patients with severe colitis.
- **Distribution:** Vancomycin is widely distributed in the body, including into the CSF in the presence of inflamed meninges and high serum concentrations. The drug is 52–60% plasma protein bound and has a Vd of 0.39 L/kg.
- **Elimination:** Vancomycin is eliminated primarily by renal excretion. The half-life is 4–6 hrs in patients with normal renal function but is prolonged to an average of 147 hrs in patients with CrCl <10 mL/min.

Dosing and Administration
The usual dose of vancomycin is 15 mg/kg IV q12h.
Dosing adjustments:
- **Renal failure:** Patients with CrCl of 35–60 mL/min, 15–34 mL/min, and <15 mL/min should receive the usual dose q24h, q48h, and randomly, respectively, when serum levels decline to <15 μg/mL.
- **HD/PD:** Patients should receive an initial 15-mg/kg dose and be subsequently redosed at 15 mg/kg when the concentration drops below 15 μg/mL.
- **CVVHD:** A total of 57–75% of the drug is removed. Patients should receive 15 mg/kg q24h (i.e., approximately four times the anuric dose), with close serum level monitoring and dose titration.

Safety
- **Adverse effects:** The main side effects of vancomycin are phlebitis and rash. Ototoxicity and nephrotoxicity may also occur, as can leukopenia and red man syndrome (flushing of the upper body with rapid administration of the drug).
- **Drug interactions:** Concurrent administration of vancomycin with other potentially nephrotoxic or ototoxic drugs may potentiate these side effects.
- **Other key safety issues:** Vancomycin does cross the placenta and is rated as pregnancy category C; it is also distributed into breast milk. The drug should be avoided if possible in these settings.
- **Monitoring:** Serum level monitoring is indicated in patients who are expected to receive ≥5 days of therapy. Trough levels should be obtained one to two times weekly. Patients with rapidly changing renal function may need more frequent serum level monitoring. Serum creatinine should also be regularly monitored to assess dosing appropriateness. Patients should also be queried about the possibility of hearing disturbances. Doses should be adjusted to maintain the trough concentration at ≥ 10–15 μg/mL. Peak levels should generally only be measured in critically ill patients with severe infection, with a goal of 30–45 μg/mL.

ANTIMYCOBACTERIAL AGENTS

ETHAMBUTOL

Ethambutol diffuses into actively growing mycobacterial cells and inhibits cellular metabolism by an unknown mechanism. This leads to the arrest of multiplication and cell death. Ethambutol's effects are bacteriostatic.

Microbiology: Key Spectrum Aspects
Strains of *M. tuberculosis*, *M. marinum*, and *M. kansasii* are sensitive to ethambutol, whereas strains of *M. avium* are consistently resistant. However, ethambutol may be useful with certain combinations of drugs against *M. avium*.

Pharmacokinetics
- **Absorption:** 75–80% of an orally administered dose is absorbed. Concomitant administration of aluminum salts and ethanol may decrease absorption.

- **Distribution:** Ethambutol is widely distributed into most body tissues, including the lung. It localizes in pulmonary alveolar and axillary lymph node macrophages. The Vd of ethambutol is approximately 56 L.
- **Elimination:** The elimination half-life of ethambutol is 3–4 hrs, with 75% of the drug excreted unchanged in the urine via glomerular filtration and tubular excretion. 15% is metabolized to two metabolites: a dicarboxylic acid derivative and an aldehyde derivative.

Dosing and Administration

Dosing interval	Weight range (kg)		
	40–55	**56–75**	**76–90**
Daily mg (mg/kg)	800 mg	1200 mg	1600 mg[a]
3×/wk mg (mg/kg)	1200 mg	2000 mg	2400 mg[a]
2×/wk mg (mg/kg)	2000 mg	2800 mg	4000 mg[a]

[a]Maximum dose irrespective of body weight.

Dosing adjustments:
- **Renal failure:** With CrCl of <10 mL/min, it is recommended to increase the dosing interval from 24 to 48 hrs.
- **HD:** 15–20 mg/kg postdialysis.
- **PD:** 15–20 mg/kg q48h.
- **CVVHD:** 15–20 mg/kg q24–36h.

Safety
- **Adverse effects:** The primary adverse effect of ethambutol is optic neuritis, which may manifest unilaterally or bilaterally as decreased red/green perception, decreased visual acuity, and visual field defects. This adverse effect is dose dependent, occurring in approximately 15% of patients treated with doses of 50 mg/kg/day and in <1% of patients treated with doses of 15 mg/kg/day. Other adverse effects include pruritus, joint pain, GI upset, malaise, headache, dizziness, and mental confusion.
- **Drug interactions:** Absorption may be decreased with coadministration of aluminum salts.
- **Other key safety issues:** Ethambutol has been used to treat TB in pregnancy. No adverse effects on the fetus have been reported, but long-term effects are unknown. Ethambutol is considered to be compatible with breast-feeding.
- **Monitoring:** At baseline, patients receiving ethambutol should have visual acuity and color perception tested. This should be tested monthly, with each eye tested separately. Ethambutol is not recommended in children in whom visual acuity cannot be monitored.

ISONIAZID

The proposed mechanism of action of isoniazid is the inhibition of synthesis of mycolic acids in the cell wall of mycobacteria. Isoniazid is bacteriostatic in nondividing mycobacteria and bactericidal in rapidly dividing organisms.

Microbiology: Key Spectrum Aspects
Strains of *M. tuberculosis* are sensitive to isoniazid, whereas those of *M. kansasii* are as well but at higher concentrations. Both *M. avium* and *M. marinum* are resistant to isoniazid.

Pharmacokinetics
- **Absorption:** Isoniazid is readily absorbed with a time to peak concentration of 1–2 hrs and a Cmax of 3–5 μg/mL. Aluminum-containing antacids may reduce the bioavailability.

- **Distribution:** Isoniazid is widely distributed through the body, with a Vd of approximately 43 L. It can be detected in the CSF (similar concentrations to that of the plasma), pleural effusions, feces, saliva, placenta, breast milk, peripheral nerves, and RBCs. High concentrations are found in the lungs and skin.
- **Elimination:** Isoniazid can be acetylated to acetyl-isoniazid or hydrolyzed to iso-nicotinic acid by the liver. The acetylation of isoniazid displays genetic polymorphism. In fast acetylators (an autosomal-dominant trait found in Asians and Inuits), the half-life is approximately 70 mins. For slow acetylators (45–65% of American and northern European populations), the half-life is approximately 2–5 hrs. 75–95% of a dose of isoniazid is excreted in the urine within 24 hrs, mostly as metabolites.

Dosing and Administration
For the treatment of *M. tuberculosis*, the recommended daily dose is 5 mg/kg up to a maximum dose of 300 mg/day. For twice-weekly regimens, the recommended dose is 15 mg/kg/dose up to a maximum of 900 mg/dose.
Dosing adjustments:
- **Renal failure:** No dosage adjustment is required.
- **HD:** No dosage adjustment is required, but the daily dose on dialysis days should be administered after the dialysis session.
- **PD:** No dosage adjustment is required.
- **CVVHD:** No dosage adjustment is required.
- **Hepatic:** The drug should be avoided in severe liver disease. Dosage reduction in milder forms of liver impairment is warranted.

Safety
- **Adverse effects:** The incidence of hepatitis with isoniazid increases with age and alcohol consumption. Increases in transaminase levels may be seen, but this generally does not necessitate holding the medication unless the transaminase levels are three to five times the upper limits of normal. Peripheral and optic neuritis may also occur with isoniazid. These may occur more frequently in slow acetylators, patients with diabetes mellitus, and patients with poor nutrition. The concurrent administration of pyridoxine (vitamin B_6) at doses of 25–50 mg PO qd may help avoid these toxicities. Other toxicities of isoniazid include hypersensitivity reactions (e.g., fever and rash), hematologic reactions (e.g., agranulocytosis, eosinophilia, thrombocytopenia, and anemia), arthritic symptoms, encephalopathy, and convulsions.
- **Drug interactions:** Aluminum salts may decrease the absorption of isoniazid. Isoniazid has a direct inhibitory effect on peripheral and central dopa decarboxylase, and can increase in parkinsonian symptoms in patients taking levodopa. The hepatotoxicity of isoniazid may be increased by the concurrent administration of rifampin.
- **Other key safety issues:** It is currently recommended that pregnant women who have positive tuberculin skin tests without evidence of clinical TB should receive therapy with isoniazid for latent TB infection if they are likely to have been infected recently or have high-risk medical conditions (e.g., HIV). Congenital abnormalities have not been observed in mammalian reproductive studies. When administered during pregnancy, concomitant administration of pyridoxine is recommended. Isoniazid is distributed in breast milk. Breast-fed infants of isoniazid-treated mothers should be monitored for adverse effects.
- **Monitoring:** Baseline and monthly LFTs should be performed in patients receiving isoniazid. Patients should be monitored for signs and symptoms of liver toxicity, such as weakness, jaundice, dark urine, decrease in appetite, nausea, and vomiting. Patients should also be monitored for peripheral and optic neuritis (e.g., numbness, tingling, burning, pain in hands or feet, blurred or loss of vision).

PYRAZINAMIDE

Pyrazinamide (PZA) is a synthetic pyrazine analog of nicotinamide with activity against *M. tuberculosis*. Its exact mechanism of action is unknown.

Microbiology: Key Spectrum Aspects
PZA exhibits *in vitro* bactericidal activity against *M. tuberculosis* within monocytes at drug concentrations of 12.5 μg/mL. Resistance develops rapidly if used alone.

Pharmacokinetics
- **Absorption:** PZA is nearly completely absorbed from the GI tract after oral administration. Peak plasma concentrations of 30–50 μg/mL are achieved within 2 hrs after doses of 20–25 mg/kg.
- **Distribution:** The Vd of PZA is approximately 0.7 L/kg, with 10% plasma protein bound. It is widely distributed into body tissues and fluids, including the liver, lungs, and CSF.
- **Elimination:** PZA is hydrolyzed in the liver to pyrazinoic acid and subsequently to 5-hydropyrazinoic acid, the main excretory metabolite, after hydroxylation. Approximately 70% of a oral dose is excreted in the urine, primarily by glomerular filtration. Its half-life range is 9–10 hrs but may be increased in patients with hepatic or renal insufficiency.

Dosing and Administration

Dosing interval	Weight range (kg)		
	40–55	56–75	76–90
Daily g (g/kg)	1.0 g	1.5 g	2.0 g[a]
3×/wk g (g/kg)	1.5 g	2.5 g	3.0 g[a]
2×/wk g (g/kg)	2.0 g	3.0 g	4.0 g[a]

[a]Maximum dose irrespective of body weight.

Dosing adjustments:
- **Renal failure:** In patients with an estimated CrCl <50 mL/min, a dosage reduction to 12–20 mg/kg/day has been recommended.
- **HD:** PZA is highly dialyzable. Dosage recommendations vary from no adjustments in patients receiving HD to doses of 25–30 mg/kg three times weekly after dialysis. Practitioners experienced in treating patients with TB should supervise treatment of these patients.
- **PD:** No dosage adjustments are recommended for patients undergoing PD.
- **CVVHD:** No data exist regarding the use of PZA in patients undergoing CVVHD.
- **Hepatic:** The drug should be avoided.

Safety
- **Adverse effects:** The most common adverse effects of PZA include nausea and vomiting. Another common, more serious adverse effect of this agent is hepatotoxicity manifested as increases in serum aminotransferases, jaundice, hepatitis, fever, anorexia, malaise, liver tenderness, hepatomegaly, and splenomegaly. Hepatotoxicity appears to be dose related and may occur at any time during therapy. Patients with hepatic dysfunction or risk factors for chronic liver disease (e.g., previous hepatitis A or B infection, hepatosteatosis, alcohol or parenteral drug abuse, or other drugs associated with liver injury) may be at higher risk. PZA also causes hyperuricemia by inhibiting the renal excretion of uric acid and should be avoided in patients with acute gout. Nongout polyarthralgia has been reported to occur in up to 40% of patients receiving PZA. More rare side effects of PZA include thrombocytopenia, rashes, urticaria, and photosensitivity.
- **Other key safety issues:** It is not known whether PZA can cause fetal harm when administered to pregnant women. Small amounts can be found in the breast milk. PZA should only be used during pregnancy or in nursing mothers when the potential benefits outweigh the possible risks to the fetus or the infant.

- **Monitoring:** Baseline LFTs as well as uric acid levels should be obtained before initiation of therapy. These lab tests should be repeated at periodic intervals and if clinical signs or symptoms of toxicity occur during treatment. Patients should be advised to watch for potential signs of hepatotoxicity, such as jaundice, right upper quadrant pain, pale stools, pruritus, or dark urine. They should also be counseled on the importance of completing therapy to prevent the development of resistance.

RIFAMPIN

Rifampin is a semisynthetic derivative of rifamycin B, a complex macrocyclic antibiotic. It inhibits DNA-dependent RNA polymerase activity in susceptible cells by interacting with bacterial RNA polymerase. Its activity does not affect mammalian RNA polymerase.

Microbiology: Key Spectrum Aspects

Rifampin is active *in vitro* against a number of mycobacterial species, including *M. tuberculosis*, *M. bovis*, *M. marinum*, *M. kansasii*, and some strains of *M. fortuitum*, *M. avium*, *M. intracellulare*, as well as *M. leprae* in experimental leprosy in mice. It also has *in vitro* activity against many gram-positive bacteria, including *S. aureus* and *Bacillus anthracis*. *In vitro* activity is also seen against gram-negative bacteria, including *Neisseria meningitidis*, *H. influenzae*, *Brucella melitensis*, and *L. pneumophila*. Activity has also been seen against *Ehrlichia phagocytophila*.

Pharmacokinetics

- **Absorption:** Rifampin is almost completely absorbed after oral administration. Peak plasma levels of approximately 7 μg/mL (range, 4–32 μg/mL) are achieved within 2–4 hrs after a dose of 600 mg PO. Absorption has been reported to be reduced by 30% when administered with food.
- **Distribution:** The Vd of rifampin is approximately 0.9–1.0 L/kg, with 60–90% plasma protein binding. Rifampin is widely distributed and is present in effective concentrations in many organs and body fluids, including the CSF, abscesses, bone, pleural fluid, and bile.
- **Elimination:** After absorption from the GI tract, rifampin is eliminated in the bile and undergoes enterohepatic recirculation. During this time, the drug does undergo deacetylation in the liver. The deacetylated metabolite retains full antibacterial activity. Intestinal reabsorption is reduced by deacetylation; thus, hepatic metabolism facilitates removal of the drug through the biliary tract. The half-life is 1.5–5 hrs and is increased in patients with hepatic dysfunction. Up to 30% of the drug is eliminated in the urine and 60–65% in the feces.

Dosing and Administration

The usual dose of rifampin for the treatment of TB is 600 mg once daily IV or PO or 600 mg twice weekly as part of a multidrug therapy. A dose of 600–900 mg/day in divided doses is recommended for synergistic use of rifampin for treatment of staphylococcal prosthetic valve endocarditis.

Dosing adjustments:

- **Renal failure:** Recommendations for dosage adjustments in renal insufficiency vary. Some recommend no adjustment provided that the daily dose does not exceed 600 mg and liver function is normal. Others recommend reducing the dose by 50% in patients with a CrCl <10 mL/min.
- **HD:** No dosage adjustment is required.
- **PD:** 50% of the normal dose has been recommended for patients undergoing PD.
- **CVVHD:** Recommendations for patients undergoing CVVHD have ranged from no adjustment to 50% of the regular dose.
- **Hepatic:** Some authors recommend dosage adjustments in patients with serum bilirubin levels >50 μmol/L. Doses of 6–8 mg/kg twice weekly have been recommended in patients with severe liver impairment. Others suggest rifampin therapy be deferred in patients with jaundice.

Safety

- **Adverse effects:** The most common adverse effects of rifampin are GI disturbances, including heartburn, nausea, vomiting, anorexia, abdominal cramps, flatulence, and diarrhea. CNS effects may occur during the first 2 wks of therapy. These include headache, drowsiness, fatigue, ataxia, dizziness, confusion, inability to concentrate, visual disturbances, fever, generalized numbness, and psychosis. Rifampin may also cause increases in serum AST, ALT, bilirubin, and alkaline phosphatase concentrations. Hepatitis and fatalities associated with jaundice have been reported in patients with preexisting liver disease or in those who have received concomitant hepatotoxic agents. Severe hepatic injuries have been reported in patients receiving rifampin in combination with pyrazinamide for the treatment of latent TB infections. Thrombocytopenia, leukopenia, hemolytic anemia, hemolysis, hemoglobinuria, and decreased hemoglobin concentrations have occurred with rifampin therapy. Hypersensitivity reactions characterized by a flu-like syndrome have also occurred, as has renal failure. Rarely, edema of the face and extremities, decrease in BP, and shock have also been reported. Red-orange discoloration of body fluids, including urine, sputum, sweat, and tears, occurs with rifampin. This may lead to permanent staining of soft contact lenses.
- **Drug interactions:** Rifampin is a potent inducer of cytochrome P450 3A4 as well as 1A2, 2C9, 2C18, 2C19, and 2D6. Decreases in plasma concentrations are seen with calcium channel blockers (verapamil, diltiazem, nifedipine), methadone, digitalis, cyclosporine, corticosteroids, oral anticoagulants, haloperidol, theophylline, barbiturates, chloramphenicol, azole antifungal agents, oral or systemic hormonal contraceptive agents, various benzodiazepines, enalapril, some beta-blockers, doxycycline, fluoroquinolones, levothyroxine, nortriptyline, tacrolimus, zidovudine (ZDV), protease inhibitors, and nonnucleoside reverse transcriptase inhibitors (RTIs). The patient's medication profile should be screened for potential drug interactions before rifampin is initiated. Antacids may decrease the absorption of rifampin. Other hepatotoxic agents may potentiate the liver toxicity of rifampin and should be used with caution.
- **Other key safety issues:** A drug-induced lupus-like syndrome characterized by malaise, myalgias, arthritis, and peripheral edema has been reported in a few patients. Rifampin does cross the placental barrier and appears in cord blood. It has been shown to be teratogenic in rodents leading to congenital malformations, such as spina bifida and cleft palate. It should be used during pregnancy only when the potential benefits outweigh the possible risks. Rifampin is excreted into breast milk. Whether to continue or discontinue the medication in nursing women should be based on the importance of the medication to the mother.
- **Monitoring:** Baseline LFTs should be performed and repeated periodically during therapy with rifampin to assess for hepatotoxicity. This may be especially important in patients receiving other agents with liver toxicity. Patients should be advised to take rifampin on an empty stomach either 1 hr before or 2 hrs after a meal or antacids. However, if GI disturbances do occur, rifampin may be taken with a small amount of food. They should also be told of the discoloration of body fluids that occurs and advised not to wear soft contact lenses. Medication profiles should be prospectively reviewed for potential drug interactions, specifically medications metabolized by the cytochrome P450 enzyme system.

ANTIFUNGAL AGENTS

Amphotericin B Preparations

Amphotericin B is active against a wide range of fungi, including yeasts and molds. *In vitro* activity is seen against *Aspergillus* species, *Blastomyces dermatitidis*, *Coccidioides immitis*, *Cryptococcus neoformans*, *Histoplasma capsulatum*, *Paracoccidioides brasiliensis*, and most species of *Candida*. High minimal inhibitory concentration values and clinical resistance have been seen with *Pseudallescheria boydii*, *Fusarium* species, *Candida lusitaniae*, *Trichosporon* species, and, occasionally, with isolates of *Candida krusei*, *Candida glabrata*, and *Aspergillus* species. The drug is available as a conventional deoxycholate formulation and as three different lipid formulations, which have been designed to minimize toxicity while preserving the therapeutic efficacy of amphotericin B.

Infusion-related **adverse effects** may occur and include fever, chills, rigors, malaise, generalized aches, nausea, vomiting, and headache. These may be mediated by tumor necrosis factor alpha, interleukin-6, interleukin-1, and prostaglandin E. Premedication with aspirin, ibuprofen, and acetaminophen may blunt response. Meperidine may be used to treat rigors but is ineffective as prophylaxis and should be used with caution in patients with decreased renal function. Antihistamines may also be useful due to the sedating effect. Other infusion-related adverse effects include hypotension, hypothermia, and bradycardia. Thrombophlebitis may also be seen at the site of infusion.

Two types of **nephrotoxicity** may be seen: pretubular (i.e., glomerular) and tubular. Pretubular toxicity results from a decrease in GFR and renal blood flow and may be due to a tubuloglomerular feedback mechanism. Increased delivery and reabsorption of chloride ions in the distal tubule initiates a decrease in the GFR of nephrons. This effect is amplified by sodium deprivation. Decreases in GFR occur early during therapy and may occur in up to 80% of patients. Renal function may return to normal but may take months in some patients. This form of nephrotoxicity may be prevented with sodium loading. Prehydration with NS (500–1000 mL) has been used. Tubular toxicity may also occur and is manifest as hypokalemia, hypomagnesemia, and renal tubular acidosis. These effects may be the result of increased renal tubular cell membrane permeability. Electrolytes (especially potassium and magnesium) should be closely monitored during therapy.

A normocytic, normochromic **anemia** may occur. Patients may experience an 18–35% decrease in hemoglobin, which may not occur until 10 wks after initiation of therapy. The anemia may be related to direct inhibition of erythrocyte and erythropoietin production.

Other adverse effects that may rarely occur with amphotericin B include ventricular arrhythmias as well as neurotoxic effects. Ventricular arrhythmias have been seen in patients with hypokalemia, those receiving rapid infusions, and patients with renal failure. Neurotoxic effects include confusion, incoherence, delirium, depression, psychotic behavior, convulsions, tremors, blurred vision, and loss of hearing. Administration during pregnancy has resulted in increased serum creatinine levels in infants. Renal function should be closely monitored in neonates born to mothers who have received amphotericin B.

Patients should be monitored for infusion-related **toxicities** as well as hypotension, bradycardia, and hypothermia during the administration of amphotericin B. Premedication may help blunt the infusion-related effects, and meperidine can be used to treat rigors once they begin. Renal function and electrolytes should also be monitored during the course of therapy. Sodium loading with NS infusions before daily doses may help prevent some of the nephrotoxicity. Electrolyte disturbances should be corrected to prevent other serious toxicities from developing, such as ventricular arrhythmias.

Nephrotoxic agents (e.g., aminoglycosides, cyclosporine, tacrolimus, pentamidine) may result in **acute deterioration of renal function** when given in combination with amphotericin B preparations. Agents causing electrolyte disturbances, such as hypokalemia seen with loop diuretics, should be used cautiously in patients being treated with amphotericin B. Hypokalemia induced by this antifungal agent may potentiate digitalis toxicity.

AMPHOTERICIN B COLLOIDAL DISPERSION

ABCD is a complex of amphotericin B and cholesteryl sulfate in a 1:1 ratio. This forms disc-like structures approximately 115 nm in diameter. Amphotericin B binds to ergosterol in the cell membrane of fungal cells, resulting in increased permeability through the formation of channels and pores. This allows leakage of cellular contents leading to cell death.

Pharmacokinetics
- **Absorption:** Absorption from the GI tract is negligible.
- **Distribution:** The Vd is increased (7.9 L/kg with a dose of 1.5 mg/kg) as compared to conventional amphotericin B deoxycholate (4 L/kg with a dose of 1 mg/kg). Maxi-

mum serum concentrations are somewhat decreased as compared to the conventional deoxycholate formulation. ABCD distributes to the liver, spleen, and bone marrow, with redistribution to the plasma in the identical form and at comparable levels as achieved with conventional amphotericin B.
- **Elimination:** As with the conventional deoxycholate formulation, the exact means by which the body eliminates amphotericin B are not completely understood. The initial half-life is approximately 28 hrs. However, as with the deoxycholate formulation and the other lipid formulations, the terminal half-life is much longer.

Dosing and Administration
The usual recommended dose is 5 mg/kg IV once daily infused over ≥4 hrs.
Dosing adjustments:
- **Renal failure:** No dosage adjustments are required for patients with renal insufficiency or those undergoing dialysis.

Safety (See Amphotericin B Preparations section)
Infusion-related adverse effects, including fever, chills, and hypotension, occur commonly with ABCD. Rates of these adverse effects are similar to those of conventional amphotericin B deoxycholate. Hypoxia has also been associated with infusions of ABCD. These events were usually associated with fever and chills and were reversible. Other toxicities that have been reported with lipid formulations include abnormalities in hepatic function, as manifested by elevations in alkaline phosphatase and conjugated bilirubin and renal failure.

AMPHOTERICIN B DEOXYCHOLATE

Amphotericin B deoxycholate is a polyene antifungal agent. It binds to ergosterol in the cell membrane of fungal cells, resulting in increased permeability through the formation of channels and pores. This allows leakage of cellular contents leading to cell death.

Pharmacokinetics
- **Absorption:** Absorption from the GI tract is negligible. After repeated daily IV administrations of 0.5 and 0.6 mg/kg/dose, plasma concentrations of 1.0–1.5 and 1.0–3.0 μg/mL, respectively, are achieved. These levels fall to 0.2–0.5 μg/mL after 24 hrs.
- **Distribution:** The Vd is approximately 4 L/kg. The drug is released from its complex with deoxycholate in the bloodstream, and 91–95% becomes protein bound, primarily to lipoproteins, erythrocytes, and cholesterol in plasma. The drug is highly distributed to many tissues, including the lungs, spleen, liver, and kidneys. Concentrations in the peritoneal, pleural, and synovial fluids are approximately half those found in the serum. Levels in the CSF are minimal, ranging from undetectable to 4% of those found in the serum.
- **Elimination:** Approximately 2–5% of each dose appears in the urine during daily therapy. Elimination of the drug appears to be unchanged in anephric patients and those on HD. Hepatic or biliary disease has no known effect on metabolism. Detectable levels have been demonstrated in the bile and urine for up to 12 days and 27–35 days, respectively, after administration. Amphotericin B is believed to follow a three-compartment model of distribution. After an initial half-life of 24–48 hrs, a terminal half-life of 15 days is seen. This reflects slow release of the drug from the peripheral compartment.

Dosing and Administration
Usual daily doses are 0.5–1.0 mg/kg, with escalation from lower doses to higher doses at the start of therapy. Infusions should be over a period of ≥4–6 hrs. Prehydration with NS is recommended to reduce nephrotoxicity (posthydration may be used in conjunction with prehydration). A 1-mg test dose may be given before the initial dose in an attempt to avoid immediate adverse reactions. However, such test doses may be given as a small portion of the first regular dose and should not delay therapy.
Dosing adjustments:
- **Renal failure:** No dosage adjustments are required for patients with renal insufficiency or those undergoing dialysis.

Safety (See Amphotericin B Preparations section)
Infusion-related reactions and nephrotoxicity are common.

AMPHOTERICIN B LIPID COMPLEX

Amphotericin B lipid complex (ABLC) consists of amphotericin B complexed to L-alpha-dimyristoylphosphatidylcholine and L-alpha-dimyristoylphosphatidylglycerol in a nonliposomal structure of lipid bilayers. This formulation results in a ribbon structure. Amphotericin B binds to ergosterol in the cell membrane of fungal cells, resulting in increased permeability through the formation of channels and pores. This allows leakage of cellular contents leading to cell death.

Pharmacokinetics
- **Absorption:** Absorption from the GI tract is negligible.
- **Distribution:** ABLC (at a dose of 0.5 mg/kg) has similar Vd (3.9 L/kg) compared to standard amphotericin B deoxycholate. Blood levels of amphotericin B are lower after a single-dose infusion of ABLC than after infusion of conventional amphotericin B. The lipid complex is believed to be rapidly taken up by the reticuloendothelial system and concentrated in the liver, spleen, lungs, and other tissues. Relatively high concentrations have been detected in the spleen (290 μg/g), liver (196 μg/g), and lungs (222 μg/g) during autopsy studies. Minimal distribution to the liver is seen with ABLC (6.9 μg/g). Lower concentrations have also been detected in the lymph nodes (7.6 μg/g), brain (1.6 μg/g), and heart (4.9 μg/g).
- **Elimination:** As with the conventional deoxycholate formulation, the exact means by which the body eliminates amphotericin B are not completely understood. The lipid complex is readily taken up by the reticuloendothelial system after administration. Here, amphotericin B may be liberated from lipid bilayers. The initial half-life of ABLC is approximately 35 hrs. However, the terminal half-life is much longer.

Dosing and Administration
The recommended dose is 5 mg/kg/day IV at a rate of 2.5 mg/kg/hr.
Dosing adjustments:
- **Renal failure:** No dosage adjustments are required for patients with renal insufficiency or those undergoing dialysis.

Safety (See Amphotericin B Preparations section)
Other toxicities that have been reported with lipid formulations include abnormalities in hepatic function, as manifested by elevations in alkaline phosphatase and conjugated bilirubin.

LIPOSOMAL AMPHOTERICIN B

Liposomal amphotericin B (LAmB) is the only true "liposomal" preparation of the three lipid preparations available. It is made up of small, unilamellar lipid vesicles that are uniform and spherical in size and average 60–70 nm. The lipid bilayer is composed of hydrogenated soy phosphatidylcholine and distearoylphosphatidylglycerol stabilized by cholesterol and combined with amphotericin B. Amphotericin B binds to ergosterol in the cell membrane of fungal cells, resulting in increased permeability through the formation of channels and pores. This allows leakage of cellular contents leading to cell death.

Pharmacokinetics
- **Absorption:** Absorption from the GI tract is negligible.
- **Distribution:** LAmB has a decreased Vd (0.22 L/kg at a dose of 5 mg/kg) as compared to conventional amphotericin B deoxycholate (4 L/kg at a dose of 1 mg/kg). Peak concentrations in the serum are higher for LAmB (57.6 μg/mL at a dose of 5 mg/kg) as compared to the deoxycholate formulation as well as ABLC and amphotericin B colloidal dispersion (ABCD). High tissue concentrations in autopsy studies have been found in the liver (175.7 μg/g) and spleen (201.5 μg/g). Lower concentrations have been documented in the lungs (16.8 μg/g), kidneys (22.8 μg/g), brain (0.56 μg/g), and heart (4.3 μg/g). After IV administration, the liposomes are rapidly

taken up by the reticuloendothelial system. It has also been hypothesized that monocytes or macrophages in peripheral blood take up the liposomes and transport them and the drug to the sites of inflammation or infection.

- **Elimination:** As with the conventional deoxycholate formulation, the exact means by which the body eliminates amphotericin B are not completely understood. The liposome is readily taken up by the reticuloendothelial system after administration. Here, amphotericin B may be liberated from liposomes. The initial half-life of LAmB is 7–10 hrs. However, the terminal half-life is 100–153 hrs.

Dosing and Administration

The recommended dose of LAmB is 3–5 mg/kg/day for the treatment of systemic fungal infections. Infusions may be given over 1 hr. Doses of 3 mg/kg/day have been used for empiric therapy of suspected fungal infections in febrile neutropenia.

Dosing adjustments:

- **Renal failure:** No dosage adjustments are required for patients with renal insufficiency or those undergoing dialysis.

Safety (See Amphotericin B Preparations section)

Infusion-related adverse effects associated with LAmB are reduced compared to those of the deoxycholate formulation. Other toxicities that have been reported with lipid formulations include abnormalities in hepatic function, as manifested by elevations in alkaline phosphatase and conjugated bilirubin. Transaminases may also rise with LAmB therapy.

Azoles

FLUCONAZOLE

Fluconazole is a triazole antifungal that inhibits sterol 14-alpha-demethylase, a microsomal cytochrome P450–dependent enzyme system. Inhibition of 14-alpha-demethylase leads to impaired biosynthesis of ergosterol and accumulation of 14-alpha-methylsterols. Accumulation of the methylsterols may disrupt the packing of the cell plasma membrane, making the fungus vulnerable to further damage.

Microbiology: Key Spectrum Aspects

Fluconazole is generally considered to be a fungistatic agent, with its principal activity against *Candida* species and *Cryptococcus* species. However, *C. krusei* is intrinsically resistant to fluconazole, and *C. glabrata* is considered to have dose-dependent sensitivity. Fluconazole does have activity against *C. immitis*, but it has limited activity against *H. capsulatum*, *B. dermatitidis*, and *S. schenckii* and no activity against *Aspergillus* species or other molds.

Pharmacokinetics

- **Absorption:** Fluconazole is almost completely absorbed after oral administration, with a bioavailability >90%. Plasma concentrations are nearly identical whether given PO or IV. A single oral dose of 400 mg results in a Cmax of 6.7 μg/mL (range, 4.1–8.1 μg/mL).
- **Distribution:** The Vd approximates that of body water, with a range of 0.7–1.2 L/kg. Fluconazole distributes well into many body fluids, including CSF and urine.
- **Elimination:** Fluconazole is principally eliminated by renal excretion. Approximately 60–80% of a single PO or IV dose is eliminated unchanged in the urine, and 11% is excreted in the urine as metabolites. Small amounts are eliminated in the feces. The elimination half-life in patients with normal renal function is approximately 30 hrs (range, 20–50 hrs).

Dosing and Administration

The usual dosage is 100–400 mg/day. A single 150-mg oral dose is effective for vaginal candidiasis.

Dosing adjustments:

- **Renal failure:** Patients with CrCl ≤50 mL/min should receive 50% of the usual daily dose.

- **HD:** HD decreases plasma fluconazole levels by approximately 50%. Various recommendations have been made for patients on HD receiving fluconazole, including administration of 100% of the usual daily dose after each dialysis session or administration of 50% of the usual daily dose administered daily (after dialysis session on dialysis days).
- **PD:** 50% of the usual daily dose q24h has been recommended.
- **CVVHD:** Fluconazole is effectively removed by CVVHD. 100% of the usual daily dose q24h may be used.
- **Hepatic:** The drug should be used cautiously in this setting.

Safety
- **Adverse effects:** Fluconazole is generally well tolerated. However, some serious adverse effects have been reported to occur, including serious hepatotoxicity. Clinical hepatitis, cholestasis, and fulminant hepatic failure have been reported to occur rarely in patients receiving fluconazole. Mild increases in LFTs have been reported to occur and are generally reversible. However, elevations to more than eight times the upper limit of normal also have been reported, as have rare fatalities. Other, less serious adverse effects include nausea, vomiting, headache, dizziness, rash, and anorexia. Reversible alopecia has also been seen with the use of this agent.
- **Drug interactions:** Fluconazole is a substrate of CYP 3A4 isoenzyme and may also inhibit metabolism of other medications going through this isoenzyme. Coadministration with ZDV has been associated with increases in the AUC, peak serum concentrations, and half-life of ZDV (74%, 84%, and 128%, respectively). Patients receiving these agents concurrently should be monitored for ZDV-associated adverse effects. Rifampin has been shown to decrease the AUC and half-life of fluconazole (25% and 20%, respectively). Use of these agents together may also increase the risk of hepatotoxicity. Fluconazole may also decrease the metabolism of TCAs, carbamazepine, certain benzodiazepines, warfarin, cyclosporine, tacrolimus, phenytoin, and oral sulfonylurea agents.
- **Other key safety issues:** According to the manufacturer, fluconazole should only be used during pregnancy if the potential benefits outweigh the possible risks. Rare cases of congenital abnormalities and malformations have been reported in infants born to women who received fluconazole during pregnancy. Fluconazole is distributed into breast milk, with concentrations approaching those achieved in plasma. Because of this, it is recommended that fluconazole not be used in nursing women.
- **Monitoring:** LFTs should be performed at baseline and monitored during prolonged courses of fluconazole. Medication profiles should be reviewed for potential drug interactions, and appropriate monitoring for signs and symptoms of toxicity associated with fluconazole alone and those associated with potential drug interactions should be performed.

ITRACONAZOLE

Itraconazole acts on ergosterol biosynthesis at the C-14 demethylation step by inhibition of 14-alpha-demethylase, preventing the conversion of lanosterol to ergosterol. Ergosterol depletion and the accumulation of methylated sterols lead to alterations in the plasma membrane, making it vulnerable to further damage.

Microbiology: Key Spectrum Aspects
Itraconazole's spectrum of activity is similar to that of fluconazole. However, it does have activity against clinically important *Aspergillus* species. Itraconazole has activity against *Candida albicans*, *Candida tropicalis*, and *Candida parapsilosis*. Its activity against *C. glabrata* and *C. lusitaniae* is usually dose dependent, whereas the susceptibility of *C. krusei* may be dose dependent or resistant. Itraconazole also has *in vitro* activity against *B. dermatitidis*, *H. capsulatum*, *Histoplasma duboisii*, *C. immitis*, *Sporothrix schenckii*, and *C. neoformans*.

Pharmacokinetics
- **Absorption:** The bioavailability after oral administration is approximately 55%. There are differences between the absorption of the capsule and oral solution formulations. The absorption of the capsules requires an acidic environment and is

increased when taken with food or a cola beverage. The oral solution should be taken on an empty stomach to maximize bioavailability.

- **Distribution:** The Vd after IV administration is 796 ± 185 L (10–11 L/kg), with 99.8% bound to plasma proteins. Itraconazole is highly lipophilic and extensively distributed in human tissues, with high concentrations being found in skin, liver, adipose tissue, bone, endometrium, cervical mucus, and the vagina. It is also incorporated into the nail matrix. Relatively high concentrations have also been found in pulmonary fluids and tissues.
- **Elimination:** Itraconazole is extensively metabolized to hydroxyitraconazole, the major metabolite that has some activity, as well as several other minor metabolites, by the CYP 3A4 isoenzyme system. <0.03% of unchanged drug is eliminated in the urine, whereas approximately 40% is eliminated via this route as inactive metabolites. After IV administration, 80–90% of hydroxypropyl-beta-cyclodextrin, the vehicle used to keep itraconazole in solution, is eliminated in the urine. This is not the case after administration of the oral solution, which also contains hydroxypropyl-beta-cyclodextrin, as this vehicle is not appreciably absorbed from the GI tract.

Dosing and Administration
The usual dose is 200–400 mg/day. During acute illness, loading doses of (a) 200 mg twice daily for four doses with the IV formulation, or (b) 200 mg three times daily for the first 4 days with the PO formulation may be used.

Dosing adjustments:
- **Renal failure:** IV itraconazole is not recommended for use in patients with CrCl <30 mL/min. No dosage adjustments are required for patients with renal insufficiency receiving capsules or the PO solution.
- **HD:** 100–200 mg q12–24h.
- **PD:** 100–200 mg q12–24h.
- **CVVHD:** 100–200 mg q12h.
- **Hepatic:** The drug should be used cautiously in this setting, and serum itraconazole levels should be obtained to assess dosing.

Safety
- **Adverse effects:** Itraconazole is usually well tolerated. However, some serious adverse effects have been reported to occur. Congestive heart failure, peripheral edema, and pulmonary edema have been reported secondary to a dose-related negative inotropic effect. Serious hepatotoxicity, including liver failure, has been reported rarely in patients receiving triazole antifungal agents with or without preexisting liver disease. Hypokalemia ranging from mild to severe has also been reported in patients receiving IV and PO itraconazole for systemic fungal infections. Other, less severe adverse effects include nausea, vomiting, diarrhea, headache, rash, fatigue, malaise, and increases in hepatic enzymes.
- **Drug interactions:** Itraconazole may inhibit the metabolism of other drugs metabolized by the CYP 3A4 isoenzyme. Concomitant use of itraconazole with quinidine or dofetilide is contraindicated due to potential increases in plasma concentrations of these agents leading to arrhythmias. Itraconazole is also contraindicated in patients receiving atorvastatin, lovastatin, and simvastatin due to the potential for rhabdomyolysis and in patients receiving certain benzodiazepines due to the potential for prolonged sedative and hypnotic effects. Itraconazole should be used with caution with other agents that are metabolized by CYP 3A4 or with medications that may induce or inhibit the metabolism of itraconazole through effects on this isoenzyme.
- **Other key safety issues:** Itraconazole has been shown to be teratogenic and embryotoxic in animals. It should be used for the treatment of systemic fungal infections in pregnancy only when the benefits outweigh the risks to the fetus. Itraconazole is contraindicated for the treatment of onychomycosis in pregnant women or women contemplating pregnancy. Itraconazole is distributed into breast milk.
- **Monitoring:** Patients receiving oral itraconazole should have LFTs performed at baseline and at regular intervals throughout the course of therapy. Potassium levels should also be monitored due to the risk of hypokalemia. Monitoring of signs and symptoms of congestive heart failure should also occur in patients receiving prolonged courses of

therapy or in those patients with predisposing risk factors. The medication profiles of patients receiving itraconazole should also be reviewed for potential drug interactions.

VORICONAZOLE

Voriconazole is a triazole antifungal agent that inhibits fungal cytochrome P450–dependent 14-α-lanosterol demethylase, which is responsible for the removal of the methyl group on the C14 site of lanosterol. Inhibition of this enzyme causes ergosterol depletion and accumulation of sterol precursor compounds. Voriconazole also inhibits 24-methylene dihydrolanosterol demethylation in certain yeasts and filamentous fungi, giving it activity against certain molds.

Microbiology: Key Spectrum Aspects

Voriconazole is active against *Aspergillus* species, including *Aspergillus flavus*, *Aspergillus fumigatus*, *Aspergillus niger*, and *Aspergillus terreus*. Voriconazole is more potent against *Candida* species. *In vitro* activity is also seen against *C. neoformans*, *B. dermatitidis*, *C. immitis*, *H. capsulatum*, *P. brasiliensis*, and *S. schenckii*.

Pharmacokinetics

- **Absorption:** Oral bioavailability has been reported to be 90%. However, the AUC and Cmax have also been reported to be 30% and 37% lower, respectively, after multiple oral doses of 200 mg as compared to those obtained after IV administration (3 mg/kg). Peak concentrations after administration of 200 mg twice daily have been reported to be 1.7 μg/mL in healthy volunteers to 2.12–4.8 μg/mL in AIDS patients with esophageal candidiasis. The time to maximum concentration is reported to be 1–2 hrs. A high-fat meal may decrease the AUC and Cmax of voriconazole as well as delay the time to peak concentration. It is recommended that voriconazole be given 1 hr before or after meals.
- **Distribution:** Voriconazole is distributed widely, with a steady-state Vd of 2 L/kg. It is moderately bound to plasma proteins (51–67%). Voriconazole does penetrate the blood-brain barrier, with concentrations 42–67% of corresponding serum levels.
- **Elimination:** Voriconazole undergoes extensive hepatic metabolism by cytochrome P450 enzymes, especially 2C9 and 3A4. Voriconazole is a substrate and inhibitor of these isoenzymes. After IV administration, approximately 80% is recovered in the urine (as unchanged drug and metabolites), with the remaining found in the feces. The elimination half-life is dose dependent, as voriconazole displays nonlinear pharmacokinetics. After a single 200-mg oral dose, the half-life is 6 hrs but increases to up to 12 hrs after a 400-mg dose.

Dosing and Administration

For invasive aspergillosis and infections caused by *Fusarium* spp. and *Scedosporium apiospermum*, a loading dose of 6 mg/kg IV every 12 hrs for two doses followed by 4 mg/kg IV every 12 hrs is recommended by the manufacturer. Oral doses of 200 mg every 12 hrs may be given once the patient is able to tolerate oral medications.

Dosing adjustments:

- **Renal failure:** Moderate renal impairment (CrCl of 30–50 mL/min) does not affect the pharmacokinetics of voriconazole. Accumulation of the IV-excipient sulfobutyl ether beta-cyclodextrin sodium may occur in patients with moderate to severe renal failure. Because of this, the IV formulation should not be used in patients with CrCl <50 mL/min unless the benefits outweigh the risks. In these circumstances, the oral formulation may be used instead.
- **HD:** No dosage adjustments are necessary.

Safety

- **Adverse effects:** Transient visual disturbances, including blurred vision, changes in light perception, photophobia, and visual hallucinations, have been reported to occur in clinical trials. These may be dose related and occur with the first few doses. Other adverse events, as with other azoles, include elevations in LFTs, skin rash, and GI disturbances.
- **Drug interactions:** *In vitro* studies have indicated voriconazole to be both a substrate and inhibitor of CYP 2C9, 2C19, and 3A4 isoenzymes. Caution should be

used when administering voriconazole with agents that are metabolized or inhibited/induced by the same pathways. Rifampin, rifabutin, and phenytoin have been shown to induce the metabolism of voriconazole. The metabolisms of cyclosporine, sirolimus, tacrolimus, warfarin, and omeprazole are inhibited by voriconazole.

- **Other key safety issues:** Other azole antifungal agents have been shown to be teratogenic and embryotoxic in animal studies. Caution should be used, and voriconazole should only be used in pregnancy when the potential benefits outweigh the risks to the fetus.
- **Monitoring:** Patients receiving voriconazole should have LFTs performed at baseline and at regular intervals, specifically if a long course of therapy is undertaken. Patients should be warned of the possible visual disturbances associated with the use of this agent. Monitoring for potential drug interactions should also be performed prospectively.

Other Antifungals

CASPOFUNGIN

Caspofungin is a member of the echinocandin class of antifungal agents. It noncompetitively inhibits the synthesis of beta-(1,3)-D glucan, an essential component of fungal cell walls.

Microbiology: Key Spectrum Aspects

Caspofungin has *in vitro* activity against *Aspergillus* spp. (*A. fumigatus*, *A. flavus*, *A. niger*, and *A. terreus*) as well as many *Candida* spp., including *C. albicans*, *C. glabrata*, *C. krusei*, *C. parapsilosis*, *C. lusitaniae*, and *C. tropicalis*. It may also have some activity against dimorphic fungi; however, no clinical data are available. Caspofungin lacks activity against *C. neoformans*.

Pharmacokinetics

- **Absorption:** Caspofungin is poorly absorbed after oral administration and is only indicated for IV administration.
- **Distribution:** Caspofungin has a Vd of approximately 9.7 L and is extensively bound to albumin (approximately 97%). It distributes well into the liver, kidneys, and large intestines, with tissue levels exceeding those of plasma concentrations. In the lung, small intestine, and spleen, tissue concentrations are similar to those found in the plasma. Caspofungin has minimal penetration into the CSF. After repeated administration, moderate accumulation may occur.
- **Elimination:** The major metabolic pathway involves peptide hydrolysis and *N*-acetylation with some spontaneous chemical degradation. The two major metabolites are without antifungal activity and are excreted in the urine (41%) and the feces (35%). Small amounts of unchanged drug (approximately 1.4%) are eliminated in the urine. Clearance is reduced in patients with mild or moderate hepatic insufficiency, with a reported increase in the AUC of 76% in patients with a Child-Pugh score of 7–9.

Dosing and Administration

Caspofungin is administered as a loading dose of 70 mg IV on day 1, followed by 50 mg IV daily thereafter. Infusions should be given over approximately 1 hr.

Dosing adjustments:
- **Renal failure:** No adjustments for decreased renal function are recommended.
- **HD:** No adjustments are needed.
- **PD, CVVHD:** No data are available.
- **Hepatic:** Patients with moderate hepatic insufficiency (Child-Pugh score 7–9) should receive the initial loading dose of 70 mg and then 35 mg IV daily thereafter.

Safety

- **Adverse effects:** The most common adverse effects associated with caspofungin have included infusion-related toxicities (pruritus, erythema, induration, pain) and headache. Toxicities associated with histamine release—including dermatologic reactions (flushing, erythema, wheals, rash), facial edema, and respiratory symptoms (wheezing, bronchoconstriction)—are rare but have been reported to occur in

approximately 1.8% of patients in clinical trials. Increases in LFTs are the most commonly reported lab adverse effects.
- **Drug interactions:** When administered concurrently with cyclosporine, the AUC of caspofungin has been reported to increase 35%. Due to elevations in LFTs observed with concurrent administration of cyclosporine, the manufacturer does not recommend coadministration. Tacrolimus levels have been reported to decrease during concomitant administration, with the AUC reportedly reduced by 20% and peak blood concentrations by 16%. Reduced caspofungin levels have been observed with concomitant administration of enzyme inducers or mixed enzyme inducers/inhibitors. Reduced concentrations have been observed with efavirenz, nelfinavir, nevirapine, phenytoin, rifampin, dexamethasone, or carbamazepine.
- **Other key safety issues:** Eosinophilia along with decreases in Hgb, Hct, neutrophils, and platelets have been reported in clinical trials. Hypokalemia has also been noted to occur. Caspofungin is pregnancy category C, and it is recommended to avoid its use in the first trimester.
- **Monitoring:** Patients should be monitored initially for allergic reactions as well as infusion-related toxicities. LFTs as well as platelets, neutrophils, Hgb, Hct, and potassium should be monitored during therapy. Patients who are concurrently taking tacrolimus should have these levels monitored closely, as concomitant administration of these two agents has been reported to decrease tacrolimus levels.

FLUCYTOSINE

Flucytosine is converted to 5-fluorouracil by susceptible fungi. 5-Fluorouracil is then metabolized to 5-fluorouridylic acid by uridine monophosphate pyrophosphorylase. 5-Fluorouridylic acid can either be incorporated into RNA in the triphosphate form or metabolized to 5-fluorodeoxyuridylic acid, which is a potent inhibitor of thymidylate synthetase that acts as a potent inhibitor of DNA synthesis.

Microbiology: Key Spectrum Aspects

Flucytosine is active *in vitro* against some strains of *C. albicans*, *C. glabrata*, *C. parapsilosis*, *C. tropicalis*, and *C. neoformans*, whereas *C. krusei* and *C. lusitaniae* are usually resistant. Resistance to flucytosine may develop during treatment and can result in clinical deterioration.

Pharmacokinetics

- **Absorption:** Flucytosine is well absorbed after oral administration. The bioavailability is 75–90%. Food may decrease the rate but not the extent of absorption. Peak plasma concentrations of 70–80 μg/mL are achieved 1–2 hrs after an oral dose of 37.5 mg/kg.
- **Distribution:** Flucytosine is minimally bound to plasma proteins and has a Vd of 0.68 L/kg. It is widely distributed into tissues, including liver, kidney, spleen, heart, aqueous humor, and bronchial secretions. CSF concentrations are 60–100% of those achieved in the serum.
- **Elimination:** Approximately 80% of a dose is excreted unchanged in the urine, with urinary concentrations of 200–500 μg/mL. The half-life is 3–6 hrs in patients with normal renal function but may increase to 30–250 hrs in patients with CrCl <10 mL/min.

Dosing and Administration

The recommended dose is 100–150 mg/kg/day divided q6h.
Dosing adjustments:
- **Renal failure:**

CrCl (mL/min)	Dosage (mg/kg)	Interval (hr)	Total daily dose (mg/kg)
>40	25	6	100
20–40	25	12	50
<20	25	24	25
<10	—	—	—

- **HD:** Flucytosine is effectively removed by HD. The recommended dose in patients undergoing HD is 25 mg/kg after each dialysis session.
- **PD:** The recommended dose is 0.5–1 g q24h.
- **CVVHD:** Flucytosine should be empirically dosed as in patients with CrCl of 10–40 mL/min and adjustments made with serum peak levels.

Safety

- **Adverse effects:** Bone marrow suppression, including leukopenia and thrombocytopenia, is the main serious complication of flucytosine. This may occur more frequently in patients with peak concentrations >100 μg/mL. It may also occur more commonly in patients with underlying hematologic disorders, those with concurrent myelosuppression, or those receiving nephrotoxic agents that may decrease the clearance of flucytosine. Because of its effects on rapidly proliferating tissues, flucytosine may also cause GI adverse effects. Severe nausea, vomiting, diarrhea, and anorexia may occur. Elevations in LFTs may occur but appear to be dose related and are generally reversible. Rash and eosinophilia have also been reported. CNS side effects (e.g., headache, confusion, hallucinations) have rarely been reported.
- **Drug interactions:** Nephrotoxicity agents may decrease the renal clearance of flucytosine, leading to accumulation and toxicity. When given in combination with such agents, flucytosine peak serum levels should be monitored along with renal function, and dosage adjustments should be made accordingly.
- **Other key safety issues:** Flucytosine has been shown to be teratogenic in animal studies. No human studies have been performed with flucytosine in pregnant women. Because of the concern for possible teratogenic effects, flucytosine should only be used in pregnancy when the potential benefits outweigh the possible risks. It is not known whether flucytosine is distributed into breast milk. Flucytosine should be used with caution in patients with hematologic disorders, those undergoing myelosuppressive therapy, and patients receiving nephrotoxic agents due to the potential for bone marrow suppression.
- **Monitoring:** Hematologic tests, renal function tests, and LFTs should be performed before and at frequent intervals during therapy. Peak serum levels should be obtained after the fifth dose. Concentrations of 25–100 μg/mL should be maintained. Peak serum levels should be monitored throughout therapy, especially in patients with signs of toxicity or a change in renal function or those with myelosuppression.

GRISEOFULVIN

Griseofulvin is an antifungal derived from a species of *Penicillium*. It is deposited in the keratin precursor cells and has a high affinity for diseased tissue. Griseofulvin produces multinucleate fungal cells by binding to microtubular protein. This causes disruption of the mitotic spindle and inhibits fungal mitosis. The infected tissue is gradually exfoliated and replaced by noninfected tissue. Griseofulvin persists as the precursor keratin cells differentiate into keratin, making this substance resistant to fungal invasion.

Microbiology: Key Spectrum Aspects
Griseofulvin is effective *in vitro* against dermatophytes. It is indicated for the treatment of ringworm infections caused by *Trichophyton rubrum*, *Trichophyton tonsurans*, *Trichophyton mentagrophytes*, *Trichophyton interdigitalis*, *Trichophyton verrucosum*, *Trichophyton megninii*, *Trichophyton gallinae*, *Trichophyton crateriform*, *Trichophyton sulphureum*, *Trichophyton schoenleinii*, *Microsporum audouinii*, *Microsporum canis*, *Microsporum gypseum*, and *Epidermophyton floccosum*.

Pharmacokinetics
- **Absorption:** After PO administration of a 500-mg dose of the microsized preparation, peak plasma concentrations of approximately 1 μg/mL (0.5–1.0 μg/mL) are reached in approximately 4 hrs. However, the levels achieved in the blood are variable. Serum levels may be increased by administering with a high-fat meal. The bioavailability of the ultramicrocrystalline preparation is believed to be 50% higher than the conventional microsized powder, but this may also be variable.

- **Distribution:** Griseofulvin is deposited in keratin precursor cells. It can be detected within the stratum corneum of the skin within 4–8 hrs after administration. Only small fractions of a dose of the drug are present in body fluids and tissue.
- **Elimination:** Griseofulvin is metabolized extensively in the liver. The primary metabolite is 6-methylgriseofulvin. The plasma half-life is approximately 1 day. 50% of an oral dose can be detected in the urine within 5 days.

Dosing and Administration

In the treatment of tinea corporis, tinea cruris, and tinea capitis, a single or divided daily dose of 500 mg of the microsized formulation or 330–375 mg of the ultramicro-crystalline formulation may be used. For tinea pedis and tinea unguium, higher doses of 750 mg to 1 g of the microsized formulation or 660–750 mg of the ultrami-crocrystalline formulation per day in divided doses is required. The duration of therapy may range from 2–4 wks for tinea corporis to >6 mos for tinea unguium of the toenails.

Dosing adjustments:

- **Renal failure:** No dosing adjustments are required.
- **HD:** No dosing adjustments are required.
- **PD:** No dosing adjustments are required.
- **CVVHD:** No dosing adjustments are required.
- **Hepatic:** No specific dosing adjustments have been recommended.

Safety

- **Adverse effects:** The most common adverse effects of griseofulvin include hypersensitivity reactions, such as skin rashes and urticaria. Other hypersensitivity reactions (e.g., erythema multiforme-like reactions) may also occur and necessitate withdrawal of therapy. Such reactions occur because griseofulvin is derived from *Penicillium*. Patients with PCN-hypersensitivity reactions may be more prone to have such reactions to griseofulvin. Lupus-like syndromes or exacerbations of lupus erythematosus have been seen in patients receiving griseofulvin. This agent may also cause photosensitivity reactions. Rare side effects that have been reported include leukopenia, hepatic toxicity, nephrosis, and paresthesias of the hands and feet.
- **Drug interactions:** Barbiturates have been shown to decrease the absorption of griseofulvin. Griseofulvin may also decrease the effects of anticoagulant agents (e.g., warfarin), reduce the efficacy of oral contraceptive agents, and decrease levels of cyclosporine.
- **Other key safety issues:** Griseofulvin has been shown to be embryotoxic and teratogenic in animal studies. Cases of conjoined twins, abortion, cleft palate, and heart failure have been reported in patients taking this medication during the first trimester of pregnancy. **Griseofulvin should not be given to pregnant women or those contemplating pregnancy. Griseofulvin may also cause fertility impairment. Men should wait ≥06 mos after completing therapy to father a child.**
- **Monitoring:** Patients on prolonged therapy should be closely observed for renal, hepatic, and hematologic side effects. They should also be monitored for hypersensitivity reactions, and the medication should be discontinued, if these are severe or worsen. Patients should also take protective measures against exposure to ultraviolet light and sunlight. Women taking oral contraceptives should use a second form of birth control while taking griseofulvin.

TERBINAFINE

Terbinafine is a synthetic allylamine derivative. It inhibits squalene-2,3-epoxidase, causing the blockage of ergosterol biosynthesis, an essential component of fungal cell membranes.

Microbiology: Key Spectrum Aspects

- Terbinafine has *in vitro* activity against most *Candida* species, *Aspergillus* species, *S. schenckii*, *Penicillium marneffei*, *Malassezia furfur*, *C. neoformans*, *Trichosporon* species, and *Blastoschizomyces*. However, the safety and efficacy of terbinafine in treating clinical infections caused by these fungi are not established. It is currently indicated for the treatment of onychomycosis of the toenail or fingernail caused by dermatophytes (tinea unguium).

Pharmacokinetics

- **Absorption:** Terbinafine is well absorbed after oral administration (>70%). Due to first-pass metabolism, the absolute bioavailability of the oral formulation is only 40%. Peak plasma concentrations of 1 μg/mL appear approximately 2 hrs after a single 250-mg dose.
- **Distribution:** Terbinafine is highly lipophilic and widely distributed, with accumulation in the skin, nails, and fat. The Vd is >2000 L, with 99% plasma protein bound.
- **Elimination:** Terbinafine is extensively metabolized in the liver before excretion. Approximately 70% of the administered dose is eliminated in the urine. Due to its lipophilicity and extensive distribution to adipose tissue, terbinafine persists in the plasma for 4–8 wks after dosing due to subsequent release from these sites. Its terminal half-life range is 200–400 hrs. Clearance is decreased with altered renal and hepatic function.

Dosing and Administration

For onychomycosis of the fingernail, 250 mg once daily may be administered for up to 6 wks. For infections involving the toenail, the duration may be increased to 12 wks.

Dosing adjustments:
- **Renal failure:** The use of terbinafine in patients with CrCl <50 mL/min has not been adequately studied. The use of this agent in patients with this level of renal dysfunction is not recommended.

Safety

- **Adverse effects:** Terbinafine is generally well tolerated. The most commonly reported side effects include rash, pruritus, diarrhea, dyspepsia, nausea, and abdominal pain. Rare cases of hepatic failure causing death or leading to liver transplantation have been reported. These have occurred in patients with and without preexisting liver disease. The severity may be worse in patients with active or chronic liver disease. Isolated cases of agranulocytosis have also been reported with terbinafine. These cases are generally reversible with discontinuation of the drug.
- **Drug interactions:** Terbinafine is an inhibitor of CYP 2D6. Drug interactions may occur with other agents that are metabolized through this isoenzyme, including SSRIs, TCAs, and MAOIs. Rifampin has been shown to increase the clearance of terbinafine significantly, whereas cimetidine has been reported to decrease the clearance. Terbinafine may increase the clearance of cyclosporine while decreasing the clearance of caffeine.
- **Other key safety issues:** There are no well-controlled studies of the use of terbinafine during pregnancy. Because the treatment of onychomycosis may be delayed until after delivery, it is not recommended for use in pregnancy. Terbinafine is excreted into breast milk; it is not recommended for nursing mothers.
- **Monitoring:** Baseline LFTs should be conducted and repeated during therapy. Patients should be instructed to monitor for symptoms such as persistent nausea, abdominal pain, fatigue, vomiting, right upper abdominal pain, jaundice, dark urine, or pale stools. Patients should also be monitored for signs and symptoms of infections during therapy due to the potential risk of severe neutropenia.

ANTIVIRAL AGENTS

ACYCLOVIR

Acyclovir is converted by thymidine kinase to acyclovir monophosphate, which is subsequently converted to the diphosphate form and ultimately to the active triphosphate form via cellular enzymes. Acyclovir triphosphate acts as an irreversible inhibitor of viral DNA synthesis by competing with 2'-deoxyguanosine triphosphate as a substrate for viral DNA polymerase.

Microbiology: Key Spectrum Aspects

Acyclovir's antiviral activity is limited to herpes viruses. Its greatest activity is against HSV-1, HSV-2, and VSV. *In vitro* acyclovir may inhibit the replication of EBV but has no clear role in the management of infections due to this virus. High concentrations are required for the inhibition of CMV *in vitro*.

Pharmacokinetics

- **Absorption:** Approximately 10–20% is absorbed after oral administration.
- **Distribution:** Acyclovir is widely distributed into body fluids, including vesicular fluid, aqueous humor, CSF (mean CSF:plasma ratio, 0.5), lungs, liver, vagina, and uterus. The Vd is 0.69 L/kg.
- **Elimination:** 60–90% reaches the urine as unchanged drug. Renal excretion of unchanged drug by glomerular filtration and tubular secretion is the primary route of elimination. The plasma elimination half-life ranges from 1.5 to 6 hrs but increases to 20 hrs in anuric patients.

Dosing and Administration

The usual dose is 200–800 mg three to five times daily or 5–10 mg/kg IV q8h.

Dosing adjustments:
- **Renal failure:**

CrCl (mL/min)	5 mg/kg IV	Oral
>50	q8h	q8h
25–50	q12h	q8–12h
10–25	q24h	q12–24h
<10	50% q24h	q24h

- **HD:** 50–100% dialyzable; administer after HD.
- **PD:** Dose as for CrCl <10 mL/min.
- **CVVHD:** Dose as for CrCl <10 mL/min.

Safety

- **Adverse effects:** Reversible nephropathy due to crystallization of the drug in the renal tubules is an uncommon adverse effect seen after IV administration. Preexisting renal insufficiency, dehydration, and bolus dosing may increase the risk of nephrotoxicity. This may be avoided by appropriately adjusting for renal dysfunction. CNS toxicity has been reported in the form of tremors, delirium, and seizures. This may be seen with high doses, in patients with impaired renal function, and in the elderly. Phlebitis has been associated with IV infusions. GI disturbances may be seen with valacyclovir and PO acyclovir.
- **Drug interactions:** Probenecid has been reported to increase serum concentrations of acyclovir by impairing renal clearance. However, no changes in acyclovir dosage appear to be necessary. Acyclovir in combination with ZDV has been reported in one case to produce excessive fatigue. Another case report stated that the addition of acyclovir to a regimen containing phenytoin and valproic acid resulted in decreased concentrations of the antiepileptic medications leading to seizure activity.
- **Other key safety issues:** Parenteral acyclovir is recommended in pregnant women with varicella associated with extensive cutaneous disease, high fever, or systemic symptoms. Whether acyclovir prevents congenital varicella syndrome in the neonate is unknown. The CDC does recommend that PO acyclovir be used for first clinical episodes of genital herpes during pregnancy; however, routine administration to pregnant women with a history of recurrent genital herpes is not recommended. IV acyclovir may also be used for the treatment of life-threatening maternal HSV infections (i.e., disseminated infections, encephalitis, pneumonitis, or hepatitis). Acyclovir is distributed into breast milk. Concentrations may be higher than concurrent maternal plasma levels. Acyclovir should be used with caution in nursing mothers and only when clearly indicated.

- **Monitoring:** Renal function should be monitored at baseline and during therapy. Patients should also be monitored for seizure activity, especially those undergoing high-dose therapy, those with renal dysfunction, or those with a history of a seizure disorder.

AMANTADINE

Amantadine blocks an ion channel formed by the M2 protein, which spans the viral membrane. This blockade prevents hydrogen ions from entering the viral particle, thus blocking the acid-mediated dissociation of the M1 protein from the ribonucleoprotein complex. The ribonucleoprotein then cannot enter the cell nucleus and initiate replication of influenza A virus.

Microbiology: Key Spectrum Aspects
Amantadine is active only against influenza A virus. It lacks activity against influenza B virus.

Pharmacokinetics
- **Absorption:** Amantadine is well absorbed after oral administration. Peak plasma levels of 0.5–0.8 μg/mL after a 100-mg twice-daily regimen are seen in healthy adults.
- **Distribution:** Amantadine is distributed widely, with a Vd of 4.5–4.8 L/kg. Concentrations found within nasal secretions approximate those found within the serum. 60–67% is bound to plasma proteins.
- **Elimination:** Amantadine is excreted largely unmetabolized in the urine via glomerular filtration and, to a lesser degree, tubular secretion. The half-life in adults is 12–18 hrs but doubles in elderly patients. It may also increase in patients with decreased renal function.

Dosing and Administration
The usual dose of amantadine in the prophylaxis and treatment of influenza A for persons aged 10–64 is 200 mg PO once daily. For persons ≥65 yrs, the dose should be reduced to 100 mg PO once daily. Duration of treatment is usually 5–7 days. For treatment, amantadine needs to be started within 48 hrs of symptom onset. For prophylaxis in nursing homes or other institutions housing high-risk patients, amantadine should be initiated as soon as possible after recognition of the outbreak and continued ≥2 wks or until approximately 1 wk after the end of the outbreak.
Dosing adjustments:
- **Renal failure:**

CrCl (mL/min/1.73 m^2)	Dose (mg)/interval
≥80	200 qd
79–35	100 qd
34–25	100 qod
24–15	100 q3d
<15	100 q7d

- **HD:** In patients on chronic HD, the half-life has been reported to be 8 days. The recommended dose is 100–200 mg every 7 days.
- **PD:** The recommended dose is 100–200 mg once every 7 days.
- **CVVHD:** In patients undergoing CVVHD, the recommended dose is 100 mg q48–72h.

Safety
- **Adverse effects:** Amantadine stimulates the release of catecholamines. This may account for its CNS side effects. Anxiety, depression, insomnia, lightheadedness, and difficulty concentrating may occur. As plasma concentrations rise, hallucina-

tions and seizures may occur rarely. Other adverse effects include nausea, vomiting, urinary retention, and rash.

- **Drug interactions:** Concurrent administration with medications having anticholinergic effects may increase the adverse effects of amantadine. The use of TMP-SMX and triamterene-hydrochlorothiazide may increase the risk of side effects due to reducing the renal clearance of amantadine.
- **Other key safety issues:** Amantadine has been reported to be teratogenic in some animal studies. Because no controlled studies have been conducted in pregnant women, it should not be used unless the potential benefits outweigh the possible risks. It is recommended that amantadine not be used during breast-feeding, as it is distributed into breast milk.
- **Monitoring:** Amantadine should be used with caution in patients with CNS or seizure disorders, patients with uncontrolled psychosis, and those with liver disease or renal impairment. Due to its potential visual disturbances and other CNS side effects, patients should be warned about use of this medication when performing hazardous activities requiring mental alertness and physical coordination.

CIDOFOVIR

Cidofovir is a synthetic acyclic purine nucleotide analog of cytosine. It is converted to the active diphosphate by cellular enzymes. The diphosphate acts as a competitive inhibitor and an alternative substrate of viral DNA polymerase. Incorporation slows chain elongation and ends chain elongation if two cidofovir molecules are introduced consecutively. The inhibitory activity is highly selective due to a greater affinity for viral DNA polymerase than for human DNA polymerase.

Microbiology: Key Spectrum Aspects
Cidofovir has *in vitro* and *in vivo* inhibitory activity against a broad spectrum of herpes viruses, including HSV-1, HSV-2, VZV, CMV, EBV, papillomaviruses, polyomaviruses, and adenoviruses.

Pharmacokinetics
- **Absorption:** Cidofovir is poorly absorbed after oral administration, with <5% absorbed. Absorption is also minimal after topical administration.
- **Distribution:** The Vd is 0.54 L/kg, approximating that of total body water. <6% is protein bound. Cidofovir does not significantly cross into the CSF.
- **Elimination:** Cidofovir is cleared via glomerular filtration and tubular secretion, with >90% found unchanged in the urine. Renal clearance is 130 mL/kg/hr. High-dose probenecid blocks tubular secretion, resulting in higher peak plasma concentrations. The elimination half-life of cidofovir is 2.5 hrs. However, the clinical duration is longer than the plasma elimination half-life, which is related to intracellular concentrations of the active diphosphate form. Cidofovir diphosphate has a plasma elimination half-life of 17 hrs.

Dosing and Administration
The induction dose of cidofovir is 5 mg/kg infused over 1 hr once weekly for 2 consecutive weeks. This is followed by a maintenance dose of 5 mg/kg infused over 1 hr once every other week. To reduce the risk of nephrotoxicity, probenecid must be used concomitantly. The recommended dose is 2 g 3 hrs before the cidofovir dose, followed by 1-g doses administered at 2 and 8 hrs after the completion of the infusion for a total dose of 4 g. Patients should also receive 1 L 0.9% sodium chloride over 1–2 hrs immediately before each cidofovir infusion. For patients who can tolerate it, a second infusion of 1 L 0.9% sodium chloride should be initiated concomitantly with or immediately after the cidofovir dose and should be infused over 1–3 hrs.

Dosing adjustments:
- **Renal failure: Cidofovir is contraindicated in patients with a serum creatinine of >1.5 mg/dL, a CrCl of ≤55 mL/min, or a urine protein concentration ≥100 mg/dL.** If renal function changes during therapy, the dose should be reduced to 3 mg/kg for an increase in serum creatinine of 0.3–0.4 mg/dL above baseline.
- **HD, PD:** No data are available.

- **CAVHD, CVVHD:** Cidofovir should be avoided.

Safety
- **Adverse effects:** Dose-related nephrotoxicity is the principal side effect of IV cidofovir and is characterized by proteinuria, azotemia, glycosuria, and metabolic acidosis. Fanconi's syndrome may also occur. Proteinuria may occur in up to 50% of patients receiving maintenance doses of 5 mg/kg every other week; elevated serum creatinine may occur in 15%. Neutropenia may occur in 20% of patients. Other adverse effects when combined with probenecid include fever, nausea, emesis, diarrhea, headache, rash, asthenia, anterior uveitis, and ocular hypotony. Topical application is associated with burning, pain, pruritus, and occasionally ulceration.
- **Drug interactions:** Concurrent use of nephrotoxic agents increases the risk of nephrotoxicity.
- **Other key safety issues:** Cidofovir has mutagenic, gonadotoxic, embryotoxic, and teratogenic effects and is considered a potential human carcinogen. It may cause infertility in humans. It is unknown whether cidofovir is excreted in breast milk.
- **Monitoring:** Serum creatinine concentration and urine protein should be determined within 48 hrs before each dose. Proteinuria may be an early sign of nephrotoxicity. Due to neutropenia associated with cidofovir, it is recommended that leukocyte counts with differentials be monitored during therapy. It is also recommended that signs and symptoms of uveitis be monitored for along with intraocular pressure and visual acuity.

FAMCICLOVIR

Famciclovir is a prodrug of penciclovir and is rapidly metabolized to penciclovir in the gastrointestinal tract, blood, and liver after oral administration. Penciclovir is then converted by viral thymidine kinase to the monophosphate form, which is further converted to the diphosphate and finally the active triphosphate form by cellular enzymes. The triphosphate form stops viral replication by competing with deoxyguanosine triphosphate for viral DNA polymerase.

Microbiology: Key Spectrum Aspects
The active triphosphate form has activity against HSV-1 and HSV-2, VZV, and EBV. Limited activity has been demonstrated *in vitro* against CMV.

Pharmacokinetics
- **Absorption:** After oral administration, the bioavailability is approximately 77%. Although food may delay the absorption of famciclovir, the extent of absorption is not affected.
- **Distribution:** Penciclovir has been reported to have a Vd ranging between 1.08 and 1.50 L/kg.
- **Metabolism/excretion:** After oral administration of famciclovir, approximately 82% is recovered in the urine as penciclovir via tubular secretion and glomerular filtration. The plasma elimination half-life of penciclovir ranges between 2.3 and 3.0 hrs after oral administration of famciclovir but may increase to 13 hrs in patients with decreased renal function (CrCl <20 mL/min).

Dosing and Administration
- **Acute localized herpes zoster infections:** 500 mg PO q8h for 7 days.
- **Recurrent episodes of genital herpes infections:** 125 mg PO bid for 5 days beginning at the first signs of infection.
- **Chronic suppressive therapy of recurrent genital herpes episodes:** 250 mg PO q12h for up to 1 yr in duration.
- **Mucosal and cutaneous herpes simplex infections in HIV-infected patients:** 500 mg PO q12h for 7 days. When used for chronic suppressive or maintenance prophylaxis in HIV-infected adults with frequent or severe recurrences, 500 mg PO bid may be used.

- **Renal adjustments:**

Indication and regimen	CrCl (mL/min)	Dose (mg)	Interval (hrs)
Herpes zoster	40–59	500	q8
	20–39	500	q12
	<20	250	q24
	HD	250	After each HD session
Recurrent genital herpes	20–39	125	q24
	<20	125	q24
	HD	125	After each HD session
Suppression of recurrent genital herpes	20–39	125	q12
	<20	125	q24
	HD	125	After each HD session
Recurrent mucosal and cutaneous HSV infections with HIV	20–39	500	q24
	<20	250	q24
	HD	250	After each HD session

- **PD:** No data available.
- **CVVHD:** Dose for CrCl between 10 and 50 mL/min.

Safety
- **Adverse effects:** Famciclovir appears to be well tolerated in both immunocompetent and immunocompromised patients. The most common adverse effects reported include headache, nausea, and diarrhea, which are generally mild to moderate in severity. Other adverse effects that may occur include abdominal pain, vomiting, pruritus, and mild increases in ALT/AST levels.
- **Drug interactions:** Concurrent administration with probenecid or other drugs excreted extensively by active renal tubular secretion may result in increased plasma levels of penciclovir.
- **Other key safety issues:** Although animal studies have not demonstrated adverse effects in embryo-fetal development, no adequate well-designed studies have been conducted in pregnant women. Famciclovir should only be used during pregnancy when the benefits to the woman clearly exceed potential risk to the fetus.
- **Monitoring:** Renal function should be monitored at baseline and during therapy. Due to potential decreases in clearance and increases in exposure of penciclovir with increasing age, geriatric patients should be monitored and the dosage adjusted accordingly.

FOSCARNET

Foscarnet is an organic analog of inorganic pyrophosphate. It noncompetitively blocks the pyrophosphate binding site of the viral polymerase and inhibits cleavage of pyrophosphate from deoxynucleotide triphosphate. It has approximately 100-fold greater inhibitory effects against herpesvirus DNA polymerase than against cellular DNA polymerase alpha.

Microbiology: Key Spectrum Aspects
Foscarnet is active against HSV-1, HSV-2, VZV, CMV, EBV, influenza A and B, hepatitis B, and HIV. Because it does not require phosphorylation by thymidine kinase, foscarnet remains active against many HSV thymidine-deficient strains and resistant strains of CMV.

Pharmacokinetics
- **Absorption:** Foscarnet must be administered IV. After doses of 5 mg/kg IV, peak and trough plasma concentrations average 8–11 and 0.6–1.2 μg/mL, respectively.

- **Distribution:** Foscarnet has a Vd of 0.3–0.74 L/kg, with 14–17% bound to plasma proteins. 3–28% of the cumulative dose has been suggested to be deposited in the bone; however, the extent of bone accumulation has not been determined. CSF concentrations are 13–103% of plasma levels, with an average of 66% of plasma values at steady state. Vitreous concentrations average 1.4 times those of concurrent plasma values.
- **Elimination:** Approximately 80% is excreted unchanged in the urine by glomerular filtration. Renal clearance is 5.6–6.4 L/hr, and total body clearance is 6.2–7.1 L/hr. Foscarnet displays triphasic compartment pharmacokinetics. The distribution half-life is 0.14–16.7 hrs and reflects distribution into bone. Foscarnet is slowly released from bone, with a half-life of 18–196 hrs. Once released from bone, the elimination half-life is 3–6 hrs.

Dosing and Administration

CMV Retinitis

The recommended dose is 60 mg/kg infused over 1 hr q8h or 90 mg/kg infused over 1.5–2 hrs q12h for 14–21 days. This is followed by a maintenance dose of 90–120 mg/kg/day infused over 2 hrs.

Acyclovir-Resistant Mucocutaneous HSV

The recommended dose is 40 mg/kg q8–12h for 14–21 days.

Herpes Zoster in Immunocompromised Patients

The recommended dose is 40 mg/kg q8h for 10–21 days or until complete healing occurs. Higher doses of 60 mg/kg q8h have also been used.

Dosing adjustments
- **Renal failure:** See Tables 27-1 and 27-2.
- **HD:** Foscarnet is highly removed by dialysis. Doses should be administered postdialysis. Administration of 60–90 mg/kg/dose postdialysis followed by 45 mg/kg/dose postdialysis (three times/wk) has been recommended by some clinicians.
- **PD:** Dose for CrCl of <10 mL/min.
- **CAVHD, CVVHD:** Dose for CrCl of 10–50 mL/min.

Safety
- **Adverse effects:** The major dose-limiting side effect of foscarnet is nephrotoxicity with azotemia, mild proteinuria, and sometimes acute tubular necrosis. Based on serum creatinine measurements, renal impairment usually begins during the sec-

TABLE 27-1. INDUCTION DOSING OF FOSCARNET IN PATIENTS WITH ABNORMAL RENAL FUNCTION

| CrCl (mL/min/kg) | Herpes simplex virus | | CMV | |
	Equivalent to 40 mg/kg q12h	Equivalent to 40 mg/kg q8h	Equivalent to 60 mg/kg q8h	Equivalent to 90 mg/kg q12h
>1.4	40 q12h	40 q8h	60 q8h	90 q12h
>1–1.4	30 q12h	30 q8h	45 q8h	70 q12h
>0.8–1	20 q12h	35 q12h	50 q12h	50 q12h
>0.6–0.8	35 q24h	25 q12h	40 q12h	80 q24h
>0.5–0.6	25 q24h	40 q24h	60 q24h	60 q24h
≥0.4–0.5	20 q24h	35 q24h	50 q24h	50 q24h
<0.4	NR	NR	NR	NR

NR, not recommended.

TABLE 27-2. MAINTENANCE DOSING OF FOSCARNET IN PATIENTS WITH ABNORMAL RENAL FUNCTION

CrCl (mL/min/kg)	Equivalent to 90 mg/kg once daily	Equivalent to 120 mg/kg once daily
>1.4	90 q24h	120 q24h
>1–1.4	70 q24h	90 q24h
>0.8–1	50 q24h	65 q24h
>0.6–0.8	80 q48h	105 q48h
>0.5–0.6	40 q48h	80 q48h
≥0.4–0.5	50 q48h	65 q48h
<0.4	NR	NR

NR, not recommended.

ond week of therapy and is reversible within 2–4 wks after cessation of the medication in most patients. Metabolic abnormalities may include hypocalcemia or hypercalcemia, hypophosphatemia or hyperphosphatemia, hypomagnesemia, and hypokalemia. CNS side effects include headache, tremor, irritability, seizures, and hallucinations. Other side effects may include fever, rash, diarrhea, nausea, vomiting, abnormal LFTs, anxiety, fatigue, and genital ulcerations. Anemia and granulocytopenia have been reported in AIDS patients receiving foscarnet for CMV retinitis.

- **Drug interactions:** Concurrent administration with other nephrotoxic drugs (e.g., amphotericin B, cidofovir, aminoglycosides, IV pentamidine) may result in additive nephrotoxicity. There are case reports of seizure activity with concomitant administration of foscarnet and ciprofloxacin. Concurrent use with IV pentamidine also may increase the risk of hypocalcemia.
- **Other key safety issues:** There are no adequate and well-controlled studies in pregnant women, and the drug should only be used when the potential benefits outweigh the potential risks. It is not known whether foscarnet is distributed in breast milk.
- **Monitoring:** Foscarnet should be administered by an infusion pump at a rate not exceeding 1 mg/kg/min. Patients should be adequately hydrated before and during administration to minimize the risk of nephrotoxicity. 750–1000 mL NS or 5% dextrose should be administered before the first dose. With additional doses of 90–120 mg/kg, 750–1000 mL of fluid should be administered concurrently with each dose; 500 mL of fluid should be administered with each dose of 40–60 mg/kg. Patients' renal function, electrolytes, and CBCs should be monitored at least two to three times a week during induction therapy and at least once every 1–2 wks during maintenance therapy.

GANCICLOVIR

Ganciclovir is converted to the monophosphate form by viral thymidine kinase in herpes simplex virus (HSV)–infected cells and by viral phosphotransferase during CMV infection. The monophosphate is then converted to the diphosphate and then to the triphosphate via cellular enzymes. Ganciclovir triphosphate competitively inhibits the incorporation of deoxyguanosine triphosphate into elongating viral DNA, which prematurely terminates DNA synthesis and ultimately arrests viral replication.

Microbiology: Key Spectrum Aspects
Ganciclovir is a potent inhibitor of CMV replication, with inhibitory concentrations 10- to >50-fold lower than acyclovir for CMV strains. Ganciclovir also has inhibitory activity against HSV-1, HSV-2, EBV, and VZV.

Pharmacokinetics

- **Absorption:** Oral bioavailability averages 6–9% when administered with food and 5% when administered on an empty stomach. With doses of 1000 mg PO q8h, the peak and trough concentrations are 1.2 and 0.2 μg/mL, respectively. IV administration of doses of 5 mg/kg result in peak and trough concentrations of 8–11 and 0.6–1.2 μg/mL, respectively.
- **Distribution:** The Vd at steady state is 0.8–1.4 L/kg, with only 1–2% plasma protein bound. Ganciclovir does cross the blood-brain barrier, with CSF levels of approximately 41% of those in the plasma. Ganciclovir also distributes to the kidneys, lungs, liver, aqueous and vitreous humor, and testes.
- **Elimination:** Ganciclovir is not appreciably metabolized in the body, with 90–99% of an IV dose eliminated unchanged in the urine. Renal excretion occurs principally by glomerular filtration, with a smaller portion by tubular secretion. The elimination half-life is 2–4 hrs after IV administration and 4.8 hrs after oral administration. This half-life increases in patients with renal impairment, ranging from 4.4–30 hrs depending on the degree of renal impairment.

Dosing and Administration

For the treatment of CMV disease, the induction dose is 5 mg/kg q12h for 2–3 wks, followed by a maintenance dose of 5 mg/kg/day IV; 6 mg/kg IV 5 days/wk; or 1000 mg three times daily PO with food. For prophylaxis, the dose in AIDS patients with CD4 <100/mm^3 is 1000 mg PO three times daily; the dose is 5 mg/kg q12h IV for 2 wks followed by 5 mg/kg/day in transplant recipients. Ganciclovir implants may also be used for the treatment of CMV retinitis. Each implant contains 4.5 mg of ganciclovir and is designed to release the drug over a 5- to 8-mo period.

Dosing adjustments:
- **Renal failure:**

CrCl (mL/min)	% IV dose (5 mg/kg)	Interval (hr)	Oral dose (mg)	Interval
≥70	100	12	1000	tid
50–69	50	12	1500	qd
25–49	50	24	1000	qd
10–24	25	24	500	qd
<10	15	tiw	500	tiw

- **HD:** 50% of the drug is removed by dialysis. Ganciclovir should be dosed postdialysis.
- **PD:** Dose for CrCl <10 mL/min.
- **CVVHD:** Administer 2.5 mg/kg/dose q24h.
- **Hepatic:** No dosing adjustments are required.

Safety

- **Adverse effects:** Myelosuppression is the principal dose-limiting toxicity, with neutropenia occurring in 15–40% of patients and thrombocytopenia in 5–20%. These effects are usually reversible with drug cessation. CNS side effects (e.g., headache, behavioral changes, convulsions, coma) may occur in 5–15% of patients. Other side effects include infusion-related phlebitis, azotemia, anemia, rash, fever, LFT abnormalities, nausea, vomiting, and eosinophilia.
- **Drug interactions:** Concomitant use with ZDV may increase the risk of hematologic toxicity. Ganciclovir antagonizes the anti-HIV effects of didanosine (ddI) and ZDV *in vitro*, and ZDV antagonizes the anti-CMV effects of ganciclovir *in vitro*; however, the clinical significance of these effects is unknown. Probenecid may lead to increased levels of ganciclovir secondary to inhibition of renal tubular secretion.
- **Other key safety issues:** It is not known whether ganciclovir is distributed in breast milk. Because of the potential for serious adverse reactions in breast-fed infants, it is recommended that nursing mothers discontinue nursing while they

are receiving the drug and that they do not resume nursing until ≥72 hrs after the last dose.
• **Monitoring:** Neutrophil counts and platelet counts should be monitored every 2 days during twice-daily dosing of ganciclovir and at least weekly thereafter. Neutrophil counts should be monitored daily in patients who have previously experienced leukopenia. Ganciclovir should not be administered if the absolute neutrophil count falls below 500 cells/mm^3 or if the platelet count falls below 25,000/mm^3.

OSELTAMIVIR

Oseltamivir is a neuraminidase inhibitor that binds to the active site of influenza virus neuraminidase, preventing the cleavage of N-acetylneuraminic acid (sialic acid) from the hemagglutinin receptor on epithelial cells. By leaving this receptor intact, viral aggregation occurs, which prevents the virus from entering into epithelial cells. Intact hemagglutinin receptors also cause aggregation of new virus particles on the cell surface, inhibiting viral release.

Microbiology: Key Spectrum Aspects
Oseltamivir is active against both influenza A and B virus.

Pharmacokinetics
• **Absorption:** Oseltamivir phosphate is the ethyl ester prodrug of oseltamivir carboxylate. Oseltamivir phosphate is well absorbed after oral administration from the GI tract, with approximately 80% of an oral dose reaching the systemic circulation after conversion to the active drug.
• **Distribution:** The Vd of oseltamivir carboxylate is 23–26 L, with approximately 3% bound to plasma proteins. Concentrations in the lung have been reported as high as five times those of corresponding plasma levels.
• **Elimination:** Oseltamivir phosphate is extensively converted by esterases in the liver and blood to the active carboxylate form. Oseltamivir carboxylate is eliminated unchanged in the urine. <20% of an oral dose of oseltamivir phosphate is eliminated in the feces.

Dosing and Administration
The recommended dose of oseltamivir is 75 mg PO twice daily for a total of 5 days. It should be initiated within 48 hrs of symptom onset.
Dosing adjustments:
• **Renal failure:** In patients with CrCl <30 mL/min, the frequency should be reduced to q24h. No data exist on the pharmacokinetics of oseltamivir in patients with renal failure (CrCl <10 mL/min).
• **Hepatic:** No data are available.

Safety
• **Adverse effects:** The main side effects are nausea and vomiting. These GI side effects usually occur after the first dose and resolve after 1–2 days with continued dosing. They may be reduced by taking oseltamivir with food.
• **Other key safety issues:** Oseltamivir should only be used in pregnancy when the potential benefits outweigh the possible risks. In animal studies, both the prodrug and active drug have been found distributed in breast milk. Caution is recommended if used in nursing mothers.
• **Monitoring:** Patients should be instructed to take oseltamivir with food to try and reduce the occurrence of GI side effects. Caution should be used in patients with renal failure.

PENCICLOVIR

Penciclovir, a synthetic acyclic purine nucleoside analog of guanine, is converted by viral thymidine kinase to the monophosphate form. The monophosphate is further converted to the diphosphate form and then the triphosphate form by other cellular enzymes. The triphosphate form stops viral replication by competing with deoxyguanosine triphosphate for viral DNA polymerase and by inhibiting DNA chain elongation.

Microbiology: Key Spectrum Aspects
Penciclovir is active against HSV-1, HSV-2, VZV, and EBV. It exhibits only limited activity *in vitro* against CMV.

Pharmacokinetics
- **Absorption:** Minimal systemic absorption occurs after topical administration.
- **Distribution:** The Vd is 1.5 L/kg and is <20% plasma protein bound.
- **Elimination:** Penciclovir is excreted mostly unchanged in the urine via glomerular filtration. Penciclovir has a prolonged intracellular half-life of 7–20 hrs.

Dosing and Administration
Penciclovir is only available as a 1% topical cream. It is applied to affected lesions of the lips and surrounding skin. Therapy should be initiated at the earliest sign or symptom of herpes labialis. The cream should be applied in sufficient quantity to cover all lesions and rubbed gently into the affected area q2h while awake for 4 days.

Safety
- **Adverse effects:** Mild erythema has been associated with penciclovir. Care should be taken not to apply the cream in or near the eyes, as irritation may occur.
- **Other key safety issues:** Application to human mucous membranes is not recommended. Use during pregnancy only if clearly needed. There is no information on its safety in pediatric patients or on whether penciclovir is excreted in breast milk after topical administration.

RIMANTADINE

Rimantadine blocks an ion channel formed by the M2 protein that spans the viral membrane. This blockade prevents hydrogen ions from entering the viral particle, thus blocking the acid-mediated dissociation of the M1 protein from the ribonucleoprotein complex. The ribonucleoprotein then cannot enter the cell nucleus and initiate replication of influenza A virus.

Microbiology: Key Spectrum Aspects
Rimantadine is only effective against influenza A virus. It lacks activity against influenza B virus.

Pharmacokinetics
- **Absorption:** Rimantadine is well absorbed after oral administration. Steady-state peak and trough concentrations after doses of 100 mg bid are 0.4–0.5 μg/mL and 0.2–0.4 μg/mL, respectively. However, in elderly nursing home patients, steady-state peak concentrations were found to be 1.2 μg/mL.
- **Distribution:** Rimantadine is widely distributed with a Vd ranging between 720 and 986 L with approximately 40% bound to plasma proteins. Concentrations found within the nasal mucus average 50% higher than those in the plasma.
- **Metabolism/excretion:** Rimantadine undergoes extensive metabolism by hydroxylation, conjugation, and glucuronidation before renal excretion. The plasma half-life is approximately twofold longer than that of amantadine, ranging from 24 to 36 hrs.

Dosing and Administration
The usual dose of rimantadine in the prophylaxis and treatment of influenza A for persons 10–64 yrs of age is 200 mg PO once daily or 100 mg PO bid. For persons 65 yrs of age or older, the dose should be reduced to 100 mg PO once daily. For treatment, rimantadine needs to be initiated within 48 hrs of symptom onset, with a duration usually between 5 and 7 days. For prophylaxis in nursing homes or other institutions housing high-risk patients, rimantadine should be initiated as soon as possible after recognition of the outbreak and continued for at least 2 wks or until approximately 1 wk after the end of the outbreak.
- **Renal adjustments:** In patients with severe renal dysfunction (CrCl <10 mL/min), the dose of rimantadine should be decreased to 100 mg PO once daily.
- **HD:** HD removes only a small portion of rimantadine, so supplemental doses are not required.

- **PD:** Dosage not established.
- **CVVHD:** Dosage not established.
- **Hepatic impairment:** The dose should be reduced to 100 mg/day in the presence of severe hepatic impairment.

Safety

- **Adverse effects:** The side effect profile of rimantadine is similar to that of amantadine and includes anxiety, depression, insomnia, lightheadedness, difficulty concentrating, nausea, vomiting, and urinary retention. However, the CNS side effects of rimantadine may be less severe and/or less frequent than those seen with amantadine. Other adverse effects include anorexia, dry mouth, and rash.
- **Drug interactions:** Concurrent administration with medications having anticholinergic effects may increase the adverse effects of rimantadine. Cimetidine has been shown to decrease the clearance of rimantadine by 18%. However, no dosage adjustments are necessary.
- **Other key safety issues:** Rimantadine has been shown to be embryotoxic in some animal studies. Because no controlled studies have been conducted in pregnant women, it should not be used unless the potential benefits outweigh the possible risks. It is also recommended that rimantadine not be used by nursing mothers.
- **Monitoring:** Rimantadine should be used with caution in patients with CNS abnormalities or seizure disorders, patients with uncontrolled psychosis, and those with severe renal and hepatic impairment. CNS adverse effects may also be seen more frequently in geriatric patients than in younger individuals due to higher drug levels. Caution should also be used in this population.

VALACYCLOVIR

Valacyclovir is a prodrug of acyclovir with increased bioavailability. It is converted to acyclovir after oral administration. Acyclovir is converted by thymidine kinase to acyclovir monophosphate, which is subsequently converted to the diphosphate and ultimately to the active triphosphate via cellular enzymes. Acyclovir triphosphate acts as an irreversible inhibitor of viral DNA synthesis by competing with 2'-deoxyguanosine triphosphate as a substrate for viral DNA polymerase.

Microbiology

Key spectrum aspects: Valacyclovir's antiviral activity is limited to herpes viruses. Its greatest activity is against HSV types 1 and 2 and VSV. *In vitro* acyclovir may inhibit the replication of EBV but has no clear role in the management of infections due to this virus. High concentrations are required for the inhibition of CMV *in vitro*.

Pharmacokinetics

- **Absorption:** The bioavailability of valacyclovir after oral administration is approximately 50%. Valacyclovir is then converted rapidly and completely to acyclovir by first-pass intestinal and hepatic enzymatic hydrolysis.
- **Distribution:** Acyclovir is widely distributed into bodily fluids, including vesicular fluid, aqueous humor, cerebrospinal fluid (mean CSF to plasma ratio, 0.5), lungs, liver, vagina, and uterus.
- **Metabolism/elimination:** Between 60 and 90% of acyclovir reaches the urine as unchanged drug. Renal excretion of unchanged drug by glomerular filtration and tubular secretion is the primary route of elimination. The plasma elimination half-life ranges from 1.5 to 6.0 hrs but increases to 20 hrs in anuric patients.

Dosing and Administration

- **Treatment of herpes zoster infections:** 1000 mg PO q8h for 7 days.
- **Treatment of genital HSV infections:** 1000 mg PO q12h for 10 days for initial episodes and 500 mg PO qd for 5 days for recurrent episodes.
- **Renal adjustments:**
  - CrCl 30–49 mL/min, administer 1000 mg q12h.
  - CrCl 10–29 mL/min, administer 1000 mg q24h.
  - CrCl <10 mL/min, administer 500 mg q24h.

- **HD:** Approximately 33% is removed by hemodialysis. Patients should be dosed after dialysis.
- **PD:** Dose for CrCl <10 mL/min.
- **CVVHD:** Dose for CrCl <10 mL/min.

Safety
- **Adverse effects:** CNS toxicity has been reported in the form of tremors, delirium, and seizures. This may be seen with high doses, in patients with impaired renal function, and in the elderly. Gastrointestinal disturbances may also be seen.
- **Drug interactions:** Probenecid has been reported to increase serum concentrations of acyclovir by impairing renal clearance. However, no changes in acyclovir dosage appear to be necessary. Acyclovir in combination with zidovudine has been reported in one case to produce excessive fatigue. Another case report stated that the addition of acyclovir to a regimen containing phenytoin and valproic acid resulted in decreased concentrations of the antiepileptic medications, leading to seizure activity.
- **Other key safety issues:** Thrombotic thrombocytopenic purpura with hemolytic uremic syndrome has occurred in immunocompromised patients receiving high doses of valacyclovir.
- **Monitoring:** Renal function should be monitored at baseline and during therapy. Patients should also be monitored for seizure activity, especially those undergoing high-dose therapy, those with renal dysfunction, and those with a history of a seizure disorder.

VALGANCICLOVIR

Valganciclovir is an L-valyl ester (prodrug) of ganciclovir. It consists of two diastereomers that, after oral administration, are converted to ganciclovir by intestinal and hepatic esterases. Ganciclovir is then converted to the monophosphate form by viral thymidine kinase in HSV-infected cells and by viral phosphotransferase during CMV infection. The monophosphate form is then converted to the diphosphate form and then to the triphosphate form via cellular enzymes. The triphosphate form competitively inhibits the incorporation of deoxyguanosine triphosphate into elongating viral DNA.

Microbiology: Key Spectrum Aspects
Ganciclovir is a potent inhibitor of CMV replication, with inhibitory concentrations 10- to >50-fold lower than acyclovir for CMV strains. Ganciclovir also has inhibitory activity against HSV-1, HSV-2, EBV, and VZV.

Pharmacokinetics
- **Absorption:** Valganciclovir is well absorbed from the GI tract and rapidly metabolized in the intestinal wall and liver to ganciclovir. The absolute bioavailability is approximately 60% after administration with food, with a Cmax of 5.61 μg/mL and a time to peak concentration of 1–3 hrs.
- **Distribution:** The Vd at steady state is 0.8–1.4 L/kg, with only 1–2% plasma protein bound. Ganciclovir does cross the blood-brain barrier, with CSF levels of approximately 41% of those in the plasma. Ganciclovir also distributes to the kidneys, lungs, liver, aqueous and vitreous humor, and testes.
- **Elimination:** Valganciclovir is rapidly hydrolyzed to ganciclovir. No other metabolites have been detected. The major route of elimination is by renal excretion as ganciclovir through glomerular filtration and active tubular secretion. The elimination half-life of valganciclovir is 4.08 ± 0.76 hrs. The systemic clearance of valganciclovir is 3.07 ± 0.64 mL/min/kg, whereas the renal clearance is 2.99 ± 0.67 mL/min/kg.

Dosing and Administration
For the treatment of active CMV retinitis in patients with normal renal function, the induction dose is 900 mg (two 450-mg tablets) twice daily for 21 days with food. After the induction dose, or in patients with inactive CMV retinitis, the recommended maintenance dosage is 900 mg once daily with food.

Dosing adjustments:
- **Renal failure:**

CrCl (mL/min)	Induction dose	Maintenance dose
≥60	900 mg bid	900 mg qd
40–59	450 mg bid	450 mg qd
25–39	450 mg qd	450 mg q2d
10–24	450 mg q2d	450 mg twice weekly

- **HD:** Valganciclovir should not be prescribed to patients receiving HD.

Safety
- **Adverse effects:** Severe leukopenia, neutropenia, anemia, thrombocytopenia, pancytopenia, and aplastic anemia have been observed in patients treated with valganciclovir. Valganciclovir should not be administered if the absolute neutrophil count is <500 cells/μL, the platelet count is <25,000/μL, or the hemoglobin is <8 g/dL. Other adverse effects associated with valganciclovir include diarrhea, nausea, vomiting, abdominal pain, headache, and pyrexia.
- **Drug interactions:** Concomitant use with ZDV may increase the risk of hematologic toxicity. Ganciclovir antagonizes the anti-HIV effects of ddI and ZDV *in vitro*, and ZDV antagonizes the anti-CMV effects of ganciclovir *in vitro*; however, the clinical significance of these effects is unknown. Probenecid may lead to increased levels of ganciclovir secondary to inhibition of renal tubular secretion.
- **Other key safety issues:** It is not known whether ganciclovir is distributed in breast milk. Because of the potential for serious adverse reactions in breast-fed infants, it is recommended that nursing mothers discontinue nursing while they are receiving the drug and that they do not resume nursing until ≥72 hrs after the last dose. Due to the mutagenic and teratogenic effects seen in animals, women of childbearing potential should be advised to use effective contraception during treatment. Similarly, men should be advised to practice barrier contraception during and for ≥90 days after treatment with valganciclovir. Because valganciclovir is also considered a potential teratogen and carcinogen in humans, caution should be observed in handling broken tablets. Tablets should not be broken or crushed. Direct contact of broken or crushed tablets should be avoided with the skin and mucous membranes.
- **Monitoring:** Secondary to the adverse effects of neutropenia, anemia, and thrombocytopenia, it is recommended that CBCs be performed frequently, especially in patients in whom ganciclovir or other nucleoside analogs have previously resulted in leukopenia or in whom neutrophil counts are <1000 cells/μL. Patients should also have serum creatinine values monitored to prevent overdosage with decreased renal clearance.

ZANAMIVIR

Zanamivir is a neuraminidase inhibitor that binds to the active site of influenza virus neuraminidase, preventing the cleavage of N-acetylneuraminic acid (sialic acid) from the hemagglutinin receptor on epithelial cells. By leaving this receptor intact, viral aggregation occurs, which prevents the virus from entering into epithelial cells. Intact hemagglutinin receptors also cause aggregation of new virus particles on the cell surface, inhibiting viral release.

Microbiology: Key Spectrum Aspects
Zanamivir is active against both influenza A and B virus.

Pharmacokinetics
- **Absorption:** Because zanamivir is a zwitterion, it is poorly absorbed after oral administration. It is delivered as a dry powder by oral inhalation. 70–87% of the

inhaled dose is deposited in the oropharynx, resulting in 7–21% reaching the lungs. Only 4–17% of an inhaled dose is absorbed systemically.

- **Distribution:** The Vd is approximately 16 L, with <10% bound to plasma proteins. Zanamivir is found in the sputum and nasal washings up to 24 hrs after the administration of a dose.
- **Elimination:** Absorbed zanamivir is excreted unchanged in the urine. The plasma half-life is approximately 2.5–5.1 hrs. Unabsorbed zanamivir is excreted in the feces.

Dosing and Administration

Zanamivir is given via two inhalations of dry powder (5 mg/inhalation for a total of 10 mg) q12h for the treatment of influenza A and B infection. A Rotadisk (GlaxoSmith-Kline, London, UK) is loaded into the supplied plastic breath-activated Diskhaler (GlaxoSmithKline) inhalation device. One blister is pierced, and zanamivir is dispersed into the airstream created by inhalation of the patient. Each Rotadisk contains four blister packets of 5 mg and supplies enough medication for 1 day. Optimal response to therapy is seen when zanamivir is initiated within 2 days of symptom onset.

Dosing adjustments:

- **Renal failure:** Dosage adjustments are not necessary in patients with impaired renal function.

Safety

- **Adverse effects:** Zanamivir is generally well tolerated. In patients with underlying airway disease, bronchospasm and allergic-like reactions have been reported. Other adverse effects that have been rarely reported include diarrhea, nausea, vomiting, and cough. Some of the adverse effects may be due to the lactose vehicle instead of the active medication.
- **Other key safety issues:** Zanamivir should only be used in pregnancy when the potential benefits outweigh the possible risks. In animal studies, zanamivir is distributed into breast milk. Caution is recommended if used in nursing mothers.
- **Monitoring:** Caution should be used when zanamivir is used in patients with underlying airway diseases, such as asthma and COPD. Some patients with such conditions may experience bronchospasm or a decline in lung function when using this agent. They should be instructed to have a fast-acting bronchodilator available when inhaling zanamivir and to discontinue use and contact their physician if they experience worsening respiratory symptoms.

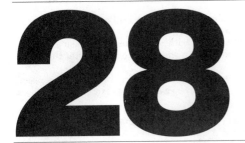

Human Immunodeficiency Virus Infection

Rebecca E. Chandler

INTRODUCTION

The epidemiology of HIV infection and its predominant mode of transmission have shifted over the course of the epidemic. HIV initially infected IV drug users and men who have sex with men. The more recent trend in the epidemic is infection of young heterosexual individuals, especially women and those of lower socioeconomic status.

As progress has been made in understanding the pathogenesis of HIV infection, the development of effective therapy has reduced the morbidity and mortality of this disease. Beginning in 1996, there has been an overall 23% decrease in AIDS-related deaths, and perinatal transmission has decreased by 26%.

PATHOPHYSIOLOGY

HIV type 1 is a member of the family of lentiviruses; it is composed of two strands of single-stranded RNA, located in a protein core, and surrounded by a lipid envelope. The genome of HIV contains genes for both structural and regulatory proteins. Three important proteins are the enzymes reverse transcriptase, protease, and integrase, which are the principal targets of current antiretroviral therapy. Two other important proteins are the glycoproteins gp120 and gp41, which are responsible for viral interactions with the human immune system.

The **life cycle of HIV** begins with the interaction of the gp120 protein of the virus with the CD4 receptor of the host T lymphocytes. Additional coreceptors, CCR5 and CXCR4, play a role in viral tropism. Once inside the cell, the virus begins replication, with reverse transcriptase protein producing large amounts of double-stranded complementary DNA forms of the genome. The viral complementary DNA enters the nucleus of the host cell and is integrated into the host DNA by the integrase protein. The viral DNA is then generally quiescent, or "latent," until activation of the host T cell; however, during this period, low levels of viral replication are occurring. A chronic, active infection is established. When triggered by activation of the host T cell, the transcription of the viral genome and construction of viral particles occur. Protease is involved in the cleavage of the viral polyprotein precursors. The viral progeny are then released, killing the host cell in the process.

An evolution occurs during which the original infecting HIV particles become a population of multiple viral genotypes as a result of the high rates and frequency of errors of the replication process. Selective pressures are exerted by the host immune system and antiretroviral therapy and further promote genetic diversity. These highly related yet genetically distinct viruses have been termed *quasispecies*. Understanding this concept is vital in choosing antiretroviral regimens and interpreting resistance testing.

Primary infection with HIV, or primary viremia, involves viral particles directly entering the bloodstream (i.e., needle stick) or infecting mucosal surfaces. Subsequent access to the bloodstream via lymphatic tissue (i.e., sexual contact) leads to large numbers of infected cells in the peripheral blood and high titers of infectious HIV in the plasma. These titers and the numbers of infected cells in the circulation fall dramatically as virus-specific immunity develops. Although undetectable levels of virus in the periphery may result, as mentioned above, viral replication continues unabated in infected cells, primarily in lymphoid tissues.

HIV infection is chronic and persistent. In most individuals, progressive immuno-deficiency and rising titers of virus develop. The **course of infection** varies among individuals: Some will be severely immunosuppressed in a few years (rapid progressors), and others will have intact immune systems 15 yrs after infection (long-term nonprogressors), with a median progression to AIDS being 10–12 yrs. This is dependent on various host and viral factors. Current treatment allows for prolongation of the periods of low viral loads and stabilization of immunologic function; however, it does not bring about eradication of the disease. Additionally, if used inappropriately, treatment exerts selective pressures that promote the development of resistant species and thus may actually be more detrimental than beneficial.

CLINICAL MANIFESTATIONS

The major **routes of transmission** of HIV are sexual contact, parenteral exposure to blood and blood products, and vertical transmission during pregnancy.

Primary infection with HIV usually manifests as a constellation of constitutional symptoms approximately 2–4 wks after exposure, coinciding with the widespread dissemination of the virus. The diagnosis of acute primary HIV infection requires a high index of suspicion and must be included in the differential diagnosis of at-risk individuals presenting with a compatible, acute illness. Clinical evaluation may reveal fever, generalized lymphadenopathy, pharyngitis, arthralgias, myalgias, malaise, nausea, vomiting, diarrhea, erythematous maculopapular rash, and oral or genital ulcerations. Lab evaluation may reveal lymphopenia, thrombocytopenia, detection of the HIV p24 antigen, absence of the HIV-specific antibody, and high HIV RNA viral loads. Serum HIV p24 antigenemia is the most widely used method to diagnose primary HIV infection; however, HIV RNA PCR or branched DNA may be more sensitive. Opportunistic infections have been reported during primary HIV infection. Medical management with antiretrovirals may be considered. A key focus should be on counseling; patients may need emotional assistance in coming to terms with their diagnosis and education assistance in understanding the disease and its transmission. The differential diagnosis of primary HIV infection includes viral hepatitis, toxoplasmosis, rubella, mononucleosis, disseminated gonococcal infection, secondary syphilis, herpes simplex virus, Lyme disease, drug reactions, and connective tissue diseases.

Asymptomatic HIV infection represents early-stage disease. The patient does not have any symptoms related to HIV infection and has a CD4 count >500 cells/mm^3. Clinical features include persistent generalized lymphadenopathy and various dermatologic conditions, such as seborrheic dermatitis. Lab tests reveal mild abnormalities in CBC; increases in transaminases may be seen. Viral loads detect varying levels of HIV in the plasma and should be repeated q6mos to reveal evidence of disease progression. Toxoplasma IgG, syphilis serology (VDRL/rapid plasma reagent), and tuberculin skin testing should be performed yearly. Hepatitis serologies and HBV vaccination should be given in those patients not previously exposed. Additional vaccinations to administer include pneumococcal, *Haemophilus*, and yearly influenza. Women should undergo pelvic exams and Pap smears at least annually. Patients should be educated about their illness and future treatment options with antiretrovirals. The average duration of this stage of disease is 7–10 yrs.

In **early symptomatic HIV disease,** most patients remain asymptomatic, with CD4 counts of 200–500 cells/mm^3. However, some patients have mild features of HIV-induced immunosuppression. Constitutional symptoms include fever, unexplained weight loss, fatigue, recurrent diarrhea, and headache. Cutaneous manifestations of herpes zoster, recurrent herpes simplex virus infections, and oral hairy leukoplakia may occur. Pulmonary conditions include sinusitis, bronchitis, community-acquired pneumonia, and pulmonary TB. Oral candidiasis and diarrheal illnesses caused by multiple organisms may occur as well. Gynecologic problems include recurrent vulvovaginal candidiasis and cervical dysplasia. Lab tests may reveal anemia, leukopenia, thrombocytopenia, mild elevations in transaminases, and hypergammaglobulinemia. CD4 counts and viral loads should be performed every 3–6 mos at this stage, and institution of antiretroviral therapy is recommended. Most experts agree in treating all patients with CD4 counts <200 cells/mm^3. The majority of experts recommend initiation of antiretroviral therapy when CD4 counts decline to <350 cells/mm^3 and plasma viral HIV RNA levels are >30,000 copies/mL. Prophylaxis against *Pneumocystis jiroveci* pneumonia (PJP) is indicated when CD4 counts decrease to <200 cells/mm^3 or when the patient has an unexplained fever for >2 wks or has had a previous episode of oral candidiasis. The regimen of choice is double-strength TMP-SMX (Bactrim), one tablet PO per day. If this drug is not tolerated, dapsone (Dapsone USP, DDS), 100 mg/day PO; aerosolized pentamidine (NebuPent), 300 mg monthly; or atovaquone, 750 mg PO twice daily, are alternatives. On reaching this stage of disease, a patient has a 20–30% chance of developing an AIDS-defining illness within the next 18–24 mos if not started on antiretroviral therapy; with such treatment, the risk is decreased by one-half.

In **late symptomatic HIV infection,** the risk of developing an opportunistic infection or malignancy increases dramatically with CD4 counts <200 cells/mm^3. With CD4 counts of 50–200 cells/mm^3, the common constitutional symptoms are fever and AIDS-related wasting. Cutaneous infections include opportunistic fungal infections and eosinophilic folliculitis with pruritus. Pulmonary infections are recurrent bacterial pneumonia; PJP; fungal pneumonia with *Coccidioides immitis, Cryptococcus neoformans, Histoplasma capsulatum*; and mycobacterial pneumonia, such as *Mycobacterium tuberculosis* and *Mycobacterium kansasii*. GI conditions include dysphagia caused by *Candida* and herpes simplex virus and diarrhea caused by *Cryptosporidium parvum, Isospora belli*, and *Microsporida* species. Oncologic diseases include cervical cancer, lymphoma, and Kaposi's sarcoma. Neurologic diseases become more significant at this stage of infection; included in this list are cryptococcal meningitis, herpes family (herpes simplex virus, CMV, and VZV) encephalitis, and *Toxoplasma* encephalitis. Lab tests reveal declining CD4 counts and may reveal pancytopenia. An elevated creatinine with protein may reveal HIV-associated nephropathy.

Management at this stage of disease is directed at the prevention, diagnosis, and treatment of opportunistic infections; antiretroviral medications are indicated in all those patients who have never received therapy. In addition to the PJP prophylaxis mentioned above, the additional organisms to protect against are *Toxoplasma* and *Mycobacterium avium* complex (MAC). *Toxoplasma* prophylaxis is indicated for CD4 <100 cells/mm^3; double-strength TMP-SMX, one tablet/day PO, is preferred. Combination therapy with dapsone, 100 mg/day PO; pyrimethamine (Daraprim), 50 mg/wk PO; and folinic acid, 25 mg/wk PO, is recommended for those patients intolerant of Bactrim. MAC prophylaxis is indicated for CD4 <50 cells/mm^3. Options include clarithromycin (Biaxin), 500 mg PO twice daily; azithromycin (Zithromax), 1200 mg/wk PO; or rifabutin (Mycobutin), 300 mg/day PO. The goal of antiretroviral therapy is to maintain HIV replication to undetectable levels. Patients should also be aggressively treated for symptomatic relief of constitutional symptoms and diarrhea; management of weight loss (e.g., Megace, Marinol) is also very significant for the patient's well-being. Patients with advanced HIV have a 50–75% chance of development of an AIDS-related condition within 18–24 mos without treatment. With the development of therapies for the opportunistic infections and the virus itself, the greatest improvements in overall survival have been revealed in patients in this stage of disease.

In **advanced HIV infection,** host CD4 cell counts are <50 cells/mm^3. Clinical features of advanced infection are mostly the same as those for late symptomatic disease. Certain conditions are more common with the profound immunosuppression of advanced disease, including disseminated MAC, CMV retinitis and encephalitis, disseminated histoplasmosis, aspergillosis, progressive multifocal leukoencephalitis, AIDS dementia complex, HIV myelitis, and CNS lymphoma. Management involves opportunistic infection prophylaxis and treatment, antiretroviral therapy, and supportive care.

There are a variety of **AIDS-related opportunistic infections and malignancies** that can occur in advanced HIV/AIDS. CNS tumors include CNS lymphoma (due to Epstein-Barr virus), progressive multifocal leukoencephalopathy (due to the JC virus), *Toxoplasma gondii*, and glioblastoma multiforme. Other malignancies include Kaposi's sarcoma. Systemic infections can occur from disseminated MAC, bacterial angiomatosis, herpes zoster, CMV, and fungal pathogens (e.g., *C. neoformans*, histoplasmosis, and blastomycosis).

DIAGNOSIS

There are two main lab markers used in combination to monitor disease progression: the **CD4 lymphocyte count** and plasma **HIV viral load.** CD4 counts are used for the determination of the need for antiretroviral therapy and for opportunistic infection prophylaxis. A CD4 count <200 cells/mm^3 indicates increased risk for opportunistic infection and AIDS-related malignancies. On average, the CD4 count decreases by 40–80 cells/mm^3/yr. Levels should be performed at least every 3–6 mos to monitor trends. Viral loads are the best indicators of long-term progression and response to treatment (e.g., plasma HIV RNA level <10,000 copies/mL in early HIV disease is associated with a decreased likelihood of early progression to AIDS). Current guidelines for this test are that measurement should be made at 3-mo intervals before the initiation of treatment, 4–8 wks after the initiation of therapy to determine initial therapeutic response, and at 3-mo intervals to assure full suppression to undetectable levels.

TREATMENT

Complete management of patients with HIV/AIDS is beyond the scope of this text; thus, what follows is a brief overview. **Effective therapy** requires near complete suppression of HIV viral reproduction to reduce the risk of developing resistance mutations concomitant with virologic failure. Potent regimens usually require the combination of three or more drugs to suppress viral replication. Suppression of viral replication permits recovery of the host's immune system. However, these regimens are complex and have many potential toxicities and drug interactions requiring close follow-up and monitoring of patients.

The currently available FDA-approved **antiretroviral medications** are targeted to two of the important proteins in the HIV life cycle: reverse transcriptase [nucleoside reverse transcriptase inhibitors (NRTIs) and nonnucleoside reverse transcriptase inhibitors (NNRTIs)] and protease [protease inhibitors (PIs)]. Adherence, side effects, and drug–drug interactions should all be considered when choosing a regimen.

The **NRTI** family includes zidovudine (Retrovir), didanosine (Videx), zalcitabine (Hivid), stavudine (Zerit), lamivudine (Epivir), abacavir (Ziagen), tenofovir (Viread), and emtricitabine (FTC, Emtriva). These compounds exert their effect by competitively inhibiting the enzyme after conversion to their active triphosphate forms. Dual NRTIs are used in a majority of treatment regimens along with an NNRTI or a PI; however, certain combinations are contraindicated. Zidovudine and stavudine may not be used together secondary to drug antagonism; didanosine should not be used with zalcitabine secondary to overlapping toxicities. Important toxicities from this family are anemia, lactic acidosis, pancreatitis, polyneuropathy, myopathy, and abacavir-induced hypersensitivity syndrome.

The **NNRTI** family includes nevirapine (Viramune), delavirdine (Rescriptor), and efavirenz (Sustiva). These compounds act by noncompetitively inhibiting the enzyme at a site distant from that involved in genomic replication. There is the potential for the development of high-level cross-resistance as a result of single reverse transcriptase mutations (the most common are K103N and Y181C). Viruses resistant to one of the NNRTIs are typically resistant to all of them. Another important concept to understand about this class of medications is their interactions with numerous other drugs that HIV patients are likely to be taking. Examples include the PIs, rifampin (Rifadin, Rimactane) and rifabutin, anticonvulsants, and benzodiazepines. The most important toxicities to know from this class are various rashes (e.g., maculopapular), erythema multiforme, and even Stevens-Johnson syndrome.

The **PI** family includes saquinavir (Fortovase, Invirase), ritonavir (Norvir), indinavir (Crixivan), nelfinavir (Viracept), atazanavir (Reyataz), amprenavir (Agenerase), fosamprenivir/ritonivir (Lexiva), and lopinavir/ritonavir (Kaletra). These compounds act by inhibiting the protease enzyme, thus preventing the production of infectious particles from viral transcripts. Each of the drugs is associated with unique mutations in the protease genes, and complete cross-resistance does not occur. However, the virus does accumulate mutations in the gene in a stepwise fashion, which results in broadening resistance to these agents. These medications are also important for drug-drug interactions, as they are potent inhibitors of the cytochrome p450 system. The most important toxicities of this class are those of lipid, glucose, and bone metabolism.

Current **standard initial regimens** include a combination of two NRTIs and one PI or two NRTIs and efavirenz. Alternative regimens are two NRTIs and one NNRTI, two PIs with one or two NRTIs, and three NRTIs. To **monitor** the success of a new treatment regimen, viral loads should be checked within 4 wks; viral levels should decrease by a minimum of 1.5–2.0 log by this time. Successful treatment is likely to obtain undetectable levels by 12–16 wks. Failures to reach these goals are due to the problems of patient nonadherence, loss of potency due to drug-drug resistance, and development of resistance. The definition of *virologic failure* generally involves a more than tenfold decrease in viral load after 8–12 wks of therapy, detectable HIV virus after 4–6 mos of therapy, and repeated detection of HIV in plasma from patients with a previously undetectable viral load. Once the possibilities of noncompliance and drug interactions have been eliminated, drug resistance testing may be performed; the current method involves genotyping the sequences of the reverse transcriptase and protease genes to uncover mutations. Phenotypic testing to determine sensitivity to particular antiretrovirals can also be performed. This information may then be used to develop a new drug regimen.

The future of drug therapy holds the development of new drugs whose targets may be at different sites in the life cycle of HIV. Vaccine development is also being aggressively pursued.

PNEUMOCYSTIS JIROVECI PNEUMONIA

PJP in homosexual men in the United States initially revealed a new epidemic: AIDS. PJP remained the most common opportunistic infection throughout the first decade of the AIDS epidemic. Institution of prophylaxis and more aggressive antiretroviral therapy have decreased the incidence of PJP in more recent years. However, PJP still remains an important opportunist especially in those unaware of their diagnosis or those nonadherent to their medications.

Pneumonia is believed most commonly to occur due to reactivation of latent infection that is typically acquired early in life. However, there are data emerging that new, exogenous infection may be more common than previously believed. The best predictor of PJP is CD4 count <200 cells/mm^3 or <15% of total circulating lymphocytes. Cytotoxic chemotherapy also increases the risk regardless of CD4 count.

Pathophysiology

Infection is limited to the lung in >95% of cases. Pneumonia is characterized by foamy eosinophilic exudates and interstitial pneumonitis. However, patients with AIDS have been described to have many "atypical" features. These include alveolar infiltrates, cystic lesions, and cavitary lesions. Pneumothorax may occur after rupture of a cystic lesion.

Clinical Manifestations

The most common manifestations are dry, nonproductive cough, fever, and shortness of breath. The illness is more insidious in patients with AIDS than in those with other immunodeficiencies that typically present more acutely. Patients with AIDS typically report dyspnea for 3–4 wks at the time of diagnosis. The physical exam is typically benign except for fever and tachypnea unless other illnesses associated with advanced immunosuppression are present (e.g., thrush). The patient may be hypoxemic on pulse oximetry or arterial blood gases. Chest x-ray is a vital part in the diagnosis of PJP. Chest x-rays are normal in <5% of cases. The most common pattern is a bilateral, fine interstitial infiltrate from the hilum to the periphery ("bat-wing" pattern). However, numerous atypical patterns may occur and illustrate the importance of including PJP in the differential diagnosis of any pulmonary disease in a patient with AIDS. CT scan can better assess the parenchymal involvement but is typically not necessary.

Diagnosis

Diagnosis requires the sampling of sputum or bronchial lavage specimens for the microorganism. Increased lactic acid dehydrogenase is a marker for PJP but is nonspecific, and no serologic test can be used to determine infection. An induced sputum is usually required as the first step, as most patients have a nonproductive cough. A sputum can be induced with aerosolized hypertonic saline. Depending on the center, the sensitivity may be 50–70% for the diagnosis of PJP. Fiberoptic bronchoscopy with bronchoalveolar lavage can also be performed. It has a sensitivity of >95% and nearly 100% specificity. Lung biopsy is now rarely required for the diagnosis. The specimen can be stained with immunofluorescent antibodies or with silver stains to look for the microorganism.

Treatment

Arterial blood gases should be routinely measured to assist in delineating the severity of disease and the appropriate therapy. In patients with mild PJP [those with a partial pressure of arterial oxygen (PaO$_2$) >70 mm Hg], outpatient therapy can be considered in reliable patients. Hospitalization is required for those patients with a PaO$_2$ <70 mm Hg, as therapy is likely to be administered IV, and careful monitoring is required, as the patients may get worse initially with therapy. The **drug of choice** for treating PJP is TMP-SMX regardless of the severity of illness. The dose is 15–20 mg/kg/day of TMP and SMX, 75 mg/kg/day IV or PO, in 3–4 divided doses for 21 days. Alternatives include pentamidine, 3–4 mg/kg/day IV; clindamycin (Cleocin), 600–900 mg/day PO, plus primaquine, 15–30 mg/day PO; trimetrexate (Neutrexin), 45 mg/m^2 PO, plus leucovorin (Wellcovorin), 20 mg/m^2 PO; and TMP, 20 mg/kg/day PO, plus dapsone, 100 mg/day PO. Atovaquone, 1500 mg/day PO, is an alternative for mild PJP. Duration of therapy is 21 days. In addition, several clinical studies have demonstrated a benefit of corticosteroids in reducing the risk of mechanical ventilation and mortality. Patients with **an initial PaO$_2$ <70 mm Hg** should be considered for a tapering dose of prednisone (Apo-Prednisone, Deltasone, Meticorten, Orasone, Prednicen-M, Sterapred, Winpred) over the 21-day course of treatment. The regimen used is prednisone, 40 mg PO q12h on days 1–5, 40 mg PO daily on days 6–10, and 20 mg PO daily on days 11–21. Care should be taken to observe for latent infections that may develop as a result of the corticosteroid therapy.

Prevention

PJP prophylaxis has been shown to be very cost effective. TMP-SMX has been shown in studies to be superior to both dapsone and aerosolized pentamidine in preventing PJP, but a statistically significant survival advantage has not been seen. The current recommendation is for prophylaxis to start with a CD4 count <200 cells/mm^3 or <15% or a history of PJP. TMP-SMX can be given as a single-strength or double-strength tablet daily or as a double-strength tablet three times/wk. Alternatives include dapsone, 100 mg PO daily; atovaquone, 750 mg PO twice daily or 1500 mg PO once daily; and aerosolized pentamidine, 300 mg every 4 wks. Prophylaxis can be discontinued in patients who have sustained increases in CD4 counts to >200 cells/mm^3 while receiving potent antiretroviral therapy.

MYCOBACTERIUM AVIUM COMPLEX

MAC is one of the most common opportunistic infections in patients with AIDS. It typically occurs as a widely disseminated disease in the setting of a patient with advanced AIDS. MAC is ubiquitous in the environment, especially in soil and water. Portals of entry are probably both inhalation of aerosols and ingestion. MAC consists of *M. avium*, *Mycobacterium intracellulare*, and other strains. The organisms are slow-growing nonphotochromogens. Nearly all the infections attributable to MAC in AIDS patients consist of *M. avium*.

Disseminated MAC was rarely reported before the first reports of the AIDS epidemic in 1981. Disseminated MAC appears to occur in 20–35% of patients with HIV each year without prophylaxis. This number has been significantly reduced with the availability of effective prophylactic regimens. The risk for developing MAC infection is greatest for patients with a CD4 count <50 cells/mm^3.

Clinical Manifestations

The most frequent symptoms are fever, night sweats, weight loss, fatigue, diarrhea, and abdominal pain. Anemia is very typical and out of proportion to that expected given other underlying conditions. The alkaline phosphatase may be elevated, and the patient may have hepatomegaly or splenomegaly on exam, possibly indicating hepatic or biliary tract disease. Intraabdominal lymphadenopathy may also be seen on imaging; however, peripheral adenopathy is uncommon. Less commonly, patients may have pneumonitis, pericarditis, osteomyelitis, skin lesions and abscesses, or CNS lesions. MAC bacteremia may transiently occur as well.

Diagnosis

Diagnosis is generally made by recovery of the organism in culture of blood or bone marrow. Recovery of MAC from other sterile sites also indicates likely disseminated disease. The easiest and most expedient means of making a diagnosis is a DNA probe species identification after the growth of mycobacteria on a liquid medium.

Treatment

Macrolides form the cornerstone of therapy for MAC. Clarithromycin, 500 mg PO twice daily, or azithromycin, 600 mg PO daily, is recommended. The regimens should also include at least one other effective agent. Ethambutol, 15 mg/kg/day PO, has been widely used as the second agent. Other agents with activity include rifabutin, 300 mg PO daily; ciprofloxacin, 750 mg PO twice daily; and amikacin, 15 mg/kg IV daily. Rifabutin has been shown to decrease the development of resistance to clarithromycin but has had no impact on survival. Therapy should be continued for life or until effective antiretroviral therapy allows sustained increases in CD4 count to >100 cells/mm^3 for 6–12 mos.

Prevention

Prophylaxis is recommended for patients with AIDS and a CD4 count <50 cells/mm^3, particularly those who have had an opportunistic infection. Due to greater efficacy, azithromycin, 1200 mg/wk PO, or clarithromycin, 500 mg PO bid, is the preferred regimen. Rifabutin, 300 mg PO daily, is an alternative. Prophylaxis may be discontinued in patients with a sustained increased in CD4 count to >100 cells/mm^3 while receiving potent antiretroviral therapy.

KEY POINTS TO REMEMBER

- HIV does not discriminate by age, sex, or race.
- The most common admitting diagnosis among hospitalized patients with previously undiagnosed HIV is PJP.
- HIV has become a very complex disease to manage, as there are multiple potential drug interactions and complications. Outcomes are improved when these patients are managed by an HIV specialist.

REFERENCES AND SUGGESTED READINGS

HIV InSite Gateway to HIV and AIDS Knowledge. http://www.hivinsite.com.
Zavasky D-M, Gerberding JL, Sande MA. Patients with AIDS. In: Wilson WR, Sande MA, Drew WL, Henry NK, eds. *Current diagnosis and treatment in infectious diseases*. New York: McGraw-Hill, 2001:315–327.

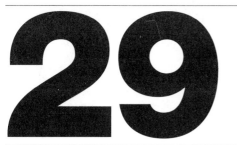

Bioterrorism

Steve J. Lawrence

INTRODUCTION

Although bioterrorism (BT)—the intentional use of biologic agents to harm others—has been encountered in the past, it has never been more important for physicians to be capable of recognizing and treating such diseases than now. Several microorganisms have been used as biologic weapons, and many more are considered to be potential agents based on a few common characteristics, including high mortality, morbidity, and infectivity and relative ease to produce, store, and disperse. The six diseases identified as the most likely to be encountered in an intentional outbreak are **anthrax, smallpox, plague, tularemia, botulism,** and **viral hemorrhagic fever** (VHF). All are capable of causing substantial disease in large populations via an aerosol route of exposure. Epidemiologic clues that should raise suspicion and subsequent investigation into a possible BT event include an unusually large number of patients presenting within a short period of time with the same syndrome, otherwise healthy patients presenting with severe disease, and identification of an unusual pathogen or syndrome for the region. More information may be found at the CDC Emergency Preparedness and Response Web site: http://www.bt.cdc.gov.

ANTHRAX

Introduction

Caused by *Bacillus anthracis*, a sporulating gram-positive bacillus, anthrax is a rare zoonotic disease in its natural state that has been used as a weapon, causing several deaths in the United States in 2001. Under poor growth conditions, the metabolically active bacillus form converts to a hardy inert spore. These spores then cause disease by germinating into toxin-producing vegetative bacilli at the site of entry into the body, primarily the pulmonary alveoli **(inhalational anthrax)** via inhalation, the skin **(cutaneous anthrax)** by direct contact, and the intestinal mucosa **(GI anthrax)** via ingestion. Although cutaneous anthrax comprises the vast majority (95%) of naturally occurring cases, the inhalational form is the most likely to be seen in an intentional release because of its delivery by aerosol and its very high *mortality of 45–89%*. Risk factors include handling the hides/carcasses of infected animals, working in wool mills (thus the historical name *woolsorter's disease*), and being exposed to delivered powders. There has been no reported person-to-person transmission of inhalational disease. Because of the rarity of naturally occurring disease and its potential as a BT agent, **any suspected or confirmed cases of inhalational anthrax should be treated as an epidemiologic emergency, prompting immediate reporting to the local health department.**

Differential Diagnosis

The differential diagnosis for inhalational anthrax primarily includes upper respiratory viral infections or gastroenteritis in the prodromal phase and severe pneumonia in the fulminant phase.

Clinical Manifestations

Inhalational anthrax usually presents as a biphasic illness, with an early prodromal phase after an incubation period of 2–4 days. **Nonspecific influenza-like symptoms** [e.g., fevers, chills, malaise, myalgias, or GI manifestations (e.g., nausea, emesis, and abdominal pain)] predominate. Usually, nasal congestion and rhinorrhea are distinctly absent. A rapidly progressive fulminant phase occurs within 3 days of symptom onset that is characterized by continued fevers, dyspnea, cyanosis, and sepsis, leading to multiorgan failure and death within 36 hrs. In most cases, a **widened mediastinum** on chest x-ray is evident during the prodromal phase and corresponds to the pathologic hallmark of hemorrhagic mediastinal lymphadenitis. Hemorrhagic pleural effusions are very common and can be of large volume requiring repeated thoracenteses. Pulmonary infiltrates are often seen but do not usually represent a true pneumonia, as the spores are carried via macrophages to the mediastinal lymph nodes where the germination and toxin production occur.

Cutaneous anthrax typically begins as a pruritic macule or papule that occurs 3–5 days after contact with spores. The lesion progresses to a vesicle or bulla with serosanguineous fluid and surrounding edema, then to a shallow ulcer, which becomes the characteristic black eschar. Systemic symptoms (e.g., fever and malaise) may occur, but severe disease leading to sepsis and death is extremely rare when treated. Through all stages, the lesion remains painless, helping to distinguish it from spider bites, ecthyma gangrenosum, and other cutaneous lesions that may have a similar appearance.

Diagnosis

There are no rapid, specific tests available to diagnose anthrax in its earliest stages; thus, a high index of suspicion is necessary to presumptively recognize cases. **Blood culture is the gold standard and is very specific when nonhemolytic, nonmotile gram-positive bacilli are isolated on blood agar.** When cultures are obtained from symptomatic individuals before antibiotic initiation, sensitivity nears 100%. Other confirmatory tests are available at reference labs and the CDC.

Treatment

Appropriate antibiotics should be administered as soon as inhalational anthrax is suspected, without waiting for confirmatory testing. **Empiric therapy,** with ciprofloxacin (Cipro) (400 mg IV q12h) or doxycycline (Monodox) (100 mg IV q12h) and one or two other antibiotics active against *B. anthracis*, is indicated until susceptibilities are known. Other antibiotics with activity against natural strains include rifampin (Rifadin, Rimactane), clindamycin (Cleocin), penicillin, amoxicillin (Amoxil), vancomycin (Vancocin), and chloramphenicol (Chloromycetin). Notably, **cephalosporins, TMP-SMX, and many macrolides are not effective.** Penicillins should not be used as monotherapy, as many strains have an inducible beta-lactamase. Patients presenting with signs or symptoms of **meningitis** should receive at least one agent with good penetration into the CSF. Therapy can be switched to oral administration after clinical improvement and should consist of ciprofloxacin (500 mg PO bid) or doxycycline (100 mg PO bid) and one other active antibiotic. The total course of therapy should be 60 days because of convincing animal and human data that spores may lie dormant before germinating and causing fatal disease. **Cutaneous anthrax** can be treated with PO agents, either ciprofloxacin (500 mg PO bid) or doxycycline (100 mg PO bid), unless (a) the lesion is on the head or neck; (b) the lesion is associated with severe edema; or (c) there is evidence of systemic disease, when the same IV regimen for inhalational disease should be used. Contact precautions should be considered if an actively draining lesion is present.

Postexposure Prophylaxis

Persons who have known or suspected exposure to anthrax spores should be given antimicrobial prophylaxis with either ciprofloxacin (500 mg PO bid) or doxycycline (100 mg PO bid). If the susceptibilities of the strain related to the possible exposure are known, then amoxicillin (500 mg PO tid) may be an alternative, especially for children and pregnant women. Duration of therapy should be 60 days for the reasons noted above. If available, administration of the licensed cell-free vaccine may be able to reduce total duration to 30 days.

SMALLPOX

Smallpox, the disease caused by variola virus, is responsible for more human deaths than any other infectious disease in history. Its global eradication in 1979 marked one of the world's greatest public health triumphs. Remaining viral stocks exist, and the potential for it to be obtained for intentional use as an aerosolized weapon is believed to be credible. Variola is **readily transmitted person to person** and would likely infect one-third of unvaccinated case contacts with a resulting *mortality of 25–30%*. Disease occurs when virus-laden droplets land on the oral or respiratory mucosa, followed by viremia and subsequent systemic disease with rash and sepsis.

Differential Diagnosis

Varicella (chickenpox) is the most likely disease to be confused with smallpox, but other acute febrile illnesses with rash must be considered.

Clinical Manifestations

The nonspecific influenza-like symptoms of the prodromal phase—predominated by high fever, myalgias, low back pain, and headache—appear 12–14 days (range, 7–17) after exposure. The eruptive phase abruptly starts with a rash, usually on the face, 3–5 days after prodrome onset. Heralding the onset of contagiousness, the rash appears in a centrifugal pattern, first affecting the face followed by distal arms and legs, including palms and soles, and relative sparing of the trunk. This pattern, along with the observation that all lesions in one region are in the same stage of development, helps to distinguish smallpox from its main consideration in the differential diagnosis, chickenpox. Lesions of the classic rash start macular and then progress through stages of deep vesicles, pustules, scabs, and permanent pitting scars. Multiorgan failure and sepsis are the usual causes of death in fatal cases, occurring during the second week of illness.

Diagnosis

The diagnosis of smallpox is primarily clinical, which is sufficient in an outbreak setting. Electron microscopy, culture, and PCR can be performed on vesicle fluid and are available at reference labs.

Treatment

There is **no specific treatment** for smallpox infection. Supportive care, including vigilant attention to volume and electrolyte status, is critical and may improve survival. **All patients with suspected or confirmed smallpox must be placed in strict contact and respiratory isolation until all scabs have separated.**

Postexposure Prophylaxis

Smallpox vaccine can reduce the risk of development of disease and subsequent mortality by >50% if given within 4 days of exposure and should be administered in this situation. Vaccinia immune globulin is also effective at preventing disease if given during the early incubation phase. Animal studies suggest that the antiviral drug cidofovir (Vistide) may provide protection if given within 2 days of exposure, but there are no human data available for correlation.

The vaccine (live vaccinia virus) is most efficacious when used as primary prevention. Near complete protection lasting at least 5–10 yrs is achieved for those who exhibit a typical vaccine reaction. Partial protection has been documented for at least 20 yrs. Revaccination may confer lifelong immunity. Serious complications occur in approximately 1/10,000 vaccinees, including one death per million.

PLAGUE

Yersinia pestis, the highly infectious gram-negative coccobacillary agent of plague, has caused three major pandemics since the fourteenth century and remains endemic in many areas of the world, including the southwestern United States. Plague is primarily a zoonotic disease, with humans becoming hosts when transmitted either directly via animal contact or indirectly through flea bites. The disease takes one of three forms: (a) **bubonic**, the most common, leading to a local lymphadenitis (bubo) and death in 14% of cases; (b) **septicemic**, with 30–50% mortality; and (c) **pneumonic**, with an over-all 57% case fatality nearing 100% when treatment is delayed. Pneumonic disease would be expected after inhalation of aerosolized *Y. pestis* and after contact with an index case. After inhalation, the highly virulent organisms cause a severe lobular pneumonia and gram-negative sepsis.

Clinical Manifestations

Pneumonic plague becomes evident 2–4 days (range, 1–6) after exposure and mimics an **acute influenza-like illness** with fevers, chills, myalgias, malaise, and headache. Within 24 hrs, signs and symptoms of a severe pneumonia appear, including dyspnea, cough, and chest pain. Rapid progression to respiratory failure and sepsis is characteristic. Hemoptysis is not uncommon and may be a diagnostic clue. Radiographic findings are variable but usually present as bilateral patchy infiltrates and consolidation.

Differential Diagnosis

The differential diagnosis includes any severe pneumonia.

Diagnosis

There are no readily available rapid and specific tests for detecting pneumonic plague. Wayson, Wright's, and Giemsa stains can provide presumptive evidence if the characteristic bipolar staining ("safety pin") is present. Blood, sputum, and CSF cultures can confirm the presence of *Y. pestis* if the appropriate biochemical tests are available. Serologic tests can provide a diagnosis retrospectively.

Treatment

Rapid antibiotic therapy is critical for survival and should be started at the first suspicion of plague. The antibiotics of choice are streptomycin (1 g IM q12h), based on its proven clinical efficacy, or gentamicin (5 mg/kg IV/IM q24h or 2 mg/kg loading dose, then 1.7 mg/kg IV/IM q8h) with appropriate monitoring of drug levels. Alternatives include doxycycline (100 mg IV q12h), ciprofloxacin (400 mg IV q12h), and chloramphenicol (25 mg/kg IV q6h; target levels, 5–20 μg/mL). **Beta-lactams, rifampin, and macrolides are ineffective.** The switch to oral therapy can be made after clinical improvement and continued for a total antibiotic duration of 10–14 days. **All patients should be isolated with respiratory droplet precautions** (face mask, gown, gloves, goggles) until 48 hrs of effective antibiotic therapy has been given and clinical improvement has occurred.

Postexposure Prophylaxis

Persons exposed to patients with pneumonic plague or to *Y. pestis* aerosol should be given doxycycline (100 mg PO bid) or ciprofloxacin (500 mg PO bid) for 7 days after last exposure.

TULAREMIA

Francisella tularensis is a small gram-negative coccobacillus responsible for the zoonotic disease tularemia, which occurs sporadically in the United States. Tick bites and direct contact with infected animals, particularly rabbits, are the most common routes of infection. The majority of cases are of the **ulceroglandular** form, characterized by a skin lesion at the point of entry and regional lymphadenopathy. Other forms include **glandular, oculoglandular, typhoidal, oropharyngeal,** and **pneumonic,** depending on the mechanism of infection. Pneumonic tularemia can be acquired via inhalation of *F. tularensis* or by secondary hematogenous spread to the lungs. There have been no reported cases of person-to-person transmission. Mortality is rare when treated but can be as high as 60% in untreated cases.

Clinical Manifestations

After a short incubation period of 2–5 days, all forms of tularemia onset suddenly with nonspecific **influenza-like symptoms,** including high fevers, profuse sweating, malaise, low back myalgias, and headache. The severity of pneumonic tularemia is variable and can range from a mild upper respiratory illness to a severe and fulminant pneumonia. Cases develop a minimally productive cough (occasionally with hemoptysis), dyspnea, and pleuritic pain. Pulse-temperature dissociation, or relative bradycardia, is not uncommon and may be a diagnostic clue. Patchy bilateral infiltrates and effusions are the most likely radiographic findings. ARDS and sepsis are the end results of the most severe cases.

Diagnosis

There are no readily available rapid, specific tests for tularemia; thus, a high index of suspicion is required to identify cases early. Culture of sputum, blood, or pleural fluid for *F. tularensis* is slow and insensitive. Sputum Gram's stain is invariably negative. The microbiology lab must be notified when tularemia is suspected because pure cultures need to be specially handled to prevent transmission to technicians. Serologic assays are more sensitive and pose no increased lab risk; however, they are generally effective for retrospective diagnosis only. Rapid confirmatory tests (e.g., PCR) are available at reference labs.

Differential Diagnosis

The differential diagnosis includes any moderately severe pneumonia, particularly those caused by atypical organisms, and other acute typhoidal-like illnesses.

Treatment

Streptomycin (1 g IM q12h) has historically been the drug of choice, demonstrating near 100% cure rates. Gentamicin (5 mg/kg IV/IM q24h or 2 mg/kg loading dose, then 1.7 mg/kg IV/IM q8h) with appropriate monitoring of drug levels is nearly as effective and easier to administer. Alternatives include doxycycline (100 mg IV q12h) and chloramphenicol (15 mg/kg IV q6h), but both have significant relapse rates. Ciprofloxacin (400 mg IV q12h) has had anecdotal success in small groups of patients exhibiting a 100% cure rate, and it is an acceptable alternative if aminoglycosides are contraindicated. Duration of therapy should be 10 days for aminoglycosides, 10–14 days for fluoroquinolones, and 14–21 days for doxycycline or chloramphenicol. Switch to an active oral agent can be accomplished on clinical improvement. **Ceftriaxone is ineffective,** despite having minimal inhibitory concentrations in the susceptible range.

Postexposure Prophylaxis

Persons with suspected or confirmed exposure to aerosolized *F. tularensis* should be given **doxycycline** (100 mg PO bid) or **ciprofloxacin** (500 mg PO bid) for 14 days.

Although a live attenuated vaccine exists, it is not recommended for postexposure prophylaxis because of slow immune response and the short incubation period.

BOTULISM

Botulism is caused by intoxication with botulinum toxin, which is produced by the anaerobic gram-positive bacillus *Clostridium botulinum*. <1 μg of botulinum toxin is necessary to cause fatal disease, making it one of the most lethal substances known. Several mechanisms of entry lead to the same neurologic disease process. Most of the sporadic outbreaks in the United States are attributed to ingestion of toxin from improperly canned foods that have been contaminated with *C. botulinum* **(food-borne botulism)**. Intoxication can also occur if *C. botulinum* infects the skin **(wound botulism)** or GI tract **(infant and intestinal botulism)** with subsequent production of botulinum toxin. Alternatively, the toxin can be inhaled directly from an aerosol source **(inhalational botulism)**. Person-to-person transmission does not occur. Once toxin enters the bloodstream, it is taken up by the motor nerve terminus, where it irreversibly blocks the release of acetylcholine. The resulting muscle paralysis lasts until axonal branches regenerate.

Clinical Manifestations

Symptoms of botulism resulting from direct inhalation of toxin appear 12–72 hrs after exposure. **Lack of fever, a clear sensorium, and a symmetric descending flaccid paralysis comprise the classic triad.** The paralysis begins with bulbar palsies, manifesting as ptosis, diplopia, dysarthria, dysphagia, and dry mouth. The weakness progresses until the gag reflex is absent and diaphragmatic function is lost and then culminates in diffuse skeletal muscle paralysis. Sensation remains intact. Paralysis may last weeks to months.

Differential Diagnosis

Guillain-Barré syndrome and myasthenia gravis are chief among other conditions on the differential diagnosis and can be distinguished from botulism by careful physical exam, electromyography, and response to anticholinesterases.

Diagnosis

Cases presenting with the classic syndrome can be diagnosed clinically. A confirmatory mouse bioassay that detects toxin in serum is available only at reference labs.

Treatment

The mainstay of treatment for botulism is supportive care, particularly ventilatory support after respiratory muscle paralysis has occurred. Although the degree of paralysis evident at time of presentation is not reversible for weeks, the progression can be halted by rapid administration of **botulinum antitoxin** (one vial administered IV per package insert).

Postexposure Prophylaxis

For asymptomatic persons with suspected exposure to botulinum toxin, the antitoxin is not recommended for prophylaxis because of the high incidence (10%) of hypersensitivity reactions as well as its limited supply. Exposed persons should be carefully monitored near critical care facilities and given antitoxin at the first sign of any neurologic deficits consistent with botulism.

VIRAL HEMORRHAGIC FEVER

VHF is a syndrome caused by many different RNA viruses, including filoviruses (Ebola and Marburg); flaviviruses (dengue and yellow fever); bunyaviruses [hantaviruses, Crimean-Congo hemorrhagic fever (CCHF), Rift Valley fever]; and arenaviruses (Argentinian, Bolivian, and Venezuelan hemorrhagic fevers and Lassa fever). All cause sporadic disease in areas of endemicity, and most have the potential to be transmitted as an aerosol. All except dengue and hantaviruses are contagious via blood and other body fluids. Lassa, CCHF, Ebola, and Marburg may be transmissible through respiratory spread. Many of the viruses are rodent zoonoses or transmitted by arthropods. Mortality is variable but can be as high as 90% for severe Ebola cases.

Clinical Manifestations

Common early symptoms mimic those of other viral diseases, including fevers, myalgias, and malaise. Disease can range from minimally symptomatic to fulminant, and symptomatology varies depending on the specific disease. However, all share the potential for severe disruption of vascular permeability and a bleeding diathesis manifested by edema, mucous membrane hemorrhage, and petechiae and accompanied by shock in the most severe cases. Thrombocytopenia, leukopenia, and hepatitis are common in many of the diseases.

Differential Diagnosis

Diseases most often misdiagnosed as VHF include malaria, typhoid, rickettsial disease, meningococcemia, hemolytic uremic syndrome, and any cause of disseminated intravascular coagulation.

Diagnosis

A confirmed diagnosis can be made for most of the VHF viral agents serologically. Some of the viruses can be cultured but require a lab with advanced safety capabilities.

Treatment

For all patients with VHF, supportive therapy is crucial. In addition to standard fluid, electrolyte, BP, and oxygenation support, hemorrhage must be addressed with specific therapy as guided by coagulation studies and by avoidance of invasive procedures if possible. IV ribavirin has been used experimentally as specific antiviral therapy for CCHF, Lassa, and Rift Valley fevers. **All patients should be placed in respiratory and contact isolation,** including the use of face mask and goggles by health care providers. Those with the highest potential of spread (e.g., severe cough, hemorrhage, diarrhea) should be placed under the stricter airborne precautions (negative pressure room and use of high-efficiency particulate air–filtered respirator).

Postexposure Prophylaxis

Other than oral ribavirin used investigationally after high-risk exposure to CCHF and Lassa fever, there is no specific prophylaxis for asymptomatic persons with suspected exposure to VHF agents. Those potentially exposed should be monitored closely for development of VHF symptoms.

KEY POINTS TO REMEMBER

- Early diagnosis is often critical to improve survival; thus, a high index of suspicion is necessary. Keep BT diseases in mind in differential diagnosis of compatible illnesses (i.e., "don't forget the zebras").
- Epidemiologic clues that suggest a BT outbreak include an unusually large number of patients presenting within a short period of time with the same syndrome, otherwise healthy patients presenting with severe disease, and identification of an unusual pathogen or syndrome for the region.

- Report any suspected BT illnesses to the local health department, the hospital epidemiologist, and infectious disease consultants immediately.
- Widened mediastinum and flu-like symptoms: Think anthrax!
- Centrifugal vesicular rash and fever: Immediately isolate!
- More information may be found at the CDC Emergency Preparedness and Response Web site: http://www.bt.cdc.gov.

REFERENCES AND SUGGESTED READINGS

Arnon SS, Schechter R, Inglesby TV, et al. Botulinum toxin as a biological weapon: medical and public health management. *JAMA* 2001;285:1059–1070.

Centers for Disease Control and Prevention. Public Health Emergency Preparedness and Response. http://www.bt.cdc.gov.

Dennis DT, Inglesby TV, Henderson DA, et al. Tularemia as a biological weapon: medical and public health management. *JAMA* 2001;285:2763–2773.

Henderson DA, Inglesby TV, Bartlett JG, et al. Smallpox as a biological weapon: medical and public health management. *JAMA* 1999;281:2127–2137.

Inglesby TV, Dennis DT, Henderson DA, et al. Plague as a biological weapon: medical and public health management. *JAMA* 2000;283:2281–2290.

Inglesby TV, Henderson DA, Bartlett JG, et al. Anthrax as a biological weapon: medical and public health management. *JAMA* 1999;281:1735–1745.

St. Louis University School of Public Health. Center for the Study of Bioterrorism. http://www.bioterrorism.slu.edu.

United States Army Medical Research Institute of Infectious Diseases. *Medical management of biological casualties handbook*, 4th ed. Frederick, MD: USAMRIID, 2001.

Infection Control

Kristin Mondy

INTRODUCTION

Within the past two decades, the discovery and emergence of infectious diseases (e.g., HIV, HCV, and multidrug-resistant bacterial pathogens) have heightened attention toward stricter, more effective infection control practices in both community and hospital settings.

UNIVERSAL PRECAUTIONS

Pathogens that are predominantly blood-borne (e.g., HIV, HBV, and HCV) can potentially cause devastating infections but are otherwise highly preventable if appropriate precautions are used. To guide communities and hospitals in the prevention and transmission of these pathogens, the CDC has defined a set of "universal precautions" that can be accessed via the Web site http://www.cdc.gov/ncidod/hip/blood/universa.htm. Unlike standard precautions, which encompass specific hospital isolation procedures (discussed below), universal precautions only address contact with blood and other bodily fluids visibly contaminated with blood, semen, and vaginal secretions (all primary modes of transmission of HIV). The CDC Web site gives instructions on the use of gloves, gowns, face masks, and other protective gear; methods to avoid percutaneous exposures; instructions on vaccination of persons at high risk for viral hepatitis exposure; and postexposure prophylaxis for those who have been potentially exposed to HIV or viral hepatitis.

PREVENTION AND CONTROL OF INFECTIONS WITHIN THE HOSPITAL ENVIRONMENT

Patient Isolation

Meticulous and up-to-date infection control practices are particularly important for the hospital-based practitioner. The CDC maintains an updated guideline for isolation precautions in hospitals that includes an appendix of type and duration of precautions needed for selected infections and conditions (available at http://www.cdc.gov/ncidod/hip/ISOLAT/isolat.htm). The various types of precautions addressed include pathogens requiring airborne, contact, droplet, or standard precautions. It is worth noting that in addition to the specific pathogens listed, any patient who is infected or colonized with a multidrug-resistant bacteria believed to be of particular significance to the physician or local infection control expert should be placed in contact isolation.

Hand-Washing and Environmental Control

Good hand-washing technique is generally regarded as the most important factor in effective control of horizontal transmission of most pathogens. Proper institution of effective techniques for the handling, cleaning, and disinfection of all patient rooms and patient-related equipment and waste is a key component of any hospital infection control program. Recommendations for proper hand-washing techniques as well as methods of cleaning, disinfecting, and sterilizing patient-related equipment; handling waste; and performing microbiologic sampling of various patient-related environmental areas (as a part of a suspected outbreak investigation) are listed at http://www.cdc.gov/ncidod/hip/guide/handwash_pre.htm.

Prevention of Specific Nosocomial Infections

Another important aspect of hospital infection control is the development of additional preventive strategies to curtail the acquisition and transmission of nosocomial infections. Generally, infections developing >48–72 hrs after admission and within 10 days after hospital discharge are considered nosocomial (the time frame may be modified for infections with very short or very long incubation periods). Nosocomial surgical site infections generally occur within 30 days after the surgical procedure or within 1 yr if prosthetic material is placed. Hospital-acquired infections are a significant cause of patient morbidity and mortality and health care cost; thus, the CDC has developed guidelines that address risk factors and prevention strategies for the most common and significant nosocomial infections (intravascular device–related infections, surgical site infections, UTIs, and nosocomial pneumonias). These guidelines are accessible at http://www.cdc.gov/ncidod/hip/Guide/guide.htm.

Surveillance

Currently, the CDC has several surveillance programs in place in which hundreds of hospitals across the United States are registered. The main purposes of these programs are to describe the epidemiology and antimicrobial resistance trends of various types of infections and to produce infection rates for certain organisms within specific hospital areas for comparison use by other hospitals (http://www.cdc.gov/ncidod/hip/SURVEILL/NNIS.HTM). Recently, reports generated from these national surveillance programs have revealed large increases in the hospital prevalence of drug-resistant pathogens (e.g., methicillin-resistant *Staphylococcus aureus*, vancomycin-resistant enterococci, and *Clostridium difficile*). As a result, numerous hospitals now have their own active or passive surveillance systems in place to detect these and other organisms. Active surveillance systems are usually specific to time (e.g., at admission) or hospital area (e.g., ICU) due to cost constraints and involve culturing patients at specific sites (e.g., nasal or rectal swabs) for problematic organisms. Patients colonized with one multidrug-resistant organism are at high risk for colonization with others, and their culture specimens are also frequently targeted for passive surveillance (e.g., stool cultures positive for one bacteria are subsequently tested for others). The purpose of these surveillance systems is to identify patient reservoirs for potential spread of problematic pathogens so that appropriate isolation precautions can be taken. Recommended infections for focused surveillance include those that are preventable, occur frequently, cause serious morbidity or mortality, are costly to treat, or are caused by multidrug-resistant organisms.

Use of the Microbiology Lab

The microbiology lab of any hospital can be a valuable tool in several areas of infection control, including surveillance, outbreak investigation, and pathogen resistance. The microbiology lab usually has data on baseline prevalence rates of specific infections throughout different areas of the hospital, the predominant pathogens involved, and the patterns of antibiotic susceptibility. The microbiologists are thus often the first personnel to notice (a) the emergence of a novel pathogen or one with an unusual resistance pattern, or (b) an increase in the incidence of a particular organism or type of infection that would cause suspicion for an outbreak. The lab also has several techniques for typing bacteria or other organisms to trace an outbreak back to a possible common source. Susceptibility patterns obtained from the microbiology lab can aid the physician in correctly choosing an initial antibiotic regimen for a particular infection, thus avoiding the further propagation of infection and emergence of drug resistance.

Other Strategies

Other control and prevention methods (infection control teaching seminars, observation and feedback on infection control technique by trained staff, antibiotic restriction policies) are often implemented by hospital and infection control committees, but these usually vary among different institutions and are beyond the scope of this chapter.

Postexposure Prophylaxis

The management of health care worker occupational exposures to HIV, HBV, and HCV and the current recommendations for prevention and postexposure prophylaxis of these and other pathogens can be found at http://www.cdc.gov/ncidod/hip/Guide/phspep.htm and http://www.cdc.gov/niosh/bbppg.html. Generally, the percentage risks for a health care worker acquiring infection after a contaminated percutaneous exposure to HBV, HCV, or HIV are approximately 30%, 3%, and 0.3%, respectively. Highrisk exposures include those from an infected source with high viremia or exposures involving a large-bore hollow needle, deep puncture, or large amount of visible blood. Other guidelines for infection control in health care personnel (including those who are pregnant or immunocompromised) can be found at http://www.cdc.gov/ncidod/hip/Occhealt/ocguide.htm.

KEY POINTS TO REMEMBER

- The CDC Web sites mentioned above are suggested guidelines only. It is important to remember that any hospital or large health-care facility should have its own guidelines, and these should be carefully reviewed by all personnel.
- Patients with recent history of colonization with multidrug-resistant bacteria should be placed on empiric isolation if readmitted to a health care facility. Isolation precautions can then be discontinued if subsequent surveillance cultures are negative.
- If an outbreak is suspected, get the infection control staff involved early.

REFERENCES AND SUGGESTED READINGS

Pottinger JM, Herwaldt LA, Perl TM. Basics of surveillance—an overview. *Infect Control Hosp Epidemiol* 1997;18:513–527.

Struelens MJ. Hospital infection control. In: Armstrong D, Cohen J, eds. *Infectious diseases*. London: Harcourt, 1999.

Index